AF183811

Issues in Contemporary International Health

Issues in Contemporary International Health

Edited by
Thomas A. Lambo
Deputy Director General (Retired)
World Health Organization
Geneva, Switzerland
and
Stacey B. Day
Founding Professor and Director
World Health Organization Collaborating Center for Community-Based Education for Health
Nashville, Tennessee

Springer Science+Business Media, LLC

Library of Congress Cataloging-in-Publication Data

Issues in contemporary international health / edited by Thomas A.
Lambo and Stacey B. Day.
p. cm.
Includes bibliographical references.

1. Public health--International cooperation. I. Lambo, Thomas A.
(Thomas Adeoye) II. Day, Stacey B.
[DNLM: 1. Public Health. 2. World Health. WA 540.1 I86]
RA441.I88 1990
362.1--dc20
DNLM/DLC
for Library of Congress 89-72169
CIP

ISBN 978-1-4899-3715-5 ISBN 978-1-4899-3713-1 (eBook)
DOI 10.1007/978-1-4899-3713-1

© 1990 Springer Science+Business Media New York
Originally published by Plenum Press, New York in 1990.
Softcover reprint of the hardcover 1st edition 1990

All rights reserved

No part of this book may be reproduced, stored in a retrieval system, or transmitted
in any form or by any means, electronic, mechanical, photocopying, microfilming,
recording, or otherwise, without written permission from the Publisher

Contributors

B. ABEL-SMITH, M.SC., PH.D.
Professor of Social Administration
London School of Economics and Political Science
London, England

S. PRINCE AKPABIO, LDS(RCS)E, FICD
Consultant, Oral Health
World Health Organization
Geneva, Switzerland;
Clinical Lecturer
University College Hospital Dental School
University of London
London, England

N. P. BOCHKOV, M.D.
Director, Institute of Medical Genetics
USSR Academy of Medical Sciences
Moscow, USSR

V. E. BULYZHENKOV, M.D.
Hereditary Diseases Programme
Division of Noncommunicable Diseases
World Health Organization
Geneva, Switzerland

J. I. COHEN, M.D., M.P.H.
Former Advisor on Health Policy
Director—General's Office
World Health Organization
Geneva, Switzerland

STACEY B. DAY, M.D., PH.D., D.SC.
Professor of International Health
Founding Director
World Health Organization Collaborating Center for Community-Based Education for Health
Nashville, Tennessee 37208

S. S. FLUSS, B.SC., M.SC.
Chief, Health Legislation
World Health Organization
Geneva, Switzerland

FRANK GUTTERIDGE, M.A., LLB, BL
Former Director
Legal Division
World Health Organization
Geneva, Switzerland

DAVID A. HAMBURG, M.D.
President, Carnegie Corporation of New York
New York, New York 10022

THOMAS A. LAMBO, M.D., FRCP, D.SC.
Deputy Director General (Retired)
World Health Organization
Geneva, Switzerland

ERNESTO MEDINA, M.D., M.P.H.
Professor of Preventive and Social Medicine and Director
School of Public Health
University of Chile
Santiago, Chile

ALLYN M. MORTIMER
Program Associate
Carnegie Corporation of New York
Washington, D.C. 20036

ELENA O. NIGHTINGALE, PH.D.
Special Advisor to the President
Carnegie Corporation of New York
Washington, D.C. 20036

D. M. Parkin, M.D.
International Agency for Research on Cancer
69372 Lyon, Cedex 8, France

Norman Sartorius, M.D., FRCP
Director, Division of Mental Health
World Health Organization
Geneva, Switzerland

L. Tomatis, M.D.
Director, International Agency for Research on Cancer
69372 Lyon, Cedex 8, France

H. Vainio, M.D.
International Agency for Research on Cancer
69372 Lyon, Cedex 8, France

Ladé Wosornu, M.D., FRCS, FRCS(E)
Professor, Department of Surgery
Director, Residency Programs
King Faisal University
College of Medicine
Dammam, Saudi Arabia

Annette M. Yonke, Ph.D.
Associate Professor, Department of Medical Education
College of Medicine
University of Illinois at Chicago
Chicago, Illinois 60612

Preface

Dr. Oliver Wendell Holmes was once asked, "When should the training of a child commence?"

"A hundred years before birth" was the reply.

Indeed it is this perspective on life through posterity that underlies the maturing field of international health, embracing as it does a responsibility for and an awareness of the needs of all peoples.

The concepts of international health are increasingly revitalizing modern medicine as it attempts to relieve mankind of the burden of disease. Curative medicine, once the paradigm, took a relatively beneficient approach to treatment. But epidemiological recognition of the frequency of disease on a global basis—and an appreciation of the vast number of those afflicted—evoked a humiliating backlash of awareness that curative medicine alone neither constrains disease nor permanently advances human health, happiness, or longevity. The growing reliance on truly international health strategies by national and international agencies, including the more definite and extended practice of preventive medicine, has provided the means to achieve significant gains in the quality of health in years to come.

A redeeming feature of contemporary failures in science and medicine is that—once intelligently studied, analyzed, and evaluated—even these failed efforts may provide real insights that can mold our capacity and determination. So it is that, more than in any bygone age, the past ten years have seen the implementation of a sound and systematic infrastructure for international health undertakings, thus paving the way for improved health for all.

Although this short monograph cannot hope to cover every current international program in medicine, public health, dentistry, or pharmacy, we hope that it will clearly demonstrate our belief that interdisciplinary integration of biopsychosocial and biobehavioral specialties within the broad disciplines of classical medicine can spearhead improvements in global health through more effective prevention of illness, through improved education and social and cultural understanding of disease, and through research and scientific investigation on behalf of the public good.

If we, and our colleagues who have herein contributed to the discussion, have succeeded in raising the threshold of interest and determination that every passing year in this field should be worth ten of those that went before, and if we can share the view that, though death may come, disease need not, then we shall have achieved our goal of furthering the influence of preventive medicine and international health—a goal to which we hope the reader can also subscribe.

THOMAS A. LAMBO
STACEY B. DAY

Contents

6 • Close-up of a Continent: Problems in South America

Ernesto Medina

II • PROBLEM AREAS IN INTERNATIONAL HEALTH

7 • International Scientific Cooperation for Maternal and Child Health

Elena O. Nightingale, David A. Hamburg, and Allyn M. Mortimer

8 • Mental Health Programs: An International Perspective

Thomas A. Lambo and Norman Sartorius

11 • Achieving Oral Health by the Year 2000

S. Prince Akpabio

12 • Trends in Managing Hereditary Diseases

N. P. Bochkov and V. E. Bulyzhenkov

III • APPROACH TO PROBLEM SOLVING IN DEVELOPING COUNTRIES

13 • Education for Health

Stacey B. Day

1

Introduction

International Health and Health for All

STACEY B. DAY AND THOMAS A. LAMBO

BACKGROUND

Few physicians, educators, or health administrators would take issue with the concept of international health; yet it has largely been only in the post-World War II era that global life has sparked such concern. This is probably due more to the impact of other survival issues, such as nuclear arms control, conflict resolutions, and trade and monetary policies, than to more humane perspectives, such as those relevant to geographic medicine or primary health care delivery in the developing world, or to educational exchanges and international participation in the training of health workers, physicians, scientists, or other personnel at various levels of management and expertise.

Curiously, the idea of using national institutions as a framework for international purposes dates back to the days of the League of Nations, when national laboratories were first designated as reference centers for the standardization of biological products.

Moreover, technical assistance by international health organizations was evident as far back as 1909, with concern over international epidemic control (*Office Internationale d'Hygiene Publique*); 1945, with the United Nations Relief and Rehabilitation Agency (UNRRA); and 1947, with the establishment of the World Health Organization.

Before 1909, voluntary help, often in social services, education, and

STACEY B. DAY • Founding Director, World Health Organization Collaborating Center for Community-Based Education for Health, Nashville, Tennessee 37208. THOMAS A. LAMBO • Deputy Director General (Retired), World Health Organization, Geneva, Switzerland.

basic health training was advanced by religious missions, university research teams, and in specialized health areas such as tropical hygiene and tropical medicine by administrative agencies regulating or controlling countries. To institute some forms of technical assistance in health and related fields was often as much in the interests of the administrative body as of the indigent population.

Governments, historically at least, seldom planned for broad adaptation to changes in the international health system. Even in 1949 when the World Health Assembly laid down the policy (which has consistently been followed since) that the organization should *not* consider "the establishment, under its own auspices, of international research institutions,"[8] the framework of international cooperation, coordination, and common action in health affairs has evolved against a backdrop of difficulties: regional conflicts, perturbation in central institutions, politicization of international health, often against prudent and better judgment, as well as critical superimposition of problems of finance, population, political ideology, basic education, environment, state-of-the-art technology, and the power leverage of the organization's aggregated institutions in the global hegemony.

It is necessary, therefore, fully to think through approaches to international health, taking into account the extraordinary variety of cultures, societies, groups, and individuals, often within one nation alone, and recognizing the dramatic changes, largely due to evolving technology, in nations, states, civilizations, economies, and their ranging political interrelations, as well as the dramatic impact disease may make upon all people and nations. One has only to remember smallpox or to refer to the current pandemic of AIDS to grasp the importance of the point.

Clearly, the issue is to find workable solutions for crises in international health in line with human needs. It is not simply to ask questions such as: "Why is it important to undertake programs in international health?"; or, "Is it *useful* to develop interaction with institutions in partner countries or in developing countries?—Or in countries in which one is in conflict on other issues?"; or, "What benefits and so forth can accrue to a parent or sponsoring institution?"

Therefore, as the mission of international health has unfolded, it is to strengthen health resources in countries in which there are needs, to develop services, research, and training, and to enhance support of national health development programs at country, intercountry, regional and interregional and global levels, as appropriate.[1] The advent of the communications era, and the advance of science and technology, as well as the dissemination of scientific information and knowledge leading towards "Health for All" has encouraged the opening up of the fields of international health. Health communications, education for health, and the biopsychosocial concept (the study of biological paradigms within sociological parameters) including general systems theory are now all part of the strategies of health care delivery in international fields.[3]

In health, we view, for society and man, a meeting point between the "inner environment" and the external environment, the integrating of the biologos in which life operates.

Man is a cultural animal. He may become sick in body, psyche, or in both. Disease may affect any or all of his configurations. The life force merges into the dynamics of all components. Where the interface is made manifest the dynamics define the nature of human action, of human behavior. Between men and between nations these biopsychosocial concepts embrace international health, including problems translating biologic or life rules between biologic levels, principally between *analyses* (scientific factorial approaches) and *syntheses* (practical modes of action between levels).

In nature, sets of translation rules arise between different domains and between different biologic levels in a given domain shaped by genetic evolutionary forces. Thus man and his environment are not to be understood as separate from each other. They are to be evaluated as interdependent parts of a united whole, a one-world. In the dynamics of the life force, change is the featured constant. *Man is always situational.*[4] His understanding must therefore be national, regional, and, above all, international.

Perception of Needs

Perception of needs in international health range from the sublime to the pragmatic,[6,9] from reflection on our responsibility for the destiny of mankind and a commitment, individually and collectively, to transform health into a bridge for peace and understanding, among all peoples and all nations, to the practical necessities. In industrialized countries we need to control, for example, excessively high dietary intakes and such risk factors as excess intake of saturated animal fats. In many countries of the developing world, especially Africa, we need to cope with problems that relate to food availability per capita; this has not increased over the past ten years and famine and malnutrition have risen as the population has increased. It is at the international level that coordination of policy and research may best facilitate care in underprivileged populations.

The touchstone of international health should be an expanding awareness and intellectual, moral, and compassionate growth of understanding in global health fields comprehending the social implications both of wellness and disease on a broad, world order. Equally, "problems" are not always to be attributed to the less developed nations, although it is certainly true that as we enter the twenty-first century, health improvement prospects inevitably are tied to the global ecosystem as well as the global econosystem. An example of international health that is truly global is exemplified by the Emergency Medical Services (EMS). The charge here is preparedness for the world community to make its populations less vulnerable to medical emergencies resulting from everyday events as well as large-scale disasters (earthquakes, floods, radiation accidents) that concern planners in *all* countries working with all populations and all agencies.

On the other hand, especially in the domain of science and technology, some developing countries are too poor or too illiterate to undertake strong efforts to involve their communities and peoples in the management of "progressive advances." Three-quarters of the global population lives in the developing world, and a reasonable projection is that by the year 2000, four-fifths of the global population will live in these areas. Further, life expectancy has increased so that in 20 years the incremental increases in the developing world have been comparable to those in the industrialized world occurring over 100 years.

It is not only science and technology that shape lives, but people and places. Often the environment may be shaped by individuals far removed in place, and international events, for better or for worse, may affect a range of lives. Often health in developing nations may affect conscious political choices and public planning, patterns of living, and social and economic outcomes that will relate to overall global situations. Food shortages, malnutrition, overpopulation, infectious and transmitted disease, and a wide variety of other parameters may all influence the health and security dynamics and balance of the well-being of nations.

Collaborative work undertaken by nations, especially when under the aegis of such reputable bodies as the World Health Organization (WHO), enhances synthesis and dissemination of information, contributes to the sharing of scientific and technical information, and enables standards to be set (nomenclature, diagnostic, therapeutic, technological, etc.), allowing for better international understanding and comparison of data on a worldwide basis.

Science and Technology for Development

Review of institutional efforts to blend modern technologies into developing societies has determined, not surprisingly, that in fact a highly technologized world cannot simply parachute "technology" onto a developing world complete with self-help labels and handbooks of instruction. Thirty years ago, U.S.-AID "thought it was only necessary to transfer technology . . . show how things are handled in Japan or in the USA . . . not to get involved in research," comments Professor Nyle Brady, Director of the Science and Technology Division of Research and University Relations (AID); and, of course, such methodology could never work. As Professor Brady pointed out, "social sciences come first, not the biological sciences," and with this refreshing light cast on international health, real advances *could* be made.[2]

Now when we consider questions of transferring technology, emphasis is placed less upon the plan than on the issues and the actors. Essential to the problem are infrastructure of knowledge, demographic transition (determinants of population in the developing world are *not* the same as those in the industrialized world of the technocracies), rural to urban relationships (migration, population sizes, trends, health, income distribution, economic growth (social factors effect technical choices), social equity and the politics of development, as well as management capabilities.

In the health area, where the burden of disease and disability has been overwhelming in the past, where data on human health are scant at best, again, initial understanding of international health was meager. In the 1960s, in the belief that all disease could be cured by an appropriate mix of policy, program direction, and delivery of health services, the Malaria Eradication program of 1965 was a prime example of misdirection. Consuming huge resources, quite without suitable research infrastructure, this approach, as was wryly observed by the British malariologist Sir Ian Macgregor, "failed to eradicate malaria, but it eradicated the malariologists.

The conceptual understanding of a need for and the application of a biopsychosocial approach to developing-world issues—the needs were for preventive, not curative medicine—improved management practices, information gathering, knowledge generation, and enhanced communication and technology education and training directed by communication. The purpose: a combining of skills and integrating of information that is contributing currently both long- and short-term benefits. Information sciences and communication technologies are as much a matter of education and literacy in the developing world now as they are in the developed world.

Notwithstanding wide-ranging interests generated for the use of science and technology (S&T) for socioeconomic development, there are severe disappointments. The Vienna Programme of Action, as reported by the United Nations Centre for Science and Technology Development (UNCSTD),[6] has experienced lack of progress due to worsening economic situations in the 1980s, lack of coherent policy frameworks, inappropriate S&T strategies, discontinuities in development of proper S & T infrastructures, and so on. Vital to successful transformation of general and global recommendations on S & T for development into activities of UN individual member states are: interactions with national, regional, and international institutions, the mobilization of both internal and external resources for their execution, and the need to monitor the quality of the results obtained over time.

Education and Health

Certainly foremost in providing encouragement and background documentation to technical discussions on education and the role of the universities in the strategies of international health has been the work of the World Health Organization.

With other agencies, investigators, and scholars, the WHO has focused on the tremendous potential that universities have for influencing the outcome of health care in different settings around the world. The work of WHO recognized the diversity in form, character, role, and function of higher educational institutions in different societies, and has sought to examine the functional relationships between these institutions, governments, and communities, especially within the context of Health for All, having regard for the fundamental imperatives of human development and social justice.

In this sense it is imperative that a few words be said on the nature of Health for All. The pledge made at Alma-Ata in 1978[10] by the members of the World Health Organization was to support the global effort to foster health for all by the year 2000. It grew out of the view that development should be based on self-reliance, community involvement, and social justice. WHO is the principal symbol of health in the world, with unique access to the various public and private institutions of the member states.

It is the single major force for sustained attention to health throughout the world and has stimulated concerted efforts to ensure at least a decent minimum of primary health care for all people by the end of the century. In this effort, far and away the most decisive factor in securing sustained national development and human well-being is investment in people and knowledge. Knowledge power—the acquired abilities of people, built up by investments that foster education, informed experience, cumulative skills, and health—are fundamental to social progress.

It is clear from this atmosphere of change that we are now witnessing a new situation in international health in which our understanding of the global imperatives of nations leads directly to heightening our understanding of the fundamental concern for an optimum use of scarce resources. It has taken the sophisticated technocracies a great time to recognize that the principal of parsimony of options is not a strategy to be reserved for economists alone, but that it is a critical force in health care management for the developing world.

Systematically, a growing interest has developed in the relationship between educational programs for the health professions and the actual practice of health care. Team care has been a vital concept. Under the guidance of WHO, critical attitudes and progressive reviews have been made of health care and strategies for better management and improved health and manpower training have been devised.

Other international agencies—e.g., the Organization for Economic Cooperation and Development (OECD), United Nations Educational, Social and Cultural Organization (UNESCO), United National Financing System For Science and Technology for Development (UNFSSTD), The World Bank—as well as national agencies—e.g., the Agency for International Development (AID) in the United States, the Association of African Universities, African Academy of Science, Third World Academy of Science, The Science, Technology and Research Commission of the O.A.U., the National Association for Equal Education Opportunity in the U.S.A. (NAFEO), national institutions in Scandinavia, France, Italy, South America, and the Eastern European bloc—have, in one way or another, over the last few years, propelled interest in enlarging and enhancing human opportunities, removing human limits, and establishing a watershed almost for a new world perspective: A perspective contributing to the fulfillment of basic human needs, including material ones, to spiritual support, and based on social and human recognition of the human biologos and the external natural environment. In effect, the biopsychosocial age has expanded human awareness, fueled by information/knowledge as a resource and space/time/location, locking societies into what has effectively become a "unit" world.

These positive advances do not, however, mean that health care does not function in an economic and political climate. The health budgeting processes in the United States Congress for the U.S. Agency for International Development is a case at point. Walsh disingenuously remarks, "Health is also politics in the Developing World,"[7] and the international dimensions of education of the physician, health team, and bureaus of policies and exchange are often themselves a tangled web of international communications, persons, policies, politics and power. Nonetheless, although much improvement is still needed, planners are learning to work within these multitiered systems, frequently discoordinated, to create pathways for improved self-sufficiency and upgrading in quality of life for the broad global community.

Contributions of This Volume

No doubt there are various ways in which a menu might be crafted of choices of subject for international health discussion. The elements of broad directions, high value content, and experience have been incorporated into the several approaches to international health offered here. Many of the authors presented might rightly be identified in their proper roles as experts surveying issues from the viewpoint of that international organization that more than any other institution is committed to international health—the WHO.

Currently there are no textbooks on international health, although basic human needs, national and international development strategies, and priorities and negotiations on behalf of economic development and the human requirements of people have been long-standing.

Further, what choices do we have in selecting from the issues that have seen a new order evolving in international health over the last decade? We might be charged with limitless concerns—water availability, food production, population growth, the price of oil, alternate fuel sources, substitutability of raw materials, marine resources, transnational migrations, women in the developing world, shifting fashions in economic theory, monetary policies, appropriate and inappropriate technologies, nuclear arms race and peace, apartheid and health, social justice, and the fact that some 50 nations change their political leadership each year.

One could develop, too, alternative sets of priority constructs for international health—world population changes, the physical environment (pollution of air and water), industrialization, world markets and trade wars, rate of use of nonrenewable resources, all of which influence variable qualities of life.

For these and related reasons we have presented this small book from a point of view of public choices. Public choices consider broad directions, not strategies. Public choices have a high content of explicit values and low technical content. Coming as they do from experts, many in the World Health Organization, these chapters generally emphasize the technique of alternative futures, a technique perhaps most familiar in the business world, especially in corporate strategic planning.

Thus, the World Health Organization has set the date of 2000 as a target in the future, and the *substance* of the chapters in general develops alternative images that might be possible in that year. For practical reasons, then, we include presentations on health policy, health management, health economics, and health education, as well as broad issues of social and medical health—cancer, mental health, mother and child, and oral (dental) health.

Clearly no list could encompass all the possibilities that might be of interest in international health. Our decision not to present a textbook was deliberate. Instead we have sought to highlight fundamental features and sometimes choices of utilitarian futures that might one day become international policy. Our intent is to consider a framework of subjects that, *if taken together,* might serve as a means to the ultimate end—improved world health and quality of life.

If these selections stimulate public discussion and can be used in formal or informal education for international health, we will have done a little more to further not only Health for All by the Year 2000, but ultimate international understanding, by encouraging nations and people to work together on problems that may affect each of them, and yet that may, not infrequently, have their origin outside the nations involved.

Finally, we present as an appendix the text of the International Health Regulations in force as of January 1982, constituting Articles 1 to 94. The original International Health Regulations were adopted by the Twenty-second World Health Assembly on 25 July, 1969 and represented a revised and consolidated version of the previous International Sanitary Regulations.

The purpose of the International Health Regulations is to ensure the maximum security against the international spread of diseases with a minimum of interference with world traffic. The new regulations "are intended to strengthen the use of epidemiological principles as applied internationally, to detect, reduce or eliminate the sources from which infection spreads, to improve sanitation in and around ports and airports, to prevent the dissemination of vectors and, in general, to encourage epidemiological activities on the national level so that there is little risk of outside infection establishing itself."[11]

It has been our experience both as teachers and as investigators committed to international health that fewer and fewer professional health workers, at all levels of training, read these guidelines. It is not uncommon for professors as well as students to be unfamiliar with fundamental protocols (the correct definition of "day" for example), in the International Health Regulations.

References

1. Bankowski Z, Mejia A (eds): *Health Manpower Out of Balance—Conflicts and Prospects.* CIMS. Geneva, WHO, 1987.
2. Brady, NC: Twenty-fifth Anniversary Commemoration of the U.S. Agency for International Development (AID). National Academy of Sciences, Washington, D.C., 1988.
3. Day, Stacey B: *Health Communications.* New York, International Foundation, 1979.
4. Day, Stacey B: Biopsychosocial Imperatives of Health Care (ed): *Soc Sci Med,* 1985; 21: 12:1335–1409.
5. Henderson, DA: Contributions of the Health Sciences. In *Science and Technology for Development: Prospects Entering the Twenty-first Century.* Washington, D.C., National Academy Press, 1988.
6. United Nations Centre For Science and Technology: *Science and Technology For Development—The Prospect Ahead of Us.* New York. UNCSTD, 1986.
7. Walsh, William B: *A Comparison of United States and Soviet Policies and Programs in International Medical Education.* Proc. Annual Meeting of the Association of American Medical Colleges. ECFMG Publication, P 41, 1984.
8. World Health Assembly Resolutions, WHA2.19 and WHA2. 32, 1949.
9. World Health Organization: *The Role of Universities in the Strategies for Health for All.* Geneva, WHO, 1984.
10. World Health Organization: *Primary Health Care.* Report of the International Conference on Primary Health Care, Alma-Ata, USSR, 6–12 September 1978. Geneva, WHO, 1978.
11. World Health Organization: *International Health Regulations.* Annotated ed 3. Geneva, WHO, 1969.

I

Management of International Health

2

Health Policy, Management, and Economics

J. I. COHEN

INTRODUCTION

The concept of health policy is of relatively recent date, with notable exceptions, such as the establishment by Bismarck in the latter half of the nineteenth century of sick funds for workers in Germany, and Chadwick's sanitary reforms in the United Kingdom. Until recently, health was considered to be an individual matter and health care a personal transaction between doctor or nurse and patient. In the course of the twentieth century it became evident that many environmental, economic, social, cultural, and educational factors affect the health of individuals and communities and that these, as well as ethical factors, influence the delivery of health care. Increasing awareness by people of the potential effectiveness of government action in improving their health made such action politically popular. For these reasons health policy has become an accepted concept in the contemporary world no less than economic or social policy, and the formulation of health policy a normal function of government.

THE NATURE OF HEALTH POLICY

Health policy is a set of decisions to pursue courses of action for achieving defined health goals; a goal being a general aim towards which to strive—for example, an environment conducive to health or universal

J. I. COHEN • Former Advisor on Health Policy, Director—General's Office, World Health Organization, Geneva, Switzerland.

access to primary health care. Such a policy determines the priorities among the goals and the main directions for achieving them, for example, to reduce the incidence and prevalence of cardiovascular diseases through modifications of life-styles. Determining priorities implies selecting from among alternatives, both between the health sector and other competing sectors and within the health sector. This implies that health policy has to be considered as part of a broader policy of social and economic development within available and potentially available resources. Moreover, socioeconomic development policy is affected by policies in other fields, such as defense.

Competition between the health and other sectors is naturally influenced by economic considerations and by social preference values. From an economic perspective, if the attainment of health is considered merely as a consumption of resources, its priority will be low; if, however, it is considered as a factor contributing to economic development, it may be accorded higher priority.

Health policy is an affair of government, but not of government alone. Individuals, communities, and other associations of people can stimulate governments to adopt health policy and can adopt their own policies if these do not conflict with legally binding national policy.

Many options for the nature and form of health policy are open to governments. The first important policy decision is whether to define a policy at all or to adopt a laissez-faire attitude. Such an attitude often prevails by default rather than being arrived at by conscious decision. Or it may result from the belief that health is too individual a matter to permit collective decision, or that governmental involvement or interference can be detrimental to the determination of health policy by individuals for themselves. Nevertheless, government policy can consist of encouraging individuals or communities to decide on their own health policies. These are fundamental issues that cannot be taken for granted.

Policies can relate to technical matters, such as the range of health care to be provided; this may be limited to high-priority issues, or may cover the whole gamut of individual and community health problems. Policies can also relate to social matters, such as the availability to the whole population of the range of care selected, or its limitation in whole or in part to selected population groups, such as mothers and children, workers, the elderly, or the poor. In addition, policies can relate to economic matters, such as methods of financing health care or different aspects of it. Policies can be promotional or prohibitive in nature, or they may consist of providing information alone. They may take the form of permitting certain measures to be taken or, on the other hand, may be legally binding in nature, or may rely solely on education and information for their implementation.

The Scope of Health Policy

The scope of health policy varies widely, depending on the health ambitions of those defining it. It may be modest in its goals, being limited to ensuring the availability of conventional medical care to the whole population or to certain sectors of it. At the other extreme, it may extend to the comprehensive goal of attaining health as described in the World Health Organization's constitution, namely, a state of complete, physical, mental, and social well-being, and not merely the absence of disease or infirmity. In the latter case the policy will have to deal with health promotion, health protection, disease prevention, medical care, and physical, mental, and social rehabilitation, with all that that implies, not only for the health sector, but also for other social and economic sectors.

If the concept of medical care is commonly understood, this may not be so for the other components of the kind of comprehensive health policy mentioned above. Thus, health promotion is an evolving concept. It encompasses fostering life-styles and other social, economic, environmental, and personal factors conducive to health. These include raising people's awareness about health matters and enabling them to cope with health problems by increasing their knowledge and providing them with valid information; encouraging adequate and appropriate diet and exercise and enough sleep; ensuring education and work in conformity with physical and mental capacity; making available suitable housing and safe water and sanitary facilities; improving the physical, economic, cultural, psychological, and social environment; and encouraging and assisting social support groups. In November 1986 the First International Conference on Health promotion adopted a charter[1] for health promotional actions. Such action includes building healthy public policy; creating supportive environments; strengthening community action for health; developing personal skills concerning health; and reorienting health services to increase their contribution to the pursuit of health.

Health protection implies guarding against potential dangers to health, such as ensuring the availability of measures to protect workers against the specific hazards of their work, or action by individuals, such as protective clothing against inclement weather. Disease prevention involves ensuring measures to prevent the occurrence of specific diseases, such as immunization against the common infectious diseases of childhood or undertaking antismoking activities to prevent or reduce the occurrence of lung cancer and certain forms of heart disease; it also involves measures to arrest the progress of disease and reduce its consequences once it is established. Comprehensive rehabilitation includes restoring function to a diseased organ, such as the heart, after a myocardial infarct, compensating for the loss of an organ, as by providing an artificial limb and restoring the function that the organic limb formerly performed, helping the individuals concerned to recover their mental equilibrium which may have been disturbed by the disease or injury, and reintegrating them into the social and economic life of the community.

The Content of Health Policy

The content of a broad health policy is fashioned by the determinants of health. These occur in the human body—endogenous factors, as well as in the environment—exogenous factors. Only very recently has it been possible and necessary for governments to take policy decisions with respect to endogenous factors, such as the control of fertility or the transplantation of human organs; ethical considerations heavily affect such policy.

Health policy can be formulated with respect to a wide variety of exogenous factors, such as habitat and housing, for example, zoning of industrial and residential areas and related questions of transport, play areas for children, location of roads to minimize noise from traffic and the danger of accidents, design of homes to prevent accidents, and housing adapted to the elderly in order to retain them in the community. Other exogenous factors amenable to health policy include the provision of safe water supply and sanitation; the control of environmental pollution from biological and chemical sources; food and nutrition policy as they affect health and related agricultural policy, for example, the balance between food crops and cash crops and the limitation of fat of animal origin. Policies may be defined for education and information as they affect health, starting in homes and schools and involving the mass media. Other issues include public policy regarding smoking, alcohol abuse, and drug abuse; the promotion of exercise and sport and their encouragement by making appropriate facilities available and the promotion of cultural pursuits conducive to mental health.

Policies may be determined concerning the collation and dissemination of information on the health situation in a country or community;

this may range from a laissez-faire attitude to the establishment of a sophisticated health information system for the collection, analysis, and storage of information on health matters and its dissemination in a forceful manner in appropriate forms for different types of audience, including health policymakers and executives, professional health workers, and the lay public.

Many different options present themselves for health research policy, including the deliberate decision to allow health research to take its own course without government or public intervention, encouraging young research workers, providing research career incentives, supporting established research workers and institutions, selectively supporting neglected areas, such as tropical disease research or research into the optimal organization of health systems, laying down technical and ethical criteria for health research from public funds, including the prohibition of certain kinds of research, such as on embryos and fetuses, or formulating a comprehensive health research policy to be adhered to by all concerned.

Economic and social policies have to be taken into account in defining health policy. Thus, selective taxation can either promote or damage health. For example, heavy taxation on tobacco and alcoholic beverages may result in a reduction in their consumption; however, it also increases government revenue and in some societies this can be a double-edged sword and can actually foster increased consumption by people in a spirit of pseudo-patriotism! An opposite example is subsidizing farmers to produce food that is conducive to health, such as low-fat meat or other foods low in cholesterol content. A laissez-faire attitude toward financing health care prevails in some societies, whereas financial policy for health may have to be decided upon in other societies. Such policy includes not only the limits to resources invested in health, but also such questions as who pays and by what means costs are distributed among the different socioeconomic groups of society or among users and nonusers of the health service.

Social policy affecting health is closely related to general policy preferences, such as preferential attention to certain geographic locations, socioeconomic groups, age groups, occupation, or degree of social deprivation. Thus, in some countries preferential care may be given to those who are politically active and influence voting patterns, such as the urban elite or a particular ethnic group. In some countries, a policy of rural development or of ensuring adequate numbers of people along the borders with neighboring countries can lead to preferential health care being provided to the periphery. If industrialization is the country's policy, the health care of industrial workers may be given higher priority than that of other economic groups. In many countries the health care of mothers and children is given top priority. Some countries give priority to the socially underprivileged in providing health care from the public purse, on the assumption that other people can more easily fend for themselves. Indeed, history has shown that social revolutions have been brought about in part as a reaction to low socioeconomic status including health status, and that introducing a policy to improve health has been one of the early and major decisions of the revolutionaries when they assumed power.

Policy concerning the administrative system of a country also affects health policy. Thus, if the country has a highly centralized administrative system, the health system is likely to be highly centralized too. If responsibilities are delegated to other administrative levels, such as provinces, districts, municipalities, or smaller communities, it is possible to adopt a parallel policy of decentralization of the health system. If decisions are taken to decentralize highly centralized administrative systems, a concomitant policy may have to be adopted of strengthening the administrative capacities of those to whom responsibility has been delegated and introducing a system of monitoring and control; this applies to the health sector no less than to other sectors.

The above kinds of health policy, each in its own way as well as in various combinations, may affect policy concerning the establishment and organization of the health care delivery system. That system will also be influenced by policy concerning the allocation of priority to care in the community at one end of the spectrum, to highly specialized hospital care at the other end, or to an appropriate balance among all constituents of the spectrum.

Resource Allocation

The ultimate expression of policy is resource allocation; otherwise the policy will remain empty phraseology. This does not imply that resource allocation necessarily dictates health policy. Ideally, health policy should dictate resource allocation, just as social policy should dictate technical policy, and not the reverse. The goal of the health policy should thus be the supreme factor in deciding on resource allocations within the defined resource ceiling for health. This goal may have to be achieved in stages because of resource constraints, and intermediate targets may have to be set on the path to the goal, resources being allocated with a view to attaining these targets. An example of a target to contribute to the goal of good child health is the immunization by the year 1990 of all the children in the country against the common infectious diseases of childhood—in conformity with the target of universal immunization of children by that date set by the World Health Organization.

A sound policy of resource allocation will reflect the policy of priority determination. Thus, the priority to be given to health within the overall national endeavor, priority health problems and measures for solving them and priority socioeconomic groups, if any, for health care, all influence resource allocation. So will decisions concerning decentralization; delegation of responsibility and authority only has meaning if it is accompanied by the related allocation of resources. Public pressure of different kinds from different sources and for different motives is also an important factor in determining priorities and related resource allocations. It can be seen that trade-offs among different social values, their expression in terms of resources and the allocation of resources accordingly are fundamental to policy-making.

Health Strategies

The existence of a health policy does not automatically mean that it will be put into effect, even if resources have been allocated to that end. Measures have to be taken to ensure the implementation of policy, and these measures depend on the nature of the policy, for example, whether it makes certain measures obligatory, or merely permits them to be taken. One way of ensuring implementation is through the preparation of an operational strategy. If policy is usually expressed in general terms, a strategy has to be more operationally specific. It lays down the main lines of action to be taken in all the sectors concerned to give effect to the policy, including the identification of obstacles to its implementation and ways of overcoming them, and the determination of the broad resource allocations for each line of action and a related financial master plan. These main lines of action will usually consist of a blend of political, economic, financial, social, legislative, educational, administrative, scientific, technical, and managerial measures in the light of the nature, scope, and content of the health policy.

A health strategy usually includes specific programs for delivery by the health infrastructure, a program being an organized aggregate of activities directed toward the attainment of defined objectives and targets that are progressively more specific than the goal to which they contribute. Each health program ought to have its specific objectives and targets, whenever possible quantified, that are consistent with those of the national health strategy. A target has been exemplified above. An objective is the end result a program seeks to achieve; for example, the objective of health education may be to ensure that people want to be healthy, know how to stay healthy, do what they can individually and collectively to maintain health, and know how to seek help when required. The health program has to set out clearly the requirements for attaining its objectives and targets in terms of health personnel, physical facilities, technology, equipment and supplies, information and intercommunication, the methods of monitoring and evaluation, a timetable of activities and ways of ensuring correlations between its various elements and other related programs, and all of these have to be costed.

A health strategy also has to define how to establish a health infrastructure, or strengthen the existing one, in order to deliver the programs devolving on it, a health infrastructure connoting the services, facilities, institutions, establishments, organizations, logistic systems and their interrelationships, as well as those operating them. The mere existence of health facilities with health personnel does not of itself constitute a health infrastructure; often these act as a suprastructure imposing their own policies. A health infrastructure as part of a health policy implies correlated action on the part of all its constituent parts with the aim of attaining the objectives of those health programs that form part of the national health strategy. These might include programs to develop the infrastructure itself, such as programs for assessing the health situation and trends on the basis of a combination of epidemiological and statistical information, for developing and organizing the health system, for assessing needs for health manpower, as well as their training and deployment, and for ensuring that the public is properly educated and informed on matters affecting their health.

Technical programs might include the promotion of relevant research; the generation, assessment, and application of medical care technology; nutrition; oral health; prevention of accidents in homes and on the roads; care of mothers and children and the elderly within the family; prevention and control of occupational diseases and promotion of occupational health; mental and environmental health; rehabilitation; control of pharmaceutical products and ensuring the availability of medicines that people need; prevention and control of infectious diseases, such as those preventable by immunization, diarrhea, acute respiratory infections, tuberculosis, and leprosy; as well as the prevention and control of parasitic and tropical diseases where these are prevalent, such as malaria, schistosomiasis, and filariasis. Technical programs might also include the prevention and control of noncommunicable diseases, such as cardiovascular disease and cancer, and access to the information required to deal with all the above.

For each of the above it may be necessary to define a program or infrastructure policy, as the case may be. For example, in the past many programs established their own infrastructure, resulting in a wasteful proliferation of infrastructures competing with one another for resources. A policy of integrating these programs within one infrastructure, or at least of ensuring their coordinated implementation by the same infrastructure, has to be defined and carried out and a strategy for doing so put into effect, often progressively. The kind of technology to be used by each program has to be decided on and that technology has to be appropriate for the country concerned. It cannot be assumed that health technology that is appropriate for one country is necessarily appropriate for another with different epidemiological and socioeconomic circumstances. In every health action the ratio of benefit to risk has to be considered, whether in relation to medicines or to the use of certain kinds of pesticides in agriculture that might have long-term effects on health. The World Health Organization (WHO) has defined health technology as methods, procedures, techniques, and related equipment and supplies in conjunction with the people using them and those on whom it is used. It has defined health technology as being appropriate if it is scientifically, technically, socially, and economically sound; that is, it is based on sound scientific evidence, it functions technically in a satisfactory manner, it is acceptable to those on whom it is used and to those who use it, and it can be afforded by the community and country concerned.

Even if all of the above had been defined and planned for in operational terms, other aspects of a health strategy are essential for its successful implementation. These include coordination within the health sector and between it and other sectors concerned, ensuring political commitment and economic support, winning over professional groups so that they can contribute to the implementation of the strategy or at least will not oppose it, and generating and mobilizing the human and financial resources required. Last but not least, they include measures to ensure that people understand the strategy and how it can contribute to the improvement of their health so that they will be adequately equipped to take part intelligently in the social control of the health system and its component parts in accordance with the means of social control that are applicable in the country concerned.

The Process of Defining Health Policies and Strategies

Health policies and strategies are normally defined in the same manner as policy in all other areas is defined in the country concerned. Countries with centrally planned economies may define health policy not only in the light of epidemiological information, but also in line with the party policy for social and economic development. Such policy is often based on ideological and technical norms, although some of the forces influencing policy in other types of country may also enter into play. In market economy countries the options are more varied; they do not exclude those in vogue in centrally planned economy countries. They include epidemiologically based estimates and forecasts of needs based on the health and economic situation as well as on socioepidemiological analysis, the assessment of popular currents, response to political, economic, and professional interests or to pressures from the public and consumer groups, public and parliamentary debate, reaction to articles on health in the popular press—particularly sensational ones—opportunistic initiatives resulting, for example, from the illness of people in power or their close relatives, recognition of needs following a health disaster—such as the need to regulate the use of medicines following the thalidomide disaster—and often a combination of many of these.

A formal way of defining health policy and strategy is through a managerial process, although it has to be admitted that management is more often the outcome of a policy than its precursor. A managerial process may be useful in generating the kind of information that will facilitate rational decision making. However, such a process may be invaluable in formulating the strategy on the basis of a defined policy. WHO has developed a managerial process for national health development of this kind.[2]

Figure 1 summarizes the process and is schematic. In practice the components of the process form a continuum and the order of action is rarely as sequential as the schema, there being different entry points, depending on current circumstances. The managerial process for national health development is a continuous process of systematically preparing plans and programs carried out in collaboration by the health sector and other sectors concerned with health. The process of translating the health policy into a strategy with clearly stated objectives and targets is known as broad programming. The preferential allocation of resources to priority activities for implementing the strategy is achieved through program budgeting, that is, defining programs by objectives and allocating budgets by programs. This differs from ordinary budgeting in that emphasis is laid on results to be achieved, rather than on unconnected budgetary items. In order to attain the program's objectives and targets, the resources required are grouped together, those who will receive them specified, and their sources determined. For each program a detailed set of activities is worked out—that is known as

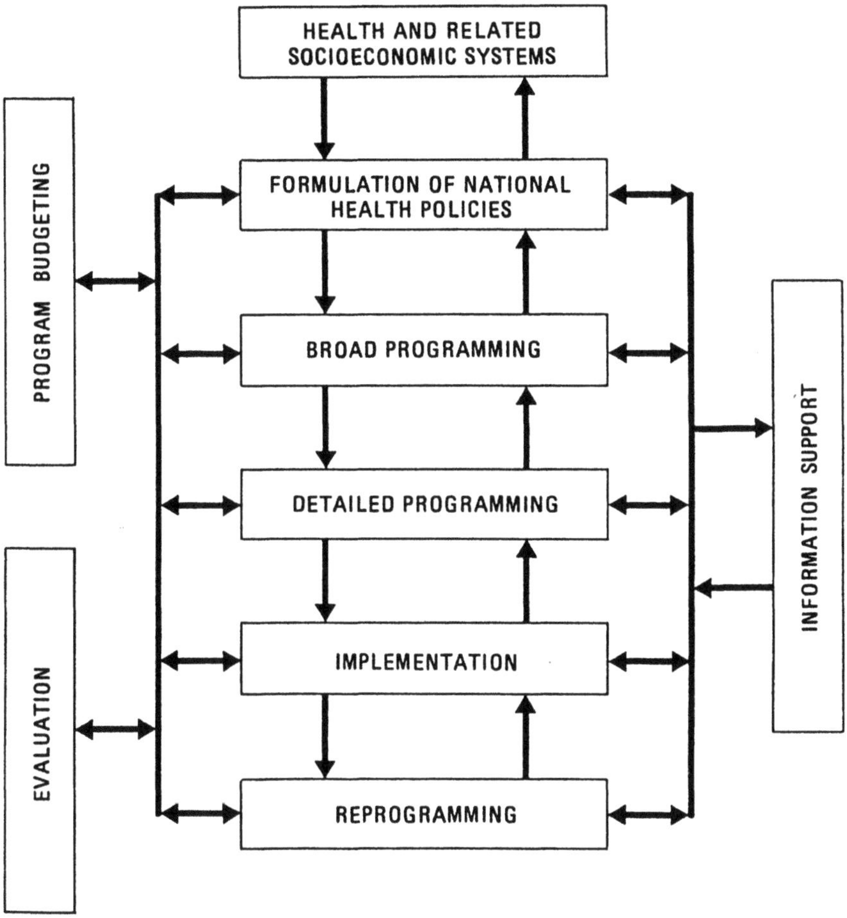

FIGURE 1. Managerial process for national health development.

detailed programming. The health infrastructure delivers the programs concerned on the basis of these detailed program activities which include a timetable and related budgetary and other resource allocations. Health systems research is applied to identify the most appropriate forms of health technology under the given circumstances and the most appropriate organization of the health system for optimal application of the technology. The health infrastructure employs sound managerial procedures for program delivery.

Programs and their delivery by the health infrastructure are monitored and evaluated with a view to ensuring that activities are proceeding as planned and that the services and institutions concerned are delivering the programs efficiently and effectively. Monitoring implies the continuous follow-up of activities to ensure that they are proceeding according to plan. It keeps track of achievements, staff movements and utilization, supplies and equipment, and the money spent in relation to the resources available, so that if anything goes wrong, immediate corrective measures can be taken.

WHO has also established a process for health program evaluation as part of the managerial process for national health development,[3] including the use of indicators and methods of collecting and analyzing the information required to that end.[4] Evaluation is the systematic assessment of the relevance, adequacy, progress, efficiency, effectiveness, and impact of a health program. A program is considered to be relevant if it answers the needs and social and health policies and priorities it has been designed to meet. It is considered to be adequate if it is proportionate to requirements. It is making good progress if its component activities are being carried out in accordance with the planned schedule. It is considered to be efficient if the effort expended on it is as good as possible in relation to the resources devoted to it, and effective if the results obtained are in accordance with the objectives and targets for reducing the dimensions of a problem or improving an unsatisfactory situation. The impact of a program is assessed by its overall effect on health status and socioeconomic development. The managerial process continues with the review of the outcomes of monitoring and evaluation with the aim of introducing any modification or improvements recommended. The process also includes ensuring the information support required for all of the above.

In view of the crucial nature of the financial master plan for a health strategy, it is worth highlighting some of its main features, although these will be elaborated in greater detail in the next part of this chapter. It is first necessary to establish the economic feasibility of the proposed health policy, taking into account resource constraints outside and inside the health sector as well as capital and recurrent expenditures. Its "opportunity cost"—that is, the value of the next best option that has to be foregone in order to carry out the proposed policy—has to be demonstrated. It is important to assess the economic feasibility of a proposed policy before political commitment to it has become too strong to be changed.

Financing the strategy has to be considered from sources inside and outside the health sector. Social values and economic systems prevailing in the country concerned will influence the ways by which health policies and strategies are financed. Alternative sources of financing have to be considered. These may include government taxation, social security schemes, and making employers responsible, for example, in mining. They may also include charging for services, which may be selective to ensure social equity or to encourage the correct use of the health service, for example, reliance first on primary health care and correct use of the referral system; or to limit excessive use of the health service, for example, of medicines; or to limit recourse to what are considered luxuries. Other sources of financing are nongovernmental organizations, which may have to be provided with certain incentives, such as tax rebates, and voluntary health insurance. In many societies the growing potential of people's financial participation in the cost of the health system must never be forgotten. To identify the extent of this may require social and economic research; there is a difference between what people are theoretically able to pay and what they are willing to pay. Their willingness will depend to a large extent on their understanding of the potentially beneficial effect of the policy on their health and on that of their children and family. External sources of financing may also be considered by developing countries.

The picture would be rosy indeed if such rationality were observed in defining and implementing health policies and strategies. In real life the process is rarely pursued with such managerial neatness; it is a messy matter, like all developmental efforts. People do not behave like passive objects when their health is concerned. They do not blindly obey mathematical models for health planning, so these have become academic tools. It is wise to encourage people to develop their own health policies and strategies in consonance with the national health policy and strategy if these are sound and hold the health and socioeconomic interests of people above all other considerations. It is their health that is at stake.

To maintain some semblance of order in the evolution of a health system that has its roots in the definition of health policies and the formulation of strategies to give them effect, this author has employed "systematic indeterminacy." The systematic part lies in the clear articulation of the goals of the policy and of the main lines of action for attaining them, as well as the clear formulation of the various options for pursuing these lines of action. The indeterminacy lies in the empirical selection of the optimal option at the opportune moment in the light of the prevailing political, social, economic, scientific, and technical circumstances, as well as the managerial capacity of the health infrastructure and the capacity of the population concerned to absorb it. Such empirical selection is often helped by "quick and dirty" health systems research to arrive at reasonable solutions for certain specific problems.

International Health Policy and Strategy

A remarkable illustration of health policy and strategy at the international level is provided by the goal of health for all by the year 2000 adopted by the member states of the World Health Organization, of which there are now 166. In 1977 the World Health Assembly, WHO's supreme policy organ composed of delegates from all member states, decided that the main social target of governments and of WHO in the coming decades should be the attainment by all the people of the world by the year 2000 of a level of health that will permit them to lead a socially and economically productive life. This is popularly known as "health for all by the year 2000." It was made clear that each country would interpret the meaning of social and economic productivity in the light of its own socioeconomic circumstances.

This goal has been the basis of a complete revolution in public health thinking. It gave rise to an international conference held in Alma-Ata in the USSR in 1978 under the auspices of WHO and UNICEF. This conference issued a declaration—the Declaration of Alma-Ata[5]—which included the following statements:

- Health, which is a state of complete physical, mental, and social well-being, and not merely the absence of disease or infirmity, is a fundamental human right; the attainment of the highest possible level of health is a most important worldwide social goal whose realization requires the action of many other social and economic sectors in addition to the health sector.
- The existing gross inequality in the health status of the people particularly between developed and developing countries as well as within countries is politically, socially, and economically unacceptable and is, therefore, of common concern to all countries.
- The promotion and protection of the health of the people are essential to sustained economic and social development and contributes to a better quality of life and to world peace.
- People have the right and duty to participate individually and collectively in the planning and implementation of their health care.
- Governments have a responsibility for the health of their people

which can be fulfilled only by the provision of adequate health and social measures.

The declaration went on to state that primary health care is the key to attaining health for all by the year 2000 as part of development in the spirit of social justice. It defined primary health care as essential health care based on practical, scientifically sound, and socially acceptable methods and technology made universally accessible to individuals and families in the community through their full participation and at a cost that the community and country can afford to maintain at every stage of their development in the spirit of self-reliance and self-determination. It forms an integral part both of the country's health system, of which it is the central function and main focus, and of the overall social and economic development of the community. It is the first level of contact of individuals, the family, and community with the national health system bringing health care as close as possible to where people live and work, and constitutes the first element of a continuing health care process.

Primary health care as defined at Alma-Ata includes at least education concerning prevailing health problems and the methods of preventing and controlling them; promotion of food supply and proper nutrition, and adequate supply of safe water and basic sanitation; maternal and child health care, including family planning; immunization against the major infectious diseases; prevention and control of locally endemic diseases; appropriate treatment of common diseases and injuries; and provision of essential drugs. It involves, in addition to the health sector, all related sectors and aspects of national and community development; in particular, agriculture, animal husbandry, food, industry, education, housing, public works, communications, and other sectors; and demands the coordinated efforts of all those sectors. It promotes maximum community and individual self-reliance and participation in the planning, organization, operation, and control of primary health care, making fullest use of local, national, and other available resources; and to this end develops through appropriate education and ability of communities to participate. In addition, it should be sustained by a referral system, leading eventually to comprehensive health care for all and giving priority to those most in need, and should rely on a variety of health personnel working as a team.

The conference urged all governments to formulate national health policies and strategies with a view of developing health systems based on primary health care and to cooperate with one another to this end.

The response has been remarkable, beyond all expectation. Governments throughout the world, poor and rich, of all political ideologies and religious creeds, with planned and market economies, have developed policies and strategies for health for all. WHO in turn developed regional strategies as a synthesis of the national strategies in each of its six regions (Africa, the Americas, Southeast Asia, Europe, Eastern Mediterranean, and Western Pacific). It then formulated a global strategy which was adopted by the World Health Assembly in 1981 as a social contact for health between governments, people, and WHO.[6]

The policy of health for all by the year 2000 is an expression of political commitment to the improvement of the health of all people everywhere. It emphasizes equity in health, the proper commitment of people to the promotion and maintenance of their own health, the involvement, in addition to the health sector, of other social and economic sectors whose activities affect health positively and negatively, and the establishment of health systems based on primary health care with suitable infrastructures for delivering health programs that use appropriate technology for health. More specifically, it incorporates the following principles:

1. Health is a fundamental human right and a worldwide social goal.
2. The existing gross inequality in the health status of people is of common concern to all countries and must be drastically reduced. A more equitable distribution of health resources, both among countries and within countries, leading to universal accessibility to primary health care and its supporting services, is therefore fundamental to the Strategy.
3. Since people have the right and the duty to participate individually and collectively in the planning and implementation of their health care, community involvement in shaping its own health and socioeconomic future, including mass involvement of women, men, youth, and children is a key factor in the Strategy.
4. Governments having a responsibility for the health of their people which can be fulfilled only by the provision of adequate health and other social measures, the political commitment of the state as a whole, and not merely the ministry of health, is essential.

Countries must become self-reliant in health matters if they are to attain health for all their people. National self-reliance implies national initiative, but not necessarily national self-sufficiency. Where health is concerned no country is self-sufficient; international solidarity is required to ensure the development and implementation of health strategies and to overcome obstacles. Such international health solidarity must respect national self-reliance.

In conformity with the recognition by the United Nations General Assembly that health is an integral part of development, the human energy generated by improved health should be channeled into sustaining economic and social development, and economic and social development should be harnessed to improve the health of people. In addition to the health sector, the coordinated efforts will be required of other social and economic sectors concerned with national and community development, as outlined in the Declaration of Alma-Ata. Ministries of health or analogous authorities have an important role in stimulating and coordinating such coordinated action for health.

Fuller and better use must be made of the world's resources to promote health and development, and thus help to promote world peace.

Technical and economic cooperation among countries is crucial to the attainment of health for all, since it will provide the mutual support required for the development and implementation of the Strategy. It is the best expression of international health solidarity that guarantees national self-reliance.

The main thrusts of the Strategy are the development by countries of their health system infrastructure, starting with primary health care, for the delivery of countrywide programs that reach the whole population. These programs include measures for health promotion and protection, disease prevention, diagnosis, therapy, and rehabilitation. The Strategy involves specifying measures to be taken by individuals and families in their homes, by communities, by the health service at the primary and supporting levels, and by other sectors. It also involves selecting technology that is appropriate for the country concerned, appropriateness being assessed in relation to WHO's criteria mentioned above. Crucial to the Strategy is making sure of social control of the health infrastructure and technology through a high degree of community involvement.

An inseparable part of the Strategy is the action required to promote and support it. This includes strengthening the Ministry of Health, or analogous authority representing the whole health sector, as the focal point for the national strategy. It is necessary to ensure political commitment at the highest level nationally and internationally, as well as the support of economic development planners. Professional groups inside and outside the health sector have to be enlisted. An appropriate managerial process for national health development has to be developed and applied, and biomedical, behavioral, and health systems research oriented to support the Strategy. Policy, technical, and popular information to ensure acceptance of an involvement in the Strategy has to be widely disseminated.

Also inseparable from the Strategy is the action required to generate and mobilize all possible resources. All human resources have to be mobilized, not only health personnel. All types of health personnel as appropriate to the country have to be motivated and mobilized. The best use has to be made of available human and financial resources, and investments in health have to be increased if necessary.

Also spelled out is the international action to be taken to support the above national action through information exchange, promoting research and development, technical support, training, ensuring international coordination within the health sector and between the health and other sectors, and fostering and supporting the essential elements of primary health care in countries.

The international transfer of resources from developed to developing countries has to be rationalized and these transfers increased if necessary.

Intercountry cooperation is an essential feature of the Strategy, because few countries will be able to formulate and implement their strategies independently. This involves both technical and economic cooperation among countries (TCDC and ECDC), and the use of WHO's regional arrangement to facilitate such cooperation.

To illustrate some of the details of the Strategy, the following are the essential characteristics of the kind of health system that is envisaged.

1. The system should encompass the entire population on a basis of equality and responsibility.
2. It should include components from the health sector and from other sectors whose interrelated actions contribute to health.
3. Primary health care, consisting of at least the essential elements included in the Declaration of Alma-Ata, should be delivered at the first point of contact between individuals and the health system.
4. At intermediate levels more complex problems should be dealt with, more skilled and specialized care as well as logistic support should be provided, and more highly trained staff should provide continuing training to primary health care workers, as well as guidance to communities and community health workers on practical problems arising in connection with all aspects of primary health care.

5. The central level should coordinate all parts of the system, and provide planning and management expertise, highly specialized care, teaching for specialized staff, the expertise of such institutions as central laboratories, and central logistic and financial support.

The Strategy indicates the following actions that have to be taken into account to develop such health systems:

1. Action to be taken in the health sector has to be identified, planned, and coordinated.
2. Action to be taken in other sectors has to be identified, and the responsible authorities approached with a view to implementation.
3. Ways have to be devised of involving people and communities in decisions concerning the health system and in taking responsibility for self-care as well as family and community care.
4. Central planning has to aim at enabling communities of different types and sizes to work out their own primary health care activities.
5. A supportive referral system has to be devised and put into effect, particular attention being paid initially to the first referral level.
6. A logistic system has to be organized and operated for the whole country.
7. Health manpower has to be planned, trained, and deployed in response to specific needs of people as an integral part of the health infrastructure.
8. Appropriate health care facilities have to be planned for, designed, constructed, and equipped so that they are readily available, accessible, and acceptable to all the population.
9. Appropriate health technology has to be selected.

Rough estimates have been made of the costs of such strategies in countries. According to these estimates, they could be carried out by developed countries well within existing costs and probably for much less. For least-developed countries, all the elements of primary health care could be introduced and maintained at a cost of about 15 dollars per person per year—5 dollars for capital expenditures and 10 dollars for recurrent ones. It has been estimated that the Strategy could be carried out in developing countries worldwide at a cost of about 50 billion U.S.

dollars a year. If 80% of that sum was covered by the developing countries, this would still leave a shortfall of 10 billion dollars from external sources. These sources currently transfer about 3 billion dollars for health to less developed countries. Nevertheless, the financial difficulties should not be insurmountable; some countries have annual budgetary deficits that greatly exceed these amounts.

WHO's member states, widely differing in their epidemiological, political, economic, social, cultural, and managerial characteristics, are acting on their honor to carry out individually and in their relationships with other countries the health policy and strategy for health for all by the year 2000 that they adopted collectively in WHO. To monitor progress in implementing the Strategy and to evaluate its effectiveness, countries are applying monitoring and evaluation processes as part of their managerial process for national health development, using collectivity agreed indicators and a common evaluation framework. At the international level WHO's structures are being used for reporting on progress and assessing the impact of the Strategy. WHO's member states are organized in six geographical regions (Africa, the Americas, Southeast Asia, Eastern Mediterranean, Europe, and Western Pacific), each region having a regional committee composed of representatives of the member states in the region concerned. Almost ninety percent of member states have now reported on their first evaluation of their strategies, and, on the basis of these, regional evaluations have been made by all six regional committees. The evaluation of the Strategy worldwide was reviewed by the World Health Assembly in May 1986, and the findings were published by WHO as the *Seventh Report on the World Health Situation,* consisting of a global review and six regional ones.[7] Progress in implementing the strategy was further monitored by the World Health Assembly in May 1989.

Is it possible to manage an internationally agreed health policy and strategy whose implementation depends on the governments of 166 countries and their more than 4 billion people carrying out national health policies and strategies that are consonant with the international one? That is precisely what WHO's member states are attempting to do collectively through the organization's highly flexible management system. The unifying force in the system is the very policy whose implementation the system is designed to manage, giving rise to an organizational complex whose "soft" component—the collective policy—holds together the "hard" component—the decentralized management system. Future social historians will judge if this was organizational genius or madness.

References

1. *Ottawa Charter for Health Promotion*. An International Conference on Health Promotion. Ottawa, Canada, 1986.
2. *Managerial Process for National Health Development—Guiding Principles*. Health for All Series, No. 5. Geneva, 1981.
3. *Health Programme Evaluation—Guiding Principles*. Health for All Series, No. 6. Geneva, 1981.
4. *Development of Indicators for Monitoring Progress Towards Health for All by the Year 2000*. Health for All Series, No. 4. Geneva, 1981.
5. Alma-Ata 1978. Primary Health Care. Health for All Series, No. 1. Geneva, 1978.
6. *Global Strategy for Health for All by the Year 2000*. Health for All Series, No. 3. Geneva, 1981.
7. Evaluation of the *Strategy for Health for All by the Year 2000*. Seventh Report on the World Health Situation, Vols 1–7.

3

Some Contributions of the World Health Organization to Legislation

S. S. Fluss and Frank Gutteridge

Introduction

In his chapter on "Public Health Law" in the latest edition of one of the classic works in the public health field, Grad has noted that "The reach of public health law is as broad as the reach of public health itself. Public health and public health law expand to meet the needs of our society."[1] Grad was writing in a United States context, but his assertion is undoubtedly valid for developed and developing countries in general. Moreover, what is true for public health is no less true in the case of personal health services. The array of subjects now covered by health legislation is vast indeed—witness any issue of WHO's quarterly journal, the *International Digest of Health Legislation*. The last two numbers for 1988, for example, contain national and international legal instruments on a very wide range of subjects, including the organization of health care systems, measures for the prevention and control of AIDS and HIV infection, new reproductive technologies, organ transplantation, food safety, drug approval and monitoring procedures, the regulation of acupuncture, mental health, measures to combat tobacco use, occupational health services, radiation protection, and environmental protection and management.

S. S. Fluss • Chief, Health Legislation, World Health Organization, Geneva, Switzerland. Frank Gutteridge • Former Director, Legal Division, World Health Organization, Geneva, Switzerland. Any views expressed are those of the authors and not necessarily those of the World Health Organization.

The *Digest* has been publishing information, not readily accessible elsewhere, on legislative policies adopted nationally and internationally in the health sector since 1948 (earlier material on the subject appeared in the Laws and Regulations section of the *Bulletin* of one of WHO's predecessor organizations, the Paris-based International Office of Public Hygiene). The resources devoted to this activity and more fundamental legislative work in line with WHO's constitution to be described below have been not inconsiderable, but would certainly appear to have been warranted in the light of a comment made in 1978 in an editorial in one of the most respected medical journals: "Public-health legislation and related measures have probably done more than all the advances of scientific medicine to promote the well-being of the community in Britain and in most other countries."[2]

It is proposed in this chapter to describe, in the first instance, the highlights of WHO's role in the formulation of what may be described as international health legislation[3] and, thereafter, to examine some of the approaches and methodologies whereby WHO can reasonably be assumed to have played a direct or indirect role in the development of national health legislation. Both aspects are vast and the original title of this chapter, "The contribution . . . ," has been modified to "Some contributions . . . ," given the impossibility of covering the topic adequately in a limited space.

The International Dimension

The text of WHO's Constitution is an amalgamation of several proposals put to the Technical Preparatory Committee in 1946. While most of the proposals contained a clause giving to a future world health conference or assembly the power to adopt international conventions, through procedures similar to those available in the International Labor Organization, an innovation was proposed in the text put forward by Dr. Thomas Parran, Surgeon General of the United States Public Health Service. Dr. Parran's draft included a provision under which the future WHO legislative body would have the authority to adopt, by simple majority vote, international regulations that would become automatically binding on the states members of the organization, except for those notifying their rejection of, or reservations to, the regulations.

This procedure differs from conventional treaty-making practice in that under conventional procedures, a positive action is required by a state in order to become bound by an international instrument, such as signature, or signature followed by ratification or acceptance, with or without some form of parliamentary endorsement. While not innovative in the historical sense, in that similar provisions had been included in the 1944 Chicago Convention on International Civil Aviation and in the 1933 International Sanitary Convention of Aerial Navigation, the inclusion of these provisions was an innovation in the constitutive instrument of an international organization.

These measures were hailed at the time as a considerable step forward. The summary report on the proceedings of the International Health Conference contains the following passage: "Probably the most significant contribution to international legislative technique in the health field made by the WHO Constitution lies in the power it confers upon the Health Assembly to adopt regulations on a broad range of technical matters." As we will see, these expectations have not been realized in practice, and the regulation-making powers enshrined in Article 21 of the WHO Constitution have only been used to replace earlier international instruments dealing with the transmission of communicable diseases with health statistics.[4]

In addition to its regulatory authority under Article 21 of the Constitution, the World Health Assembly has authority under Article 19 to adopt conventions or agreements with respect to any matter within the competence of the organization. This article has not been implemented except with regard to formal and administrative matters, such as the approval of headquarters agreements. Under Article 23 of the Constitution, the Assembly has authority to make recommendations with respect to any matter within the competence of the organization. Under Article 62, the states members of WHO are to report annually on the action taken by them with respect to such recommendations, as well as with respect to conventions, agreements, and regulations.

The regulatory powers of WHO under Article 21, as distinguished from those under Articles 19 and 23, are expressly limited. Broadly speaking, they cover requirements and procedures to prevent the international spread of disease, the international comparability of reporting for statistical purposes, and standards relating to drugs and vaccines and other biologicals. Thus, while there was an endeavor to innovate by the introduction of simplified treaty-making practices into the constitution, these were severely circumscribed, so that in the main they cover traditional matters that had been the subject of international legislation since the middle of the nineteenth century.

The avowed intention of the regulatory technique was principally to consolidate and simplify the somewhat incoherent regime of the international sanitary conventions and agreements that by 1946 had become included in 13 such instruments. In addition, it was thought that the introduction of regulatory powers with respect to biological, pharmaceutical, and similar products moving in international commerce would act to protect public health and also, by the elimination of the market for low-standard pharmaceutical and biological products, would stimulate the export market for high-quality products.[5]

The adoption of conventions and agreements requires a two-thirds vote of the World Health Assembly. Regulations are adopted by a majority of the members present and voting, as is also the case for recommendations.

The Assembly has adopted two international regulations under Article 21, paragraphs (*a*) and (*b*). The first of these were the WHO Regulations No. 1 regarding nomenclature (including the compilation and publication of statistics) with respect to diseases and causes of death. The regulations were given the short title of Nomenclature Regulations, thus compounding the unfortunate confusion in terminology in Article 21 (*b*), since the subject matter of the instrument is not in fact the nomenclature of disease, but the statistical classification of morbidity and mortality. Nomenclature is a distinct issue that is being dealt with by the Council for International Organizations of Medical Sciences (CIOMS), a nongovernmental organization in relations with WHO.

The Nomenclature Regulations represent the continuation of work commenced in the last century and entrusted in 1891 to the International Statistical Institute. Decennial revisions of the international classification were initiated in 1898 and this work was taken up by WHO after its creation.[6]

The initial regulations incorporated the work of the sixth revision of the International Statistical Classification of Diseases, Injuries, and Causes of Death, which was prepared by an international conference that met in Paris in 1948. No particular provisions were included to deal with the question of reservations permitted by Article 21 of the constitution. As a consequence of this, those reservations that were made were considered as having been accepted in advance. Despite the relatively flexible procedures of the regulation-making process, these were found to be unduly constraining in that with a decennial revision process, the international classification incorporated in the regulations would necessarily be the subject of the regulatory revision process, thus reopening the question of rejection or reservations at each decennial revision, with the consequent risk of a multiplicity of regimes.

When the regulations were reviewed by the World Health Assembly in 1966 and 1967, most of the purely technical items in the text were removed and given the status of recommendations under Article 23 of the constitution, pending the preparation of a compendium of recommendations, standards, and definitions. Subsequent revisions of the international classification, published in the *Manual of the International Statistical Classification of Diseases, Injuries, and Causes of Death,* have been adopted without any corresponding revision of the regulations.[7]

The revision and consolidation of the international conventions and agreements dealing with the international spread of disease was undertaken from 1948 onwards, and regulations were first adopted in 1951 as WHO Regulations No. 2, the International Sanitary Regulations. These regulations covered the so-called "quarantinable diseases," namely plague, cholera, yellow fever, smallpox, louse-borne typhus, and louse-borne relapsing fever.

Apart from the inconsistency of the earlier regime under the conventions and agreements (none of these entirely replaced each other), they did not take account of new methods available for the control of the diseases they covered, nor were they framed to deal adequately with the greatly increased volume and speed of international traffic. For years it had been pointed out that the need for the health control of international traffic could be obviated if the transmission of diseases was stopped or reduced in the places where it principally occurred. This is, however, a solution that cannot be obtained by an international instrument, but only by the improvement of the health conditions of the peoples of WHO's member states. Any attempt to control diseases by the imposition of barriers at frontiers is by definition fortuitous, since frontiers are political and do not constitute any natural barrier to the spread of infection. To obtain effective control of the international spread of diseases required sound epidemiological services with reliable disease surveillance and the frank and rapid exchange of information between national epidemiological services.[8]

The International Sanitary Regulations, although a considerable improvement over the earlier arrangements, did not therefore address themselves to this problem, but continued to deal with the conditions to be maintained and measures to be taken against diseases at seaports and airports open to international traffic, including measures on arrival and departure, health documents and charges, the conditions under which vaccination may be required as a condition of entry into a country, conditions entailing the handling of arriving passengers, their isolation or surveillance, measures to be taken in the case of "suspect" or "infected" ships or aircraft, etc.

The regulations have been subjected to several revisions, generally resulting from the global improvement in the knowledge and control of epidemic diseases. Thus special provisions covering the Mecca Pilgrimage adopted provisionally in 1951 were abrogated in 1956, the concept of large tropical areas being considered as perennially "yellow fever endemic zones" was dropped in 1955, louse-borne typhus and relapsing fever were removed from the scope of the regulations in 1969, when a major revision of the text was undertaken, and the regulations were renamed "International Health Regulations" and, more particularly, smallpox was removed entirely from the scope of international quarantine control in 1981, consequent upon the global eradication of this disease as a result of WHO's eradication program.

Viewed as an international instrument, the International Health Regulations contain two sets of provisions that are of special interest. The somewhat laxist position that was taken over reservations in the Nomenclature Regulations clearly would not do for the Health Regulations, in view of the problems of reciprocity arising if, despite measures having been taken in accordance with the legal provision on or before departure, travelers and means of transport were to be subject to additional measures not provided for in the text through uncontrolled reservations. The regulations therefore contain provision under which reservations are to be reviewed by the World Health Assembly before they come into effect. If the reservation is not accepted by the Assembly, then the regulations will not enter into force for the reserving state. This procedure has led in practice to a form of consultation between the reserving state and the organization, under which a number of reservations offered have been withdrawn or attenuated or accepted subject to a time limit, followed by further review. The most intractable problem with regard to reservations has been the yellow fever situation, where countries free of the disease but presenting the conditions that would be favorable to its uncontrollable spread if either the disease itself or its vectors (or both) were accidentally introduced have, understandably, been reluctant to accept modifications of the international regime without offering reservations for their own protection.

As in the case of the Sanitary Conventions and Agreements, WHO has had to face the problem of excessive measures, either prohibited by the regulations or not justified by the epidemiological situation. This problem came to the fore in the 1960s and early 1970s, following the westward spread of the El Tor strain of cholera. This led to the imposition in some cases of unjustified measures affecting travel and commerce and to the consequent reluctance of some health authorities to report the presence of the disease, or its acknowledgment as "summer diarrhea" or some equivalent euphemism. Recently, WHO has expressed its views on the imposition of health measures on international travelers in respect of HIV/AIDS transmission, pointing out that under Article 81 of the regulations, no health document other than those provided in the regulations shall be required in international traffic. There is consequently no provision for any certificate guaranteeing that a person entering any country or coming from any country is free from a given disease. A certificate stating that a person is not carrying the virus would in no way prevent the introduction and spread of AIDS and would afford no protection; the only way to protect against the disease is through proper epidemiological surveillance by competent services. The regulations therefore contain detailed provisions for dispute-settling, with an initial reference to the Director-General followed by a reference, if the dispute is not so settled, to an "appropriate committee" or "other organ" of the organization for settlement. In the practice of WHO, the vast majority of disputes have been settled by their reference to the Director-General.[9]

In the administration of the regulations, WHO produces a number of publications for the use of its member states and others. The regulations are available in an "annotated" edition, which, in addition to the text of the articles, includes the format of international certificates of vaccination and other health documents required in international travel, as well as information on interpretation given to the provisions, etc., information on the incidence of disease, including communicable diseases under surveillance, is published in the *Weekly Epidemiological Record*. Health travel information is available in "Vaccination Certificate Requirements and Health Advice for International Travel," revised annually.

Despite the early promise of this international regulatory technique, no further regulations have been drawn up or approved by the World Health Assembly. Those international regulatory regimes that have been the subject of a formal submission to WHO's governing bodies have taken the form of recommendations under Article 23 of the constitution or even of simple resolutions, the practice of the organization having not been entirely consistent in this respect. Thus, the proposal of an expert subcommittee on the definition of "stillbirth" for statistical purposes was adopted formally as a recommendation under Article 23, whereas the important texts on "Good practices in the manufacture and quality control of drugs" and the "Certification scheme on the quality of pharmaceutical products moving in international commerce" were adopted by the Assembly as a simple resolution without other formality.

Various reasons have been put forward for this apparent failure of the regulatory technique. These include the restricted scope of Article 21, as compared with the general statement of the functions of WHO under Article 2, the difficulties inherent in formalizing technical requirements in a rapidly evolving domain, the cost of maintaining centralized administrative facilities for the administration of legally binding instruments, the absence of any requirement of reciprocity in many cases, the reluctance of the organization to indulge in what might be termed the "making of official science," a reluctance shared with its forebears and epitomized by the refusal of the World Health Assembly in 1955 to endorse a particular poliomyelitis vaccine,[10] and the uneven development of states in science and technology.[11]

The position was summarized in the Report on the Second Ten Years of the World Health Organization in the following terms:

> No international conventions or regulations were adopted by the World Health Assembly during the second ten years, other than regulations modifying or supplementing the Nomenclature Regulations and the International Sanitary (now "Health") Regulations. Where it has been necessary to elaborate and promulgate international norms or standards, the tendency has been to rely on the procedure provided under Article 23 of the Constitution relating to recommendations. This procedure appears to be adequate where questions of reciprocity are not predominant, and it has the advantage of flexibility, since a recommendation may be modified or adopted without any formalities having to be observed.[12]

The possibility of the preparation and adoption of further regulations has been discussed in connection with a variety of topics, namely international maritime venereal disease control, the control of malaria, the international pharmacopoeia and pharmacopoeial formulas for potent drugs, quality control of drugs, biological standardization, and the use of breast-milk substitutes for infant feeding. However, the governing bodies have not been prepared to extend the coverage of Article 21, and these matters have been dealt with by the adoption of recommendations or technical standards.

The greater part of WHO's international regulatory activities has therefore been carried out through less formal procedures, that is to say either through the adoption by the World Health Assembly of recommendations under Article 23, or by the adoption of resolutions, or by the promulgation of technical standards, usually drawn up by expert bodies. As mentioned above, the practice has not been entirely consistent with regard to the use of Article 23. The only way in which a decision taken under this Article differs from a decision taken by way of resolution is that in the case of the former, there is an obligation placed on states to report annually, in accordance with Article 62. In practice, this distinction is insubstantial, since an annual reporting requirement is unrealistic, and has never in fact been strictly applied.

Important regulatory decisions of the World Health Assembly have encompassed the following subjects: the International Pharmacopoeia and the replacement of the obsolete 1929 Agreement respecting the Unification of Pharmacopoeial Formulas for Potent Drugs, international standards and units for biological substances, good practices in the manufacturing and the quality control of pharmaceutical products, the certification scheme on the quality of pharmaceutical products moving in international commerce, post eradication policy regarding smallpox, and the international classification of diseases and causes of death. In 1981, the Health Assembly adopted the International Code of Marketing of Breast-Milk Substitutes. This has as its purpose to promote the breast-feeding of infants as a means of improving infant and young child health and to regulate the advertising and marketing of breast-milk substitutes. The possibility of having this Code expressed in the form of international regulations was discussed. Article 21 of the Constitution, in contradistinction to Article 2(*u*), does not include food within the category of products in respect of which standards may be drawn up; nevertheless, the decision to issue the Code as a recommendation rather than as regulations was taken primarily to ensure a consensus and to avoid the likelihood of rejection of or reservations to the international regime, which would have rendered it extremely difficult to administer.[13]

WHO has also undertaken substantial international regulatory activities in collaboration with the United Nations and with other specialized agencies. In particular, the organization provides expert advice to the United Nations in the administration of the international instruments on the control of dependence-producing drugs. It also collaborates with the Food and Agriculture Organization of the United Nations (FAO) as a partner in the administration of the Codex Alimentarius program, a program initiated to promulgate food standards aimed at protecting consumers' health and ensuring fair practices in the food trade. The standards prescribe requirements pertaining to food hygiene, food additives, food contaminants, food labeling, etc. These standards are not binding per se and the members of the Codex Alimentarius Commission become bound only when they accept them.[14]

We have thus seen that while WHO has been active from its early days in promulgating international normative texts and requirements, for the most part these have not been expressed as legislative texts in the form of international treaties, but rather as recommendations, in a more or less formal manner. In this way, the legislative process has been accelerated and a multiplicity of different regimes as between its Member States avoided by using the procedure of consensus for the approval of these international norms.[15]

Information Transfer

The *International Digest of Health Legislation* and Associated Activities

WHO's work in promoting the international dissemination of information on health legislation can be traced back to a circular addressed on 30 January 1909 by the then Director of the International Office of Public Hygiene to the health administrations of all states participating in the Rome Arrangement signed on 9 December 1907.[16] Since that date, changes and improvements have been constantly introduced and the current system is based largely on the *International Digest of Health Legislation*, a journal that appears in English and French editions and is widely read by public health administrators, health lawyers, and many other interested groups in developed and developing countries alike. The *Digest* in its present form reflects the desire of WHO's member states to have access to primary health legislation texts and materials in an accessible and readable form, and also what has been aptly described as "analyzed" or "distilled" information (for example, the 300 or so books and other publications that are now covered annually in the Book Reviews and In the Literature sections of the journal). The criteria used by the editorial staff for the selection of texts for publication are those laid down by WHO's executive board in a series of resolutions, the most recent being EB65.R13, adopted in January 1980.[17] The overall orientation of this key component of WHO's health legislation program was presented in a report submitted by the Director-General of the organization to the executive board and the World Health Assembly in that year.[18] Anyone familiar with legislative materials will be aware of the sheer bulk and unwieldiness of official gazettes (the issues of the *U.S. Federal Register* for any given year would alone occupy several precious yards of shelf space). WHO's secretariat is aided in its access to this documentation, and its exploitation for the benefit of government and others, by, in particular, the libraries of the United Nations and the International Labor Organization in Geneva, the rapidly expanding library of the Lausanne-based Swiss Institute of Comparative Law, and the unrivalled Library of Congress in Washington. Similarly, WHO relies heavily on the unstinting cooperation of an informal network of centers of expertise as well as individual experts (government and nongovernmental) in health law throughout the world—a network that is constantly expanding as, following Grad's maxim, health law expands (and draws in more and more young lawyers and health administrators attracted by the challenge it offers for an area that lies at the interface between medicine, law, and science, and that touches on so many issues of interest to experts and laymen alike).

A legitimate question is whether this information is actually being utilized or are the 40 volumes of the *Digest* published to date merely gathering dust on obscure departmental shelves? It must be conceded that only in 1978 did WHO obtain direct, objective information to respond, thanks to the dispatch of a questionnaire to all 150 countries that were member states at the time. No less than 100 replies were received and it transpired from an analysis that—at the time, i.e., prior to a major restructuring of the journal that took place in 1981—40 countries were actually using the *Digest* in the elaboration of new legislation or revision of existing legislation (a further 10 countries were actively contemplating using the journal for this purpose in the future). Continuing review and revision of health legislation are essential, the main reasons being no doubt those advanced by Roemer:

> In all countries health legislation becomes outdated at times because of technological developments, newly identified health hazards, advances in education, and new directions in health policy. In the developing countries, the need for revised legislation may also be caused by laws that are vestiges from colonial times, by customary law, or by adaptations of legislation from industrialized countries that are not appropriate to current needs.[19]

Perhaps the most striking example of this is the removal of the provisions on smallpox from the communicable diseases control statutes and regulations of virtually all countries as a consequence of the global eradication of smallpox.

It should be emphasized that the material published by the *Digest* is complemented by legislative information disseminated in other fields—some with a bearing on health in the sense that this elusive concept is defined in the preamble to the WHO constitution—by other agencies. Thus, labor legislation is covered in the ILO's *Legislative Series,* food and environmental legislation in the FAO's *Food and Agricultural Legislation,* nuclear legislation in the OECD Nuclear Energy Agency's *Nuclear Law Bulletin,* and narcotics legislation in a series produced by the United Nations Division of Narcotic Drugs. Population-related policies (including texts dealing with many aspects of the status of women) are reported in the *Annual Review of Population Law,* produced by the New York-based United Nations Population Fund. It goes without saying that WHO and the other agencies concerned cooperate to avoid any duplication of effort and to ensure the sharing of information where appropriate. An optimal methodology for institutionalizing (though not bureaucratizing) such coordination remains to be developed.

Comparative Surveys of Health Legislation and Similar Studies

From the inception of WHO's activities in health legislation, it was clearly perceived that countries could gain much from comparative surveys of legislation. Such surveys, whether prepared by WHO staff or (as is most frequently the case at the present time) by outside experts, have been well received and generally regarded as an important component of the program. Owing to space constraints it is possible to cite only a few of the most noteworthy that have appeared in recent years: W. J. Curran and T. W. Harding's *The Law and Mental Health: Harmonizing Objectives* (1978); R. J. Cook and B. M. Dickens's *Abortion Laws in Commonwealth Countries* (1979); R. Roemer's *Legislative Action to Combat the World Smoking Epidemic* (1982) (an update appeared as a WHO document in 1986); M. Owen's *Laws and Policies Affecting the Training and Practice of Traditional Birth Attendants* (1983); J. Stepan's *Traditional and Alternative Systems of Medicine: A Comparative Review of Legislation* (1985); L. Porter, A. E. Arif, and W. J. Curran's *Law and the Treatment of Drug- and Alcohol-Dependent Persons* (1986); and J. M. Paxman and R. J. Zuckerman's *Laws and Policies Affecting Adolescent Health* (1987). Studies on key regulatory issues in the health sector, based partly on the legislative data base maintained by WHO, have also appeared, notably D. C. Jayasuriya's *Regulation of Pharmaceuticals in Developing Countries: Legal Issues and Approaches* (1985). One of the papers presented to the November 1985 Nairobi Conference of Experts on the Rational Use of Drugs was a review of legislation on drug marketing.[20] A global survey of legislation on the prevention and control of AIDS and HIV infection, commissioned by WHO's Global Program on AIDS, has just been completed by a team of experts at the Harvard School of Public Health. Annotated listings of all known legislation in this area are regularly prepared, the most recent being dated May 1989.

WHO has historically been and remains a decentralized agency, and it is difficult to envisage the organization without its six regional offices. The latter have also initiated major studies on diverse aspects of health legislation. Specific reference should be made to *Trends in Health Legislation in Europe* (by H. J. J. Leenen, G. Pinet, and A. V. Prims), published in 1986 under the auspices of the Copenhagen-based Regional Office for Europe. This covers the period 1970–1983 and will be of undoubted interest to health policymakers throughout the world. An important study (by H. L. Fuenzalida-Puelma and S. Scholle Connor) on the place of health in national constitutions and other fundamental laws in the countries of the Region of the Americas (with contributions by eminent legal specialists in each country) was published by the Pan

American Health Organization (the WHO Regional Office for the Americas) in early 1989 (in English and Spanish editions).

The crucial area of environmental health has not been neglected. In 1976, WHO cooperated with the United Nations Environment Program in the preparation of a survey of national legislation for the protection of the Mediterranean against pollution from land-based sources—a form of pollution that is particularly noxious as far as human health is concerned. It seems likely that this compendium has been and will continue to be useful to the Mediterranean states as they implement the 1980 Athens Protocol dealing with land-based pollution.[21]

Technical Cooperation

The thrust of WHO's technical cooperation program in the health legislation field is on the strengthening of national capacities. One of the main approaches has consisted of the dispatch of carefully selected consultants to developing countries, at the request of the latter. Such consultants must and do work with national counterparts and may be called upon to undertake a variety of tasks, ranging from the formulation of draft legal instruments covering the organization of the health care system as a whole to proposing a national strategy for implementing the International Code of Marketing of Breast-Milk Substitutes. The evaluation of the effectiveness of such missions is difficult, for obvious reasons; nor does the informal roster of potential consultants maintained and regularly updated by WHO evidently contain the names of all those with the knowledge, expertise, and sensitivity necessary to undertake successful assignments. These problems are significant, since it appears from available information that the demand for such consultant services will, if anything, increase in the future.

Another approach is to promote national and sometimes international meetings designed to clarify the role of legislation in supporting new and reoriented health policies, particularly those endorsed by the collectivity of member states that make up WHO. Thus, the organization convened or supported the following:

- A Meeting on Technical Cooperation among the ASEAN Countries on Drug Legislation, Evaluation, and Quality Assurance (Jakarta, November 26–29, 1979)[22]
- A Meeting of a Working Group on Legislation Concerning Nursing/Midwifery Services and Education (Hamburg, December 11–14, 1979)

- A Seminar on Law and Health for Development (Chonburi, Thailand, August 13–14, 1980)
- A National Workshop on Infant and Young Child Feeding (Bangui, Central African Republic, November 16–20, 1981)
- An Intercountry Consultation Meeting on Drug Legislation (Kathmandu, Nepal, April 25–29, 1983)
- A National Workshop on Food Safety Laws (Xian, China, October 13–18, 1983)
- A Workshop on Legislative Measures in Relation to the Development of Lifestyles Conducive to Health (Dresden, German Democratic Republic, April 9–10, 1984)
- A Study Group on the Strengthening of Regulatory Mechanisms for Nursing Training and Practice Relating to Primary Health Care (Geneva, December 9–13, 1985)
- A National Workshop on Health Legislation (Hangzhou, China, April 14–26, 1986)
- A Round Table on Health Legislation in the African Region of WHO (Brazzaville, Congo, October 13–15, 1986)
- The Second National Workshop on Health Legislation (Shanghai, April 4–12, 1988) and
- An International Consultation on Health Legislation and Ethics in the Field of AIDS and HIV Infection (Oslo, April 26–29, 1988).

The organization has also participated in a large number of international meetings on a wide variety of subjects at which legislative issues have been high on the agenda. A good example of technical cooperation with a group of member states is furnished by WHO's participation in an expert committee on "Health Legislation in the Arab World," established by the Council of Arab Ministers of Health. One of the issues discussed at the first meeting (Tunis, October 12–16, 1984) was the adoption of legislation that would help achieve the goal of health for all by the year 2000, popularly known as HFA/2000.

Training

In this as in many other areas of health development, training can be a powerful and cost-effective mechanism for strengthening national capacities. A rather small number of fellowships in health legislation have been awarded by WHO, and their impact remains uncertain.

With support from the government of Belgium, the WHO Regional

Office for Europe organized the First International Course on Health Legislation (Leuven, Belgium, July 2–13, 1984). Its objectives were to foster the exchange of knowledge and experience and to stimulate national cooperation to promote the understanding of legislation as a tool for developing and implementing health policy; to stimulate awareness of the role that legislation can play in achieving HFA/2000; and to provide an incentive for developing or initiating training programs at national level. This significant activity was repeated in 1986 (in the form of a French-language course held in Montpellier, France) and in 1988 (in the form of an English-language seminar held in Haifa, Israel) and will no doubt be replicated in due course in other regions.

WHO is frequently called upon to assist advanced students in the health and legal sciences in the preparation of theses and dissertations. An academic exercise, perhaps, and yet authors may go on to become health leaders in the future and their exposure to knowledge and ideas generated or disseminated by WHO may enhance their awareness of new health doctrines. Only two can be cited here, namely P. Fallet's "Revision of Health Legislation in a Developing Country" (submitted for a state doctorate in pharmacy on June 28, 1985, to the University of Paris-South) and H. Hammad's "The Right to Health in the Libyan Arab Jamahiriya: A Contribution to the Study of the Concept of the Right to Health as a Human Right" (submitted for a doctorate in law on October 8, 1985 to the Faculty of Law and Economic and Political Sciences of the University of Besançon, France). An evocative title indeed, that brings to mind the oft-quoted third paragraph of the preamble to WHO's Constitution and the no less important provisions of Article 12 of the International Covenant on Economic, Social and Cultural Rights.

Development of Guidelines and Frameworks for Policy

The current patterns of national legislation in fields as diverse as human experimentation, radiation protection, breast-feeding, pharmaceuticals, biological standardization, the control of the "smoking pandemic," food safety, blood policy, AIDS and HIV infection, occupational health, environmental protection, chemical safety, the control of drug- and alcohol-related problems, and even such "core" areas as the organization of health services and health manpower have been influenced by WHO activities, ranging from resolutions of the governing bodies to sometimes highly technical reports of expert committees, study groups, etc. Only a few examples can be cited here.

Blood Policy

A statement entitled "Legislation on Blood Transfusion: A Model for a National Blood Policy" has been issued by the International Society of Blood Transfusion. The guidelines are stated to be based upon recommendations of, in particular, WHO.[23]

Human Experimentation

WHO provided input to the 1975 revision of the World Medical Association's Declaration of Helsinki. Moreover, it worked in conjunction with the Geneva-based Council for International Organizations of Medical Sciences in the development of *Proposed International Guidelines for Biomedical Research Involving Human Subjects* (published in Geneva in 1982).

Drinking Water

The regulations on this subject in many countries have been greatly influenced by the *European Standards for Drinking-water* and the *International Standards for Drinking-water*. These have now been superseded by *Guidelines for Drinking-water Quality* (appearing in three volumes). The impact of these Guidelines is already perceptible.[24]

Pharmaceuticals

It would be quite impossible to do anything like justice to the multiplicity of WHO activities having a bearing on drug regulation. Suffice it to say that drug legislation throughout the world is increasingly influenced by WHO's important work on the safety, efficacy, and quality of drugs, as well as on its powerful advocacy of the essential drugs concept. The information transfer component has been no less important, as reflected in (inter alia) the quarterly journal *WHO Drug Information* and the monthly mailings to designated national drug officials.[25] Another significant activity has been the cosponsorship of a series of conferences of drug regulatory authorities, the most recent having been held near Stockholm on June 11–14, 1984,[26] and in Tokyo on July 6–11, 1986. The next is scheduled to be held in Paris on October 10–13, 1989.

Chemical Safety

More and more countries are giving attention to the regulation of the enormous number of chemicals encountered in the human environment. The International Program on Chemical Safety, established on the basis of decisions by the World Health Assembly in 1977 and 1978, has provided invaluable information to governments on the scientific basis for regulating individual chemicals.[27] Also highly important have been the activities of the International Agency for Research on Cancer, insofar as the regulation of carcinogens and putative carcinogens is concerned.[28]

Smoking

One cannot in this short chapter do justice to WHO's important and indeed pioneering role in stimulating governments to act in a coordinated and comprehensive manner to combat this modern scourge. Many of WHO's activities have been designed to support the legislative and other components of smoking control programs. A whole series of resolutions on the subject have been adopted by WHO's governing bodies, one of the most recent (WHA39.14) in response to a report by the director-general on this subject.[29] An Action Program on Tobacco or Health was approved by WHO's Executive Board in January 1989 and endorsed by the Forty-second World Health Assembly in May 1989.

The Health-for-All Movement

In 1977, the World Health Assembly adopted the goal for health for all by the year 2000. This was closely followed by the historic International Conference on Primary Health Care, jointly organized by WHO and UNICEF and held in Alma-Ata, USSR, in September 1978. The Declaration of Alma-Ata adopted at the Conference noted the importance of legislation in the development of primary health care in the following terms:

> In some countries, legislation will be required to facilitate the development of primary health care and the implementation of its strategy. Thus, there might be a need for new legislation or the revision of existing legislation, to permit communities to plan, manage and control primary health care and to allow various types of health workers to perform duties hitherto carried out exclusively by health professionals. On the other hand, there often exist laws which are not applied but which, as they stand, might be used to facilitate the development of primary health care.[30]

In May 1984, the Thirty-seventh World Health Assembly adopted resolution WHA37.17, in which operative paragraph 1(18) urged member states "to consider the desirability of enacting health legislation incorporating the basic principles of health for all." In fact, many countries have not waited to do so, and an increasing number of laws and regulations from many parts of the world reaching WHO are thoroughly permeated by the spirit and the letter of the health-for-all philosophies, approaches, and strategies. It would be amiss to fail to mention one of the targets formulated in the 1985 European Regional Strategy for Health for All and it is cited below in full:

> Before 1990, all Member States should ensure that their health policies and strategies are in line with health for all principles and that their legislation and regulations make their implementation effective in all sectors of society.
>
> This could be achieved if all countries were to make a systematic review of their health policies and health legislation in the light of the regional health for all strategy and targets, and to develop health for all strategies and targets and amend or extend their health legislation accordingly, taking due account of the specific legal, political and structural conditions in each Member State.[31]

The target laid down for health legislation at the global level in WHO's next General Program of Work (covering the period 1990–1995) is no less ambitious:

> By 1995 more than 50% of countries will have health legislation supportive of national strategies of health for all.[32]

Conclusion

In this chapter, we have sought to cover in a minimum of space, but with a maximum of information, the multifaceted and diverse activities undertaken by WHO in the field of health legislation. How can one judge their impact? Perhaps the best way is to look at some of the key health laws and regulations now being adopted in many of WHO's member states. In several areas WHO has exerted no discernible influence (in some instances, the work of other agencies inside and outside the United Nations system may have been significant). In others, the organization's ideas, policies, and technical output are clearly reflected.[33] It can be anticipated that the integrated range of information transfer, technical cooperation, and other activities described in this chapter will tend to augment the organization's influence in this key sector of health development in the years to come and that morbidity and mortality will be reduced and the quality of human life improved by this endeavor.

References

1. Grad, F: Public health law, in Last JM (ed): *Maxcy-Rosenau Preventive Medicine and Public Health*, ed 12. New York, Appleton-Century-Crofts, 1986, chap 64.
2. *Lancet* 1978; 2: 354–355. See also World Health Organization: *Sixth Report on the World Health Situation 1973–1977. Part I: Global Analysis.* Geneva, WHO, 1978, pp 57–63.
3. Readers seeking further information on WHO's regulatory role are referred to Leive DM: *International Regulatory Regimes, Case Studies in Health, Meteorology, and Food.* Lexington, MA, Lexington Books, 1976, Vol I.
4. For the text of the Constitution, see World Health Organization: Basic Documents, ed 37. Geneva, WHO, 1988, pp 1–18.
5. Hearings before Subcommittee No 5—National and international movements of the Committee of Foreign Affairs, House of Representatives, Eightieth Congress, first session, on HJ Res 161. A joint resolution providing for membership and participation by the United States in the World Health Organization and authorizing an appropriation therefor. June 13, 17, and July 3, 1947. Washington, DC, Government Printing Office, 1947.
6. World Health Organization: *The First Ten Years of the World Health Organization.* Geneva, WHO, 1958, p 278.
7. World Health Organization: *Manual of the International Statistical Classification of Diseases, Injuries, and Causes of Death.* Geneva, WHO, 1977.
8. Black RH, Sencer DJ: The long-term future of the International Health Regulations. WHO *Chron* 1978; 32: 439–447. Carter ID: Communication and disease. *Proc Roy Soc Edin* 82B: 101–113, 1982.
9. Vignes C-H: Le réglement sanitaire international: aspects juridiques. *Annuaire Français de Droit International* 11: 665–667, 1965.
10. WHO Off Rec 63: 272–273, 1955.
11. Gutteridge F: Notes on decisions of the World Health Organization, in Schwebel SM (ed): *The Effectiveness of International Decisions.* Leyden, Sijthoff, and Dobbs-Ferry, NY, Oceana, 1971.
12. World Health Organization: *The Second Ten Years of the World Health Organization, 1958–1967.* Geneva, WHO, 1968, p 299.
13. Shubber S: The International Code of Marketing of Breast-milk Substitutes. *Int Dig Hlth Leg,* 1985; 36: 877–908.
14. Dobbert JP: Le Codex Alimentarius: vers une nouvelle méthode de réglementation internationale. *Annuaire Française de Droit International* 1969; 15: 677–717.
15. For further information on some of WHO's international activities, see World Health Organization: *Selected Bibliography on Legal, Historical and Political Aspects.* Geneva, WHO, 1982 (unpublished document LEG/MISC/1982/1).
16. *Bull Off Int Hyg Publ* 1909; 1: 3–8.
17. World Health Organization: *Handbook of Resolutions and Decisions of the World Health Assembly and the Executive Board.* Vol II, 1973–1984. Geneva, WHO, 1985, p 63. All other resolutions cited in this chapter can be readily retrieved in this compilation.
18. World Health Organization: Executive Board, sixty-fifth session, Geneva, 9–25 January 1980. *Resolutions and decisions, annexes.* Geneva, 1980, Annex 5, pp 77–83.
19. Roemer R: *Legislative Approaches to Promote Primary Health Care: A Guide for Parliamentarians and Other Policy-Makers.* Geneva, WHO, 1989.
20. World Health Organization: Review of National Health Legislation on Drug Marketing. Geneva, WHO, 1985 (unpublished document WHO/CONRAD/WP/2.2).

21. For the text of the Protocol, see *Int Dig Hlth Leg* 31: 950–958, 1980. For an account of the role of WHO in its genesis, see an article by Dobbert JP in the same issue, pp 986–990.
22. For an article on this Meeting, see Yeap Boon Chye: *Int Dig Hlth Leg* 31: 227–229, 1980. Reports on other meetings cited in this text at this juncture will be found elsewhere in the *Digest*.
23. Transfusion International, 1985, No 40, p 11.
24. New Zealand, Board of Health: *Drinking-Water Standards for New Zealand*. Wellington, 1984.
25. World Health Organization: *The Role of WHO in the Transfer and Dissemination of Information on Drug Quality, Safety and Efficacy*. Geneva, WHO, 1985 (unpublished document WHO/CONRAD/WP/1.2).
26. National Board of Health and Welfare (NBHW), Sweden: Proc Third International Conference on Drug Regulatory Authorities. Stockholm, Department of Drugs, NBHW, 1985. An article by A. Wehrli on this Conference appears in *Int Dig Hlth Leg* 1986; 37:141–145.
27. World Health Organization: *International Programme on Chemical Safety: Progress Report by the Director-General*. Geneva, WHO, 1985 (unpublished document EB77/26).
28. See, in particular, Tomatis L: *The contribution of the IARC Monographs programme to the identification of cancer risk factors* (unpublished paper presented to the Conference on the Occupational and Environmental Significance of Industrial Carcinogens, Bologna, Italy, October 1985).
29. World Health Organization: *WHO Programme on Tobacco or Health: Report by the Director-General*. Geneva, WHO, 1986 (document EB77/1986/REC/1, pp 58–102.
30. World Health Organization: *Primary Health Care: Report of the International Conference on Primary Health Care*. Geneva, WHO, 1978 ("Health for All" Series No 1), pp 4–5. The reader is referred to R. Roemer's document mentioned in ref 19 for further amplification of this issue, as well as to Najera E et al: Health For All as a Strategy and the Role of Health Legislation: Some Issues and Views. *Int Dig Hlth Leg* 1986; 37: 362–379.
31. World Health Organization, Regional Office for Europe: *Targets for Health for All: Targets in Support of the European Regional Strategy for Health for All*. Copenhagen, 1985, p 132.
32. The World Health Organization: *Eighth General Programme of Work Covering the Period 1990–1995*. Geneva, WHO, 1987 ("Health for All" Series No 10), p 223.
33. See, in this respect, World Health Organization: *Evaluation of the Strategy for Health for All by the Year 2000: Seventh Report on the World Health Situation*. Vol 1. Global Review. Geneva, WHO, 1987, pp 45–47.

4

The Economics of Health Care

B. ABEL-SMITH

Economics is centrally concerned about the use of scarce resources, and resources of many kinds are, almost by definition, particularly scarce in developing countries. Average levels of living are low and there is a limited pool of educated and trained manpower. Morever, a lower proportion of such a nation's resources can be mobilized through taxation for communal purposes not only because a high proportion of the population is poor but also because of the administrative difficulties of collecting taxes with a low proportion of the population in regular salaried employment.

HEALTH BENEFITS IN DEVELOPING COUNTRIES

What therefore do such countries gain by devoting resources to promote the objective of better health, particularly resources collected from taxation? The use of resources to promote health objectives means that they are not available for other economic and social objectives. Health care is clearly valued as an item of consumption. It provides an important supportive function in life by the comfort and treatment of the sick. It also satisfies a deeply felt human need and may provide relief for conditions that are socially stigmatizing. Even very poor people in poor societies are prepared to pay for it in cash and kind. All societies have for generations supported their traditional medical men.

But better health is also an investment both for individuals and for societies. Ill health reduces the labor available for productive work paid

B. ABEL-SMITH • Professor of Social Administration, London School of Economics and Political Science, London, England.

or unpaid, in the home, the fields, or the factory. It reduces the amount of work that people can do. Children with stunted growth can never achieve their full economic potential. Disability may make people wholly dependent on others for economic support. In some developing countries illness may affect a tenth of the life span. The prevention of illness may also permit a saving of resources devoted to curative treatment. Finally, it may permit the exploitation of natural resources on a greater scale. For example, land in areas afflicted by malaria or onchocerciasis may be underused or abandoned.

For these reasons health is not just an individual concern, it is a collective concern. Efforts to secure better health are an investment in people—the key resource for socioeconomic development. The collective implications are particularly clear in the case of communicable disease. What the individual does to maintain his or her health is of major concern to others.

But to say that efforts to improve health can be an investment both for the individual and for society is not to say either that it is the most important investment, or that any activity that might conceivably improve health should be paid for. This is where the concept of opportunity cost is central in the consideration of alternative uses of scarce resources. Both societies and individuals must make choices between quite different types of potentially beneficial investments. Also, when resources are particularly scarce, choices will have to be made between different types of investment that have the potential to benefit health. Health economists try to help politicians and administrators in making such decisions. While it may be relatively easy to calculate the cost of undertaking a particular form of health investment, the benefits are more difficult to predict and can be assessed in a variety of different ways. It may not be possible to qualify all of them, let alone express them in money terms to facilitate comparison with costs.[1]

Under all the rhetoric, WHO's Health for All program is essentially the application of basic economic principles to health policy-making. The problem is how a society can maximize health out of limited resources and assure that health benefits are equitably distributed. It became recognized during the 1970s that certain health interventions were known to be extremely cost-effective, though not being made available to whole populations. These were listed as the eight essential elements of primary health care, packaged together as primary health care programs—the key to achieving Health for All by the Year 2000. The emphasis on community participation was also based on cost-effective principles, since in democratic societies you cannot even take the horse to water, let alone make him drink. Changes in life-style cannot be made from above. People can be given information about the ill effects of smoking, alcohol, or polluted water. Whether people take action on such information depends on individual choice, strongly influenced by social pressures within each work or home community.

Growing Concern about Cost

In more and more countries, spending on health services is becoming a subject of major concern. Even in the richest countries it is widely recognized that it is no longer economically acceptable to finance whatever level of expenditure on health services the health professions generate. And in developing countries it is increasingly recognized that the few dollars per head per year that can be found to pay for organized health services may have little impact on the health standards of the bulk of the population. However much health professionals may regret it, the hard facts of the economics of health care are now moving to the center of the stage. And however desirable it may seem to keep politics out of health, increasing economic pressures are forcing politicians to intervene.

The pattern of organizing and financing health services in the more developed countries has strongly influenced the developing countries and continues to do so long after the colonial era. Not least among these influences has been the training and role of the physician and his interpretation of the concept of clinical freedom. Another important influence has been the perception of the hospital as the center point of health activity in the training of health professionals if not also in the delivery of services. The longer-term responses of those wealthy countries that see themselves faced with a crisis in health costs may contain valuable lessons for the developing countries. Similarly, new initiatives taken by developing countries to try and secure health for all by radical rethinking, reorganization, and redeployment may well indicate new directions for richer countries grappling with their crises, even though they are of a very different scale and character—the crises of affluence.

The Problems of the More Developed Countries

In virtually all of the more developed countries, health care costs have been rising substantially faster than national resources over the past 30 years. This trend could obviously not have continued indefinitely. But it did not cause great concern when national economies were growing rapidly as they were in the 1960s. More health services were seen as part of the spoils of affluence—like more cars, more televisions, and more washing machines. This was true even where the bulk of health services were financed through the public sector—by taxes and social security contributions.

It was the lower rate of economic growth following the world oil crisis starting at the end of 1973 that brought the problem into prominence. Where social spending was allowed to continue its earlier rate of growth in the new economic context, public opinion made its voice heard and the political process responded. Health spending has been selected for particular attention because of its growing share of social spending. There is a point at which people want to keep their own money to spend in their own way. What may also be important is that the bulk of money in health care is spent on a small minority who are seriously ill. There may well be a limit to what the healthy are prepared to spend on the unhealthy, even though they know that they themselves are given protection against this risk.

Already there are several countries where spending on health services is around 10% of the gross national product.[2] This is the case in France, Sweden, and the United States. If people are now working four or five weeks a year simply to pay for their health services, it is not surprising that they wish to be reassured that they are getting value for money—that what they are gaining could not be obtained at lower cost, or that they could not obtain more for the same cost. And the "more" they are seeking is not in terms of health services but in terms of health—less premature death, less illness and disability, less pain and restricted activity, and more comfort, support, and care when disability cannot be further ameliorated.

One consequence of the reexamination of spending on health services has been to raise serious doubts as to whether the richer countries of the world have in fact gained anything like commensurate benefits for their vastly increased expenditure over the past few decades. There are four reasons for this doubt. The first three come from the crude evidence of mortality experience. It should, of course, be recognized that mortality is far from providing a comprehensive picture of the benefits of health care.

First, mortality rates among children, young adults, and the middle-aged have continued to improve—but not at an enhanced rate; and the gains in expectation of life at age 65 have been far from dramatic. In that the vast majority of effective drugs used today were first marketed in the last 40 years and the high technology machinery of the modern hospital dates from the last 20 years, the improvements in mortality have been disappointing. Of course it is harder to cut mortality rates when they are low than when they are high. But an examination of the causes of mortality suggest that further preventive efforts may be more cost-effective in health terms than further investment in curative medicine.

Second, countries that appear to spend the most on health services do not necessarily have the best health. While Sweden and the Netherlands are high spenders and have good mortality, France, West Germany, and the USA are also high spenders but do not clearly have better mortality than the low-spending United Kingdom.

Third, the spread of health services, free or nearly free at time of use to the vast majority of the population, has been accompanied by major extensions in other social programs—cash benefits to support income, to share the costs of child rearing and to help the poor, programs to help the lower-income groups obtain better housing, the extension of education before and after compulsory schooling, and a whole range of social support programs. Thirty years ago it would have been predicted that all this massive social investment would inevitably lead to a narrowing of relative social class differences in mortality rates. But while rates have generally improved among all social classes, there does not seem to have been a narrowing of relative rates between them.

What is the explanation of this phenomenon? Were our social programs not sufficiently concentrated on the poor? In the case of health services, did we make a serious mistake by assuming that the lowering of money barriers was all that was needed to secure that all social groups used health care to the extent that they should? In Britain, at least, there is clear evidence that the lower social classes use services substantially less than their health status would warrant.[3]

Fourth, there is in many, but not all, affluent countries a distorted distribution of health resources, though not on the scale to be found in developing countries. Sometimes it is the inner cities that are relatively underprovided, and sometimes it is the more remote rural areas. In general, health resources tend to be most sparse where health needs are greatest.

The Response of the More Developed Countries

The immediate response of governments has been addressed to the narrow presenting problem of containing rising costs. They have grasped such weapons as were immediately available. In countries that finance their health services out of government budgets, these budgets have been tightened. In countries operating health insurance systems, what can be most readily squeezed are hospital construction, hospital budgets, and pharmaceutical costs. In both these two systems of financing, cost-sharing by the patient has tended to be increased partly to raise revenue, but also as a price signal to the patient and, via the patient, to the doctor.[4] But these are short-term measures that can put a temporary lid on costs and postpone the time when the upward trend reasserts itself.

However, in a number of countries, more fundamental questions are being asked, and some longer-term measures are being considered or taken. To help work out options for the future, there is now a burgeoning of interest in health economics throughout Europe, North America, and Japan. The economist can assist by analyzing the effect on costs of different policy options, and attempting to identify why costs are increasing in particular sectors. Of special importance are the economic incentives to providers caused by different systems of payment and the extent to which providers respond to them. Alternative payments systems could be devised that have different underlying economic incentives, and encourage providers to be cost-conscious and make better use of existing resources.

One approach to the problem of cost containment is to restrict the supply both of hospital beds and of medical manpower, as it appears to be these elements of supply that create the major costs. Hospital beds that are provided tend to be used. Extra doctors generate more work—some of which may be "unnecessary." Hence the trend in Western Europe is to cut the output of medical schools, following the vast expansion of the 1960s. Strict controls are being operated on hospital construction and extension.

Questions are being asked about the whole pattern of organizing and financing health services. In countries where general practice has rapidly declined in the face of growing specialization, there is discussion of whether the rebirth of general practice is possible and, if so, whether it would provide as good care at lower cost. In several countries where there are specialists without access to hospital beds, there are moves to secure hospital privileges for them so that the same specialist can handle the whole of an episode of illness. In several countries where hospital-based specialists have no outpatient facilities, there has been discussion of providing them for the same reason. The incentives under fee-for-service payment systems are being reexamined. In Western Germany, for example, there are moves to pay the doctor relatively more for consultations and relatively less for pathology and X ray. In the United States, the response has been a bewildering series of regulating mechanisms (utilization review, professional standards review organizations, certificate of need approval for new health facilities and equipment, comprehensive technology assessment, and payments of hospitals by diagnostically related groups, etc.) and the encouragement of Health Maintenance Organizations.

The most fundamental changes have been in Italy. Hospitals, instead of being paid per day of care, are now financed out of a local budget that will in turn form part of a regional budget. Ten years ago, the majority of doctors practicing in the community under health insurance were paid on a fee-for-service basis. Now they are all paid on a capitation basis. It was found that the prescribing rate of doctors paid under fee-for-service was much higher than for doctors paid by capitation. It is also of interest to note that prescription items per person per year are seven or less in Denmark, the Netherlands, and the United Kingdom, where general practitioners are paid on a capitation basis (or some variant of it). This compares with a rate of 9 in Belgium, 10.5 in France, and 11 in West Germany—all countries where doctors are paid on a fee-for-service basis under health insurance.[5]

Prescribing is by no means the only area where there are wide variations in the use of services within countries and between countries. There is a massive field for research to identify and explain variations in the use of particular types of surgery, of pathology, of X ray, and of the use of the hospital for particular conditions—the admission rate, the length of stay, and the real resource use per day of care. How far are variations really explicable in terms of health needs?

Thus five questions are increasingly being asked. First, is some of what is now done unnecessary and, if it is, why is it done, and how can this waste be prevented? Second, are there current treatments and procedures that are ineffective? Third, how is it possible to ensure that new technology and new procedures are not introduced in the future until there has been full and thorough evaluation of benefits and costs? Fourth, are there ways in which effective and acceptable care can be provided at lower cost, particularly by changing the place of care (e.g., outpatient surgery) or the mix of manpower (a greater proportionate use of less highly qualified manpower)? Finally, what new steps can be taken to prevent the need for health care arising in the first place? How, for example, can life-styles be changed, and what would it cost to do so?

On top of all this, some countries are consciously establishing priorities for the development of their health services—both between types of health need and between sectors of the population. This underlies plans to redistribute health spending geographically from northern Italy to southern Italy or from southeast England towards the north. In the longer run, this may lead to conscious searches for underusers of health care. It is, of course, easier to develop this plan within a health *service* than a health *insurance* system.

Healthy policy as distinct from health service policy is now clearly coming to the forefront in the thinking of many of the highly industrialized countries. There is no longer a willingness to leave health insurance agencies to pay any bills generated in open-ended insurance simply because the premium cost is now seen as becoming intolerable. The developed countries undoubtedly have lessons to teach the developing countries from their experience. Some of the most valuable may be negative rather than positive—"Don't do it our way."

The Problems of the Developing Countries

The critical difference that dominates health policy planning in developing countries is the sheer fact of poverty. This makes the waste of health resources intolerable, including the waste of doing well at high cost what could be done equally well at low cost. But even more important is the fact that poverty is itself a predominant cause of bad health. Poverty is the key vector—more important than any worm, microbe, or parasite. As has so often been said, poverty creates illness and illness creates poverty. The key to improving health is to break out of the cycle of malnutrition, disease, unhealthy environment, lack of education, and excessive fertility. It is a fact based on human experience that birth rates tend to fall when living standards rise and mortality rates fall.

Thus health improvement is a question of economic and social planning, not just of medical planning. In some cases political changes may be a prerequisite for health improvement—particularly where land tenure systems lie at the root of rural poverty. Health for all will not be achieved by the year 2000 by regimes whose power base is built upon providing health for a privileged few, or by regimes that cannot face up to the fundamental changes required to develop an equitable health policy. While planners can show the way, politicians can choose not to take it. That is their privilege. But any effective plan for health services must be part of a wider health policy and the latter must be part of a plan for integrated socioeconomic development.

The strategy of Health for All by the Year 2000 published in 1981 called upon Ministers of Health to establish a financial master plan for the use of all financial resources, after examining all possible sources of finance.[6] Some 20 countries were encouraged to cost their plans as part of what was called a "country resource utilization review"; but in many cases the data were hurriedly put together and were difficult to relate to existing expenditures. Making cost projections was also emphasized as part of the promotion of program budgeting. Where countries did attempt to cost their plans, they often lacked credibility simply because the sources of finances were unspecified or left a future gap, often a very large one, for foreign donors to fill.

The new thrust to promote financially realistic plans for health for all has come about for two main reasons. First, it became clear during the first attempt of WHO to monitor progress towards health for all how few developing countries could even attempt an estimate of what proportion of their gross national product they were spending on health services, and that a high proportion of the estimates that were provided were unreliable or seriously incomplete. But the second and most compelling reason was the world economic crisis. Health for All was launched in 1977—still a time of economic optimism: only in the case of the countries south of the Sahara was there any doubt among international agencies about the prospect of a continuing rise in the living standards of developing countries. Moreover, there was a hidden assumption that much more financial support for the health programs of the developing countries could be attracted from richer countries if the case were well presented.

It therefore came as a shock that between 1981 and 1983 the average gross domestic product fell by about 9.5% in Latin America and by 11% in Sub-Saharan Africa, and that there were also drops in living standards in the least developed countries of Asia. During the same period, low growth in Western Europe and North America led to a massive increase in unemployment.

The decline in living standards exposed the extent to which developing countries had fallen into debt. Devaluation and high interest rates made debt charges a formidable prior charge on government budgets, amounting to up to a third or a half of export earnings. While some countries fought valiantly to maintain the level of their health budgets, or even increase them, austerity policies drove many developing countries into cutting expenditures on the health sector. In addition, balance-of-payments deficits forced many countries to cut imports of drugs and medical equipment.

At the same time, the industrialized market economies were saddled with the problem of maintaining millions of unemployed—most of them young. This created a crisis in social security financing: more people needed maintenance while there were less people at work paying taxes and contributions to support them. As mentioned earlier, containing the cost of health care became an overriding objective of policy in these countries. In such circumstances, budgets to help poor countries develop their health programs were competing with extra heavy demands on public expenditure at home. The result was virtually no increase in external aid to the health sector between 1981 and 1983, and an apparent cut in 1984.[7]

Some African countries, faced with the formidable consequences of drought, on top of all their other problems and the virtual disruption of their rural health services, began to lose faith that Health for All was possible—or at least by the year 2000. One suggested that the year 2100 might be more appropriate. There was a real danger that Health for All would remain a dream unless countries were prepared to face up to the problem of limited resources and plan within totals of what further resources could realistically be expected to be made available, both internally and internationally.

The Thrust for Financial Planning of the Health Sector

A new program was launched by WHO in 1983 to promote four messages. First, countries need to know what is being spent on the whole of the health sector, public and private, and how it is financed. Second, the extra cost of Health for All plans should be calculated as uncosted plans amounting to no more than window-shopping. Third, that countries should investigate every possible source of finance for paying for the plan. Fourth, where necessary, plans should be revised downward to fit the resources that could realistically be expected to be made available, and every step taken to make better use of existing resources and to find the most cost-effective way of achieving particular health objectives.[8]

All this may seem so obvious that it hardly needs stating, let alone promoting as a world program. But remarkably few countries have in fact a costed health plan, and by no means all that have one have faced up to the question of how it is going to be paid for. An unduly optimistic plan contains a number of dangers. First, highly qualified staff may be trained in large numbers only to find later on that they cannot all earn their living either in the public sector or in the private sector. This wastes both training costs and human resources. Second, political pressures may lead to paid jobs being found for surplus doctors and the money found by cutting both training for and staff complements at lower levels of qualification. Third, costly buildings, particularly hospitals, may be constructed, but when they are complete money may not be available to equip, staff, and supply them at an adequate level. Or, if the money is found, this may be at the expense of developments of higher priority such as extensions in primary health care. Fourth, staff may be trained and given jobs but grossly insufficient supplies of drugs, supplies, and equipment to use their skills effectively. There are many examples of each of these planning errors in developing countries today. The aim must be to avoid repeating these mistakes.

Faced with all the uncertainties, some countries are reluctant to attempt to plan for more than a few years ahead. But a longer-term plan, up to the year 2000, is needed, for three reasons. First, the number of highly trained staff that can be financed in the long run should determine the educational program for the next 5 years. Second, the number of hospital beds whose running costs can be found in the year 2000 must determine the number of beds built over the next 5 years. Third, any major redeployment of resources that may be thought too painful or politically contentious, if carried out over a short period, may be more acceptable if phased over 10 years or more, during which time vacancies caused by retirements can be left unfilled and younger staff retrained for other tasks.

The most creative part of the planning task is the search for new or further sources of finance. The essential problem is that it is unlikely that developing countries will be able to find much more money out of taxation unless the economic fortunes of the Third World change radically for the better or the health sector is given much higher priority. This is unlikely to happen in view of the demands of other sectors of development. Moreover, additional taxes that are regressive can be counterproductive to health development. Nor are there any signs that there will be a massive increase in foreign aid to the health sector. Even if donors can be found to help with capital developments, this still leaves the running costs to be met and these are the major costs in the long run.

The possibilities for further funds differ according to the way in which health services are organized, and the traditions of the different countries. In some there may be opportunities for stimulating further support for nonprofit organizations, or creating new systems of local informal insurance or revolving funds (e.g., for drugs). A further possibility is to increase the yield of existing charges or introduce new charges particularly geared to help secure a more efficient use of current resources. Some developing countries charge far below cost for the use of private rooms in government hospitals. In some countries modest charges for drugs may be the only practicable way to discourage excessive prescribing. Other charges may be geared to discourage patients going direct to the hospital, bypassing on the way their local health center. Substantial charges levied at the hospital for nonemergency cases with exemptions for cases referred from the health center may help to secure a more economic use of the health care system. If services are only well developed in urban areas and some rural areas have no services at all within reasonable access, it seems only equitable that charges levied at urban services should be used to help finance extensions of services to the rural areas, provided ways can be found of exempting the urban poor.

A further possibility that is attracting increased interest is the development of new plans or further plans of compulsory health insurance. This option has been discreditied among many public health experts in view of the unfortunate effects caused by health insurance in so many countries of Latin America. At its worst, health insurance can be extremely socially divisive: it can promote sophisticated curative services heavily weighted toward expensive hospital care for the regularly employed (mainly the urban populations) and provide such generous remuneration for doctors and others that it becomes extremely difficult for ministers of health to recruit staff to work in rural areas or provide the critical preventive services that should be of highest priority in both urban and rural areas. What does not, however, follow is that it is impossible to devise plans that do not have these adverse effects.[9]

The essential case for compulsory insurance is that if ways can be found for those in the modern sector and their employers to pay the full cost of the services they use, tax money can be released to extend rural services to those uncovered or inadequately covered at present. But what is crucial is to avoid creating financial incentives that make it harder to recruit staff for rural services. One way of avoiding this is to confine the right to work for health insurance to staff who have completed a substantial period of rural service, or to make the extent of insurance practice allowed depend upon the duration of the rural service that has been completed.

Over the past decade, new health insurance plans have been started in Korea, the Philippines, Thailand, and Indonesia, though not all meet the above criteria. There are currently new plans for health insurance in Syria and Zimbabwe. Not surprisingly, they take many different forms. Some build on earlier precedents, while others have been specially devised to meet the requirements of the particular country.

The solutions that countries choose to adopt will inevitably depend on what is politically acceptable. The question of charging for health services is politically contentious in developing countries, as it is in countries already more developed. A plan that works well in one country, such as the sale of health cards to the rural population that give rights to free health care, may never get off the ground in another. A country with strong rural cooperatives may be able to build an informal health insurance plan as one of the functions of cooperatives. Much depends on what is administratively feasible. Workmen's compensation plans are commonly found in developing countries. This may be an administrative base upon which compulsory health insurance could be developed.

Priorities within Health Services

The failings of the health services of most developing countries have long been recognized. The following list does not of course apply to every country:

- relatively high expenditure on health services in urban areas while little or nothing is available within access of the bulk of the population living in rural areas;
- concentration of resources on hospitals, including teaching hospitals using high technology, rather than on primary health care;
- these trends are reinforced when physician-based social security plans have been introduced that provide services only to the wage- and salary-earning sections of the population. In some cases it would be economically impossible to extend such services to the whole population until the real national product had multiplied by five or ten;
- heavy cost of such "free" services as are available in travel costs and waiting time;
- imbalance in providing costly training to doctors, including specialist training, who are unwilling to work in rural areas, while there is a vast relative lack of auxiliaries to work with them;
- orientation of medical education towards the curricula of more developed countries rather than one designed to train doctors for their intended role in a particular developing country;
- relative lack of funding for preventive medicine including health education compared to the funding for urban curative medicine;
- heavy expenditure on a vast range of imported specialist pharmaceuticals, some of which may even be purchased twice (once by the government and then again in the private sector after purloining from government stores);
- services are hierarchically controlled so that there is neither integration with other local development workers nor participation from the local community; and last but not least,
- the majority of the population who are denied effective access to science-based services incur heavy expenditure on herbal reme-

dies and traditional practitioners who receive neither training, support, nor supplies from the organized services.

Each of these features can limit severely the lasting gains to health from expenditure on health services. And many countries are attempting to reorient their services in line with Health-for-All objectives. In economic terms, the essential problem is to maximize the health improvement that can be obtained from any given level of expenditure. The problem is the same as in the more developed countries. And if the benefits obtained from existing levels of expenditure could be improved, and shown to have improved, the health sector would be in a stronger position to negotiate for higher appropriations in view of the proven contribution to the process of integrated development.

The health economist can help by providing a clearer quantified picture of the existing situation. What are the sources of funds and how are they being spent? Existing health budgets in developing countries so often seem to be still designed to detect the misappropriation of funds rather than to serve as tools for health planning. They do not provide answers to the critical questions. How much is spent on training different types of personnel and on constructing different types of building? How much is being spent per head of urban population and per head of rural population? How does expenditure vary between urban centers and between different regions and districts of the rural areas? How much is spent on supplies—particularly pharmaceuticals? How is the budget divided between inpatient and ambulatory services, between curative services and different fields of preventive activity? All this information the health economist can help to collect.

Once collected, it can be related to the population reached. For example, what proportion of the population has effective access to services? What proportion of children in each district are fully immunized, and at what cost? What proportion of the population actually uses a health facility in the course of a year at what cost per visit (rather than how many visits are made)?

As a tool for the construction of a health plan, the health economist can construct a whole series of costing units. What is the cost of training a doctor, a nurse, a medical assistant, and a medical auxiliary? What is the annual cost of paying personnel once they are trained? What is the cost per day of maintaining different types of hospital beds, or of a consultation, an immunization, or a health inspection (for a particular purpose) provided by different grades of personnel? What is the cost per mile of different types of modes of transport?

These costing units can be used to work out the cost of performing a list of priority tasks. This cost will, of course, depend on what level of training is really needed to perform them. For example, no training at all may be needed to provide a regular distribution of antimalaria drugs for young children. How much training is needed to carry out an immunization procedure or to teach mothers oral rehydration? What would it cost to have each task performed by the lowest level of staff who could adequately perform it? And what would it cost to provide full population coverage for the performance of that task? In this way, each potential health benefit can be compared with its cost, though the combination of tasks may, of course, bring economies.

Alternative staffing models for providing coverage of rural areas by health-trained workers can be constructed to set out the cost of different options and compare the extent of effective access to services these models could provide. If, for example, one could make a new start, and the existing expenditure on health services were divided equally among each 100,000 of the population, what staffing would be chosen? Let us assume that 300,000 currency units are available per 100,000 population and that 100,000 units are needed for supplies, transport, and all other costs, other than staff costs. Some possible staffing options are set out in Table 1.

Only Option C, or some variant of it, provides a prospect of ready access of the whole population of a rural area to primary health services. If access is given the highest priority, then the limiting factors are the tasks that are chosen for the three grades of health worker to be trained to perform ensuring that they will have the time to perform them for the whole population they are expected to serve. These tasks can then determine the training program, rather than allowing traditional training patterns to determine how many people can benefit from the performance of any task.

TABLE 1. Model for Choosing Manpower Goals from a Limited Budget

Grade	Training cost	Annual cost per staff member	Optional numbers in post		
			A	B	C
University training for 5 years	100,000	20,000	10	6	2
Secondary school for 2-year training	3,000	6,000	0	10	10
Primary school plus 6-month training	1,000	2,000	0	10	50

Of course, no country is ever in a position to make a wholly new start. Even after radical political change, there is still an inheritance of staff trained with particular types of skill, and buildings designed for particular purposes sited at particular places. But once the direction of change is decided, a step-by-step progression can be made in the desired direction. And the success of each step can be evaluated soon after it has been taken.

The only services that can be hoped to reach the whole population are low-cost services, using frontline staff with limited training and low technology. Such services can nevertheless be effective if the tasks to be performed are carefully chosen, the staff properly trained and supervised, and the necessary supplies provided.

The impact of paid staff can be widely extended by the participation of the local community. The cheapest way of providing any service is for people to provide it for themselves wherever this is possible. The basic health knowledge passed on within the family is an invaluable asset in more developed countries. Building this knowledge base in a developing country that lacks it is potentially one of the most beneficial health investments.

The search for the most cost-effective ways of improving health inevitably challenges traditional patterns of thinking and the roles and functions of health personnel as they have developed in the more developed countries. But what is really involved is a further step in the process of delegation of task that is constantly evolving in the modern hospital. Tasks that, when new, were only performed by physicians, are now routinely performed by auxiliaries with much less training. The challenge for the developing countries is to see how far the process can be taken while still providing safe and effective health care. In this process new and simpler technologies may well be developed for the delivery of services.

Conclusion

The same fundamental questions are being asked in the more affluent countries as in the developing countries. What is the most cost-effective way of improving health? How can the health effort be redirected to provide better value for money? Insofar as this involves changing behavior, how can such change be best secured? And in the case of services, what should be the priorities, how can they be equitably distributed in terms of health need, and how can they be made to secure the maximum health improvements for the money that can be devoted to them?

The physician tends to see his task as the provision of the best service he can offer the individual patient, irrespective of cost. But no longer can cost considerations be ignored. When resources are limited, service provided to one patient at greater cost than is needed to provide a good and effective service means that resources will not be available for the care of other patients or to improve health by other means—many of which may be more cost-effective. Lack of cost-consciousness of one physician in exercising his clinical freedom can severely limit the clinical freedom of another physician, simply because the resources are not available for him to exercise it. It is for this reason that health professionals cannot escape a collective responsibility for how health resources are used. Health economists can assist them in exercising this responsibility and work with them to identify the more effective way of improving the health of the different nations of the world.

References

1. For a useful discussion of the problems and summary of major studies, see Anne Mills and Margaret Thomas: *Economic Evaluation in Health Programmes in Developing Countries,* EPC, London School of Hygiene and Tropical Medicine, London, 1984.
2. See OECD, *Measuring Health Care 1960–1983,* 1985, p 12.
3. Davidson N, Townsend P: *Inequalities in Health,* London, Penguin, 1982.
4. Abel-Smith B: *Cost Containment in Health Care,* London, Bedford Square Press, 1984.
5. Abel-Smith B, Grandjeat, P: *Pharmaceutical Consumption,* Commission of the European Communities, 1977.
6. WHO: *Global Strategy for Health for All by the Year 2000,* Geneva, 1981.
7. OECD, *Twenty-Five Years of Development Cooperation,* Paris, 1985, pp 302–303.
8. Mach EP, Abel-Smith B: *Planning the Finances of the Health Sector,* WHO, Geneva, 1983.
9. Abel-Smith B: Global perspective on health service financing. *Soc Sci Med* 1985; 21: (9) 957–963.

5

Internationalizing U.S. Universities through Health for All—2000

ANNETTE M. YONKE

The aim of this chapter is to call attention to a critical problem facing today's universities—the necessity to internationalize curricula, teaching, and research. The discussion points to the symbolic significance of the World Health Organization as an international institution challenging universities to consider international health as an organizing theme for institutional development. The chapter suggests how universities might think about "Health for All—2000" as an educational model to strengthen and focus international programs within the university.

THE PROBLEM: INTERNATIONALIZING U.S. UNIVERSITIES

During the last decade, leaders in higher education have strongly advocated "world community" and have made significant statements about the university's role in educating for a global society. More than ten years ago, the American Academy of Arts published a series on the future of higher education in which writers described the university as a symbol for establishing a "world community" of peace, concord, and justice. The curriculum and teaching of higher education was called up to define and articulate a universal knowledge and system of symbols to further international understanding.[1] In more recent years, several prominent literary figures within the international community have

ANNETTE M. YONKE • Associate Professor, Department of Medical Education, College of Medicine, University of Illinois at Chicago, Chicago, Illinois 60612.

called attention to the growing transnational culture of individuals, groups of intellectuals, and universities throughout the world who are the "special bearers of internationalism." All have worked out an infrastructure of international communication, a network as dynamic and developing as an emerging nation.[2] And even more recently, educational leaders have said that new opportunities for higher education exist within this world community, that the previous decades of internationalizing our universities supported by the Ford and Rockefeller foundations need to be continued on a variety of fronts to enrich the education of American students.[3]

The record of university accomplishments in international studies is impressive. Area studies for Africa, Asia, Latin America, Studies Abroad programs, comparative education, language training, scholarly exchanges, and major research centers provide a real international dimension for major U.S. campuses. However, a closer examination reveals that international centers exist in support of faculty and students who are already captivated by the ideal of "world community" and who have cast their lots in research, development, and teaching careers outside the U.S. The typical American faculty person or student has no taste for world politics but, with other citizens, find themselves drawn into it by our special interests and national pride.[4]

Today's events challenge us seriously to modify our resistance, indifference, or even distaste for things foreign, especially within our institutions of higher education. The economic and political restructuring in all regions of the world with possibilities for new trading partners, the ever-present threat of nuclear effects and terrorism, the rise of Islam and worldwide fundamentalism, and the international health epidemic of AIDS force us to look beyond our borders for insight into the problems that are most significant for the final decade of the 20th century. The predominant issues will be international. The pressing need for universities will be to shift our academic programs from the conventional and dominant western perspectives and ideals to culturally broader, more challenging, universal, and international themes.

The challenge to internationalize U.S. universities will not come from federal or state mandates or from the urgings of major professional organizations. Recent efforts of the Association of American Universities to organize a legislative attempt for a national foundation to strengthen international programs and studies within U.S. institutions of higher education[5] have not met with consensus among the many international agencies in Washington, nor can we be sanguine of prospects for successful legislation. As with any major effort, the various constituents or interest groups will have to work out policy differences and avenues of communication prior to creating a national mechanism for furthering international education. Moreover, legislative statements usually occur after the fact; once a phenomenon has rooted itself in the consciousness of the American people, national legislation follows. The time is not yet right for Washington to say what will be.

The task of internationalizing U.S. universities is one of institutional development. Here, the Third World development literature is useful. One school departs from viewing societal development solely from an economic perspective and focuses instead on a rationale based on the images and metaphors that underlie actions and beliefs of a society.[6]

Images, metaphors, signs, and symbols play a vital role in moving people, institutions, or countries forward. Universities that are developing toward a new world perspective, or a broader social-psychological attitude, are helped and encouraged by universal and symbolic challenges. Development of U.S. universities toward a new attitude requires an image that heightens the public consciousness about the metaphor of a global society. The image must be universal, freestanding—not linked to a particular way of thought, ideology, or institution. And it must have a history that legitimizes the symbol. In spite of current skepticism around its four decades as an international institution, the United Nations and its specialized agency, the World Health Organization, function as a powerful symbol for "world community." In particular, the recent movement of WHO toward partnership with universities throughout the world in its goal of "Health for All by the Year 2000" is an excellent use of contemporary eschatology for mobilizing institutions around a metaphor or image. The symbolic value lies in an institution that is both global and technical, a special organization that represents upward of 160 nations. Through its network of scientists around the world, WHO's eradication of smallpox has produced a mythology whereby the people of many nations claim a universal advocate for soundness of body and mind.

The purpose of this chapter, then, is to examine the WHO image of "health for all" in the context of universities; to consider how a university's response to WHO could be a source for institutional development around the concept of international health; and, finally, to show that international health as an organizing theme and model makes good curricular and methodological sense.

"Health for All" and Universities

In 1978, nations of the world gathered at Alma-Ata, USSR to draw up a proclamation that would change the emphasis on health care as it was universally practiced. In simple terms, countries decided to shift policy from emphasis on technological medicine to a practice of health care that originates and thrives in the community. The approach was named "primary health care," whereby health care services would no longer focus on the few but would give greater attention to the masses—a shift in ideology from elitist to democratic or socialistic. Consistent with this orientation toward health care for the many rather than the few, there developed a motto: Health for All by the Year 2000. The slogan evolved into the HFA-2000 or H-2000, the logo that now universally capsulizes and identifies a major global enterprise. A remarkable and significant common consciousness, international language of sign, symbol, practice, and program has emerged in less than ten years.

By 1984, it was time to take the idea to the universities of the world. The World Health Organization extended an invitation to university leaders throughout the world to meet in Geneva and consider the issues of curriculum relevance, applied research, and the meaning of community service within the framework of health. The role of universities in the strategy of HFA-2000 became the topic of the World Health Assembly discussions. Education and country leaders came up with a list of recommendations for universities of which several are significant for U.S. universities.

Recommendations to universities were to reshape institutional attitudes, so that applied research on social problems would be elevated to equal status with technically sophisticated research. Universities were challenged to overcome attitudes of insularity among disciplines and to find ways that fundamental knowledge across disciplines could be related to contemporary problems. Institutions were advised to broaden their learner base to include education of the community, not only in the health sector, but in government, the financial, and communications sectors. Finally, the World Health Assembly recommended that universities develop mutually beneficial academic linkages with similar institutions at the international level.[7]

How seriously the universities of the world take the above recommendations of the World Health Assembly remains to be seen. My guess is that most universities, at least in the U.S., have not much knowledge or interest in major international agencies such as WHO. But as a technical organization for research, training, and service, the functions of WHO parallel those of the university. The work of WHO in biomedical and social research, training, and technical assistance provides an expert counterpart institution for universities entering the field of international research and education. Not only is it able to access dozens of institutions of higher education throughout the globe, but its major orientation toward primary health care provides a framework and mechanism where the university might organize new international research and training programs.

In his keynote address for the WHA Technical Discussion on the "Role of Universities in Primary Health Care," David Hamburg, President of the Carnegie Corporation of New York, talks about how he has been impressed by the impact of agricultural extension services at a time when the U.S. was a developing country. He says that it was a kind of sharply focused adult education that draws upon a high-grade applied research. His astute reference to the land-grant concept is one that is particularly significant for our discussion.[7]

> When land-grant colleges were conceived and begun, there was no science of agriculture, no training faculty, no method of instruction established. . . . It was very much a picture of a developing country in that period . . . Many farmers were suspicious; the very lack of curricula drove educators out to the farms to get the firsthand feel of the situation. Educators and farmers got to know each other, a mutual respect developed, solutions were sought by research . . . And the transfer system for getting research results to the farms became quite orderly. . . . Moreover, in that experience, we came to see the dynamic interplay between basic research and applied inquiry.

One hundred years ago, the U.S. was a developing country in agriculture. Today, it is a developing country attitudinally and intellectually in its international outlook and understanding. Only a few of our citizens have the knowledge, attitudes, and skills for interacting with people from other countries, societies, and cultures. Despite specialized university programs in international studies, the U.S. is a third-world country in international human relations, whether in our neighborhoods or in the international assembly rooms. Although always friendly and generous, we are naive, blustering, and unaware of highly sophisticated and complex cultural forces now reshaping our world.

The history of U.S. higher education written 100 years ago featured new colleges of agriculture and schools of education. In the final decade of the 20th century, our universities and colleges face another great challenge—that of making our research, curriculum, teaching, and service more completely international. The problems facing all citizens of the 21st century will be that of assimilating the now developing world with its enormous masses of people into the actual "world community." Universities will have to educate future citizens about the 10-million-people cities, the new competitors in world markets, the transnational corporations that cross borders, social, and economic barriers, the emerging nonwestern institutions. Our students will be employed in companies and agencies that will become more international as we move into the next century. They will need a greater "sense of the world" and skills enabling them to operate in an international setting. Although they will not necessarily work overseas, the volume of "international interactions" will require a high level of international expertise.

But academic leaders have not yet defined the problem, nor have they ever felt the necessity to start thinking about formulating new "sciences," training faculty, and developing new research and pedagogical models. Hamburg's description of agriculture in the land-grant colleges has its parallel for today. Historians writing about U.S. higher education 100 years from now will say that there was no science of international human relations; no trained faculty; no method of instruction; that the very lack of curricula drove educators to get a firsthand feel of the situation and to seek solutions to the problems.

The invitation set forth by the World Health Organization for universities to join in partnership in the task of health for all provides an excellent mechanism for internationalizing universities. A partnership between an international organization whose charter is concerned with research, education, and service in collaboration with institutions of higher education is a viable and promising social innovation. Universities could begin to strengthen their internationalizing process by organizing around problems and issues of international health. The World Health Assembly recommendations call for applied research; multidisciplinary curriculum, teaching, and research; and education of the community toward the relationship between health and human behavior. Informative linkages with other universities abroad and with the World Health Organization become the mechanism for internationalizing programs.

Although the case for applied research and multidisciplinary teaching and research is not a new platform in the university, structuring curriculum to address the relationship between health and human behavior is new. Traditionally, the study of health issues is rooted in the basic sciences, clinical studies, or the epidemiological method. The added variable of human behavior opens new doors for research to include attitudes, practices, and issues related to education of the public for health. Following scientific findings on the pathophysiology of disease and occurrences in populations, solution to problems of international health will come from the behavioral and social sciences. Because improvement in health is largely a matter of shift in attitude and behavior, there is great opportunity for scholars to work across disciplines. For example, issues such as population shifts and urbanization, nutrition studies on specialized populations, methods of disease prevention, health problems of special groups such as refugees, laborers, adolescents, and pregnant women—are all rich with research potential from several disciplines in the social and behavioral sciences. Up to now, the mode of research in health has been that of the experimental method or critical trials that has dominated the medical sciences. Input from the social science disciplines will breathe fresh air into old methodologies for the study of health problems.

A further consideration for innovation is that international health does not have to be an area for research that is done overseas. In clarifying the relationship between health and human behavior within an international framework, major U.S. universities have international communities often associated with the institution through community activities or employment. The communities provide excellent opportunity for a type of research based on university/community collaboration that is action-oriented. For example, in a large urban university having adjacent Hispanic and Asian populations, studies have been generated on the relationship of migration to mental health; community-based population studies have been jointly designed by university faculty and community leaders; and epidemiological research results have been the basis for planning health education programs. Linkages with universities overseas, however, provide opportunities for comparative research on populations, health practices, and educational programs, as well as the entire range of problems in the basic, clinical epidemiological and social sciences.

Universities and HFA-2000 as an Educational Model

The WHO-University agenda calling for applied research, a multidisciplinary base for teaching and research, and inclusion of the social and behavioral sciences through linkages with universities overseas is a challenging prospect, but certainly not new. At the turn of the century, when the academic disciplines branched from philosophy, Durkheim advocated a method of approaching an event or institution from more than a single discipline. He predicted that sociology, economics, and geography would become more intertwined.[8] At about the same time, Dewey argued for crossing the natural sciences and human disciplines of history, literature, economics, and politics. It makes for good pedagogy for the simple reason that outside the lecture hall students meet with scientific facts and principles all wrapped together in human behavior. Rupturing the association of facts and process breaks the continuity of intellectual development, causes unreality in studies, and deprives students of normal experiences of interest and curiosity.[9]

Just as in Durkheim and Dewey's era, educators began to think about relationships between the disciplines based on the everyday problems faced by individuals in society; the new requirement for intellectual development today will be international studies. The university's task will be to produce an international citizen with familiarity and understanding of the First, Second, and Third Worlds and their relationship to one another in economic and political terms. This international person will have capability in one or more foreign languages and will be familiar with the major cultures of the world and the religious traditions, practices, and behaviors out of which the culture flows. The international citizen will be well-grounded in the western intellectual tradition but with capacity to understand, appreciate, and respect other intellectual traditions. Some understanding of economic and social development, patterns of country development, and political-social issues related to emergence of Third World countries will be important. Finally, the international citizen will have developed a social capacity to interact comfortably with individuals from other countries or cultures in domestic settings, or under less familiar circumstances outside the U.S.

From an institutional perspective, the university will need to develop an organizational mechanism to strengthen the international curriculum. International professional education based upon international health problems would provide a convincing organizing theme and educational model with appeal to the professional schools as well as the disciplines.

Within the present structure of U.S. universities, the home of "international health" as an interdisciplinary program is now in the schools of public health or in departments of social or preventive medicine. This is because, contrary to engineering, law, or education, international health historically evolved from international medicine, and is well established with its epidemiology, biostatistics, and management core. Graduate students and faculty generally come from a health sciences background. But within the total university, one is always surprised and delighted to find individuals concerned with international health issues and research in schools of engineering, business, law, education, and departments of economics, sociology, geography, and urban planning. Within the comprehensive university, interest in international health spreads across colleges and schools. An academic program with a strong international health dimension could bring faculty, students, and research topics together in a broad interdisciplinary setting.

Some preliminary considerations for organizing an international professional curriculum are worth examining. These are based on programs that already exit within universities and may suggest workable mechanisms for organizing faculty and students prior to setting up or strengthening an international program. These institutional processes are: a renewed approach to international exchange of talent; new educational models for the professions; and establishment of an institutional matrix for international activities. Several U.S. universities are working with one or more of these strategies to strengthen their international capability.

International Exchange

Exchange of scholars has generally been studied from the perspective of institution building for Third World universities. Coleman analyzes the experience of the Rockefeller Foundation in building institutions in the developing world, in showing differences in institutional development based on university, professional, and national environments.[10] Rarely, however, is there mention of the impact of foreign Third World scholars on U.S. universities. Probably the phenomenon most closely approaching the issue has to do with the awareness of the misfit between the needs of foreign professionals in the policy, managerial, and economic sciences and the western theoretical base out of which such programs come.

The problem is that U.S. universities do not convey skills and conceptual categories that are useful to scholars or students from the developing world. Universities today reinforce the worldwide elite tradition whereby scholars from all countries have been educated in western modes of thought, analysis, and attitude. Because the educated of the world form a unique social class separate from the masses, universities sustain this class culture and cultivate dependence rather than interdependence. U.S. universities need to take seriously the variety of epistemological paradigms for understanding human and social problems. In short, we need to decolonize our curriculum.[11]

My own experience in a health professions education confirms the above. In the last decade, visiting scholars who have studied with me and who are often in leadership positions within government or universities in the developing world, have attempted to formulate new models for education. The more astute recognize that as a result of schooling in Europe or North America, their own medical education has been stamped with the western seal. The curriculum of today reinforces the medical model of their earlier training. Many feel caught between the desire to compete in the western mode and the necessity to develop their research and educational programs of their own religious, economic, and cultural tradition.

In his discussion of the dilemmas of foreign study, Weiler writes that involvement of universities in Third World "human resource development" ought to be a declining business in the long run and that we need to stop producing our own kind. He advocates centers for research and training on the periphery to become "health anti-bodies in the international bloodstream of discovery."[12] I would argue that the business of development should continue, but with a new slant—and that is the development of our own university faculty.

The exchange of foreign scholars presents a unique opportunity for two-way "decolonization" whereby our faculty expand their international outlook, and visiting scholars articulate how western methodologies may or may not apply to social problems in their countries. Particularly in the sciences and professions, collaborative analysis and development of methods for analyzing the transfer of technology would contribute to an exchange of culturally based professional knowledge. Our standard technology, whether the research methods and strategies in the medical, physical, or social sciences, equipment, data, or the software of management techniques, program planning, development, and evaluation need to be viewed with the double vision of cultural embeddedness in western practice and an eye toward feasibility and viability of transfer to a visiting scholar's country. For example, our Chinese medical scholars, after studying in our laboratories for one or more years, exist with state-of-the-art knowledge and skills in their field. Yet, they return to academic situations where the newly acquired learning is not applicable, and in some cases not culturally viable. A challenging prospect for our own university faculty would be to determine jointly the body of knowledge and skills germane to the scholars' academic and cultural environment and to collaboratively plan a program for study here and for follow-up at home. Planning for follow-up would necessarily include a series of reciprocal visits for the education of UHS faculty as well.

Faculty development through technical assistance to developing countries is a complex issue. Since it falls under the university foundation of service, only a small segment of faculty are interested. One of our deans refers to technical assistance as "missionary work" and says that his faculty will collaborate only on state-of-the-art research. Younger faculty who are attracted to the international world have no time for overseas activities unless it provides research opportunity for their tenure goals. Because reward for service abroad is not built into tenure criteria, technical assistance generally becomes the task of faculty who have reached a plateau in their careers and who wish to extend themselves by participating in international activities.

The concept of technical assistance also belongs to a bygone era when aid and technology transfer were major means of interacting with professionals from the developing world. The newer mode described by the UN as the "new international order"[13] requires an attitude of mutual interdependence rather than the dependent relation of learner to expert or apprentice to preceptor. Colleagues from Third World universities have resources and skills for collaborative research. Successful models of community health care developed in Southeast Asian countries, results of research findings on drug-free populations, study results from stable populations without migration over generations, and natural products used in clinical therapy are only several examples of notable research occurring with faculty from developing countries. These research projects, however, result from work of scientists in a single department or academic center.

Interdisciplinary research projects involving faculty from several departments and linked with universities of the developing world most closely correspond with the WHO challenge for universities in international health development. For example, one school of urban planning has assembled a group of researchers from sociology, health services research, anthropology, environmental sciences, and medicines to address common research themes on health of children in urban settings. They have linked with relevant individuals within the Pan American Health Organization for the purpose of identifying several collaborating universities in Latin America whose faculty are interested in similar research topics. Their challenge is the opportunity to meet with colleagues from other universities both here and abroad for the long or short term. Resources of the group are unique in that several members are of Latin-American origin, area studies experts, or former nationals with useful knowledge and experience from universities abroad. By participating in such a group-directed research effort, faculty are broadening their framework, concepts, and resources.

New Models for Professional Education

On a fairly universal basis within U.S. universities, international studies programs are housed within colleges of liberal arts and sciences, in special country area programs such as Latin America, Southeast Asia, African studies programs, or within special international centers. Programs vary from one university to another, depending upon local interest and resources. Those who participate in these international programs are faculty and students whose academic interests are in the liberal arts and science disciplines and whose agendas and specialties are in language or area studies.

As the importance of international programs evolves within U.S. universities, the professional schools are beginning to recognize the importance of internationalizing curriculum. The leaders in this regard have been the schools and colleges of business and commerce. In a recent study on the importance of international expertise in business, Korbin said that his findings were not encouraging for area studies and language programs. While many firms employ area study specialists or international relations graduates, the number is small and the demand is likely to remain low. With few exceptions, firms hire according to basic skills and view international expertise as enhancement of fundamental skills. The basis for international expertise is some foreign language competency; a systematic understanding of differences in political and economic systems, culture, behavior—worldwide—and interpersonal interaction. This requires some traditional academic courses, such as comparative politics, economics, and anthropology, taught in such a way that students can acquire a framework on which to build through future study and experience.[14]

International health of the future will be largely that of international business. The health sciences will play a significant role as research institutes and universities in developing countries work on indigenous diseases and begin to participate in the entrepreneurial aspects of biotechnology. Recent breakthroughs in immunology, vaccines, diagnostic technologies, and psychopharmacological innovations in drug therapy are only several examples of the current wave. Next steps will be placement of technologies within the international marketplace. Following the U.S. phenomena, universities of the developing world will shortly be involved in commercial utilization of academic science whereby the university evolves into an enterprise capable of obtaining income from research activities.[15] As the university enters into the world of commerce, and as elements of the commercial world become more closely linked internationally, new opportunities for interdisciplinary input and research will emerge for biotechnology. Issues arising in international-academic-industry relations will be information and intellectual property rights having to do with patent guarantees, publication issues, and the extent to which different countries value property rights. As universities move away from the technical assistance approach to international health, institutions will also have to think about nontraditional delivery of instruction, often relevant to the private sector goals of bringing education and the workplace together. For international health of the future, the university will find itself increasingly tied to the private sector.[16]

With international health and business linking more closely in world markets, and research institutes in the developing world (especially in India) standing at the entrance to the international entrepreneurial biotechnology scene, the specialty field of international health will have greater interaction with the professions of law, engineering, and architecture. The traditional place of area studies in the liberal arts colleges will require examination. New models for international studies will need to be developed for the professional schools whereby students or members of the community have the opportunity to acquire at least general knowledge of a culture. For example, one university has developed a Thai studies program for students in the professional schools of business and health sciences that features faculty from both U.S. and Thai universities. An added component of this joint effort is that the program offers intellectual and cultural support to members of the business community who are interested in doing business in Thailand, some of whom are in health products business. Another international effort focuses on a collaborative effort for biotechnology transfer in India in which cultural and managerial support is provided to the entrepreneurs from university faculty. In short, the future of international health as part of the international commercial enterprise will necessitate new models of education for traditional and not-so-conventional university programs.

International Institutional Matrix

As the world of business and commerce increasingly drives the international health scene, as Third World governments encourage development of the private sector, and as universities become more internationalized, institutions need to think more strategically about an institutional mechanism for storing and disseminating information on international activities. For the most part, area studies centers, special international research centers, and internal studies programs exist as independent entities on U.S. university campuses. Each is a fiefdom in itself. Within the last few years, several major universities have created an institutional focal format for international programs, activities, and studies to function as an information bank and development assistance agent for the campus and community. The purpose of a central source for information and development is to expand the prospects and potential for international activities to other than established centers within the university and to create an increased public awareness of the importance of international education. Of critical importance to this central matrix is the relationship of the institution to foreign visiting scholars; the data bank on collaborating institutions in regions of the world including inter-institutional activities with consortia; and the education of the public. These are briefly described below.

Although the foreign student issue is critical for development of the international ethos of the university, the issues are addressed elsewhere.[17] The discussion here relates to the foreign scholar, a professional visiting the campus as a fellow scholar. Reflecting the institutional structure of the university, these individuals usually remain hidden within their departments. The university community does not capitalize on the special resources of the scholars principally because the institution had not thought about them as an overall resource. The reason for this is that there is no centralized unit that disseminates information and recommends channeling of resources inside and outside the university. When, for example, a faculty or community group develops a project relating to Africa or Latin America, visiting scholars could well act as advisors. Similarly, within the international business community, the visiting scholars become an excellent resource for international ventures. But the university needs to know who these scholars are, where they are located within the university, and what their capability and interests are. Collecting and disseminating this information are the functions of a central institutional source.

Tracking scholars after their stay at the university presents an opportunity for universities to strengthen their overseas relationships with other universities. International health has an organizing theme for institutional relationships, and thereby exchange of scholars provides a critical mass of individuals within institutions who can influence the development of the university's international program. As scholars become more involved in interdisciplinary studies under the international health umbrella, there is excellent potential for influencing the international involvement of the colleges and departments.

Institutional considerations aside, the enduring relationship of one scholar to another is the personal one. We all have our individual friends overseas, and our friendships are not weakened by time or distance. We all know of occasions when colleagues have called on friends in other countries to assist with early stages of project implementation or development—a common and very human networking. But the point is that a central information source can be of great use to faculty, students, and administrators to identify who knows who at what institution in which country.

As universities increasingly take seriously their institutional research efforts, the development of a central data base on international persons and activities merits consideration.[18] Ordinarily this component is omitted from institutional research studies. The initial purpose of the data base would be to profile university-wide participation in international activities by people and programs, track the overseas institutional linkages, identify international networks and consortia in the U.S. and overseas. The data could be used by academic units and by the external community for development and support of international activities. Application of data would be directed toward institutional policy making with regard to overseas linkages, promotion, and tenure, and program development.

As U.S. universities strengthen international relations, linkages with overseas universities become an important factor in international development. Such institutional linkages are recommended by WHO in its university statement. Since universities have memoranda of understanding with overseas institutions, establishment of university policy by one institution is worth mentioning. Based on university data about current linkages and with the judgment of a university-wide international council, this university developed a linkage policy statement containing recommendations for major and secondary linkages. The policy statement is useful to academic units in planning research and educational programs.

A university international data base of faculty activities also serves the promotion and tenure issue. Although community service is one of the functions of the university, "service" is not rewarded in the tenure process. Nor do research activities with overseas universities always result in publishable works. Analysis of data on extent, depth, and impact of faculty work overseas would be instrumental in influencing promotion and tenure policy.

Finally, a major consideration within the institutional focal point for international development of the university is the education of the public. Just as the land-grant colleges formerly educated the public in agriculture and engineering, the institutions of higher education will be educating society about the international world. A centralized international agent for the university could be useful not only for the institution, but also for the larger community. Through access to educational programs, nongovernmental organizations, primary and secondary schools, as well as the university community, a forum for educating the public could be developed. Many universities have engaged in "international outreach" in community-wide educational programs, but the present global situation and the public debate on U.S. foreign policy require greater attention to major issues.

Of importance these days is the growing interconnectedness of countries in trade—economic development. Closer to the heart than the pocketbook, however, is the prospect of international country-connected disease or global threats to the health of the individual: the world's concern about AIDS is the chief example. A public forum for health-related issues from a global perspective would provide an excellent means for enhancing public awareness of how countries relate to one another. The education of the public toward an international perspective strengthened by activities that focus on international health issues could provide a springboard for other issues related to how people live together on a single planet.

Of public concern today are other health-related issues wherein nations are beginning to recognize their links. For example, the global greenhouse question wherein, since the 19th century, countries have boosted the amount of carbon dioxide in the atmosphere. The intercountry effects of the acid rain question generate great public concern related to individual and community health. Of further interest to the public are the effects of natural resource abuse and environmental mismanagement and links to nutrition, disease, and developmental opportunities. The public is also becoming more aware of alternative health care practices in ancient cultures such as Chinese or oriental medicine as practiced in a western setting. The increasing popularity of acupuncture, acupressure, yoga, and other eastern health care practices for chronic disease looks promising for developing a greater international awareness for the public.

Conclusion

Although the considerations in this chapter, may, for some institutions, be idealistic, and for others, conventional and prosaic, the time has come for U.S. universities to play a leadership role in international education. The World Health Organization has provided a sensible and well-constructed framework. By capitalizing on the current resources within universities, programs can gradually be developed to educate faculty, students, and the public toward a more global perspective, beginning with international health. As McGeorge Bundy said 10 years ago: "There is no reason why we cannot meet the test of educating ourselves to the necessary levels of new understanding—both in what students learn and say and in what statesmen preach and perform." International health opens the door to that education for a world community.

References

1. Tolkett KS: Community and Higher Education. *Daedalus,* American Higher Education: Toward an Uncertain Future, Winter 1975; 2: 278–297.
2. Konrad G: *Antipolitics: An Essay.* New York, Harcourt Brace Jovanovich, 1984, pp 208–243.
3. Bok D: *Higher Learning.* Cambridge, Harvard University Press, 1986, p 170.
4. Bundy: The Americans and the World. *Daedalus,* A New America? Winter 1978; 303.
5. *A Legislative Proposal to Strengthen the Nation's Investment in Foreign Languages and International Studies to Create a National Foundation for Foreign Language and International Studies. Draft Document.* Association of American Universities, October 1986.
6. Wordsley P: *The Three Worlds: Culture and World Development.* Chicago, University of Chicago Press, 1987, p 41–60.
7. *The Role of Universities in the Strategies for Health for All.* Report of Technical Discussions, Office of Research Promotion and Development, Geneva, 1984.
8. Durkheim E: *On Institutional Analysis.* M. Trangott (ed), Chicago, University of Chicago Press, 1978, p 89.
9. Dewey J: *Democracy and Education.* New York, Free Press, 1966, p 286.
10. Coleman JS: Professional training and institution building in the Third World: Two Rockefeller Foundation experiences, in Barber EG et al (eds): *Bridges to Knowledge: Foreign Students in Comparative Perspective,* University of Chicago Press, 1984, pp 32–54.
11. Weiler HN: The political dilemmas of foreign study, in Barber EG et al (eds): *Bridges to Knowledge: Foreign Students in Comparative Perspective.* University of Chicago Press, pp 32–54.
12. Weiler: Ibid, p 195.
13. For a discussion of the New International Order in the context of technical assistance by university faculty, see Spitzberg I (ed): *Exchange of Expertise: The Counterpart System in the New International Order,* Boulder, West Press, 1978, pp 1–17.
14. Korbin SJ: *International Expertise in American Business,* New York: Institute of International Education, 1984, p 54.
15. Etzkowitz H: Entrepreneurial Scientists and Entrepreneurial Universities in the American Academic Scene," *Minerva,* Summer–Autumn 1983; XXI: 2–3.
16. Johnson LG: *The High Technology Connection: Academic-Industrial Cooperation for Technical Development.* University of Akron, Center for Urban Studies, Monograph Series No. 14, August 1984, pp 117–25.
17. Goodwin CD, Nacht, M: *Absence of Decision: Foreign Students in American Colleges and Universities.* New York: Institute of International Education, 1983.
18. Altbach P: The international perspective: Benefitting from institutional research, in: *New Directions for Institutional Research,* Winter 1976; 12: San Francisco, Jossey-Bass, pp 57–68.

6

Close-up of a Continent
Problems in South America

ERNESTO MEDINA

INTRODUCTION

The name of South America is given to the southern part of the Americas region. It is an area of relatively low population density (14 people per square kilometer) with an area of about 18,000,000 square kilometers and 253 million population, geographically located between the parallels northern 10° and southern 53°. According to the Pan American Health Organization,[1] for a better understanding, it is advisable to separate the so-called "Tropical South America" and the "Temperate South America." Tropical South America (Tr SA) includes the countries of Brazil (123 million population), which roughly represents one-half of all South America, Colombia (31 million), Peru (20 million), Venezuela (16 million), Ecuador (9 million), Bolivia (6 million), Paraguay (3 million), Guyana, Surinam, and French Guyana, with less than one million population. Temperate South America (Te SA) includes Argentina (29 million), Chile (12 million), Uruguay (3 million), and the British territory of the Falkland Islands, with only a few thousand people. Besides the differences in climate and geographical location, further reasons to separate Tr SA and Te SA are the significantly higher level of development of the Te SA, also called the Southern Cone of America, referring to the triangular shape of the southernmost part of America.

ERNESTO MEDINA • Professor of Preventive and Social Medicine and Director, School of Public Health, University of Chile, Santiago, Chile.

The Health Level

The General Situation

According to some commonly used indicators, the health situation of South America appears to be at a worse level than that observed in the North American countries (the U.S. and Canada), as is shown in Table 1.

The life expectancy at birth, under 70 years, mainly depends on high infant mortality rates and high death rates adjusted by age. Nevertheless, the crude death rate is lower in South America than in North America. The reasons for the difference are the diverse demographic conditions; the population aging process associated with the social and economic development determines an increase in the proportion of those 65 or older and, for that reason, an increase in the crude death rate. This is the case of North America as compared with the younger countries of Tropical South America. Temperate South America, with an intermedial demographic condition, also shows intermedial crude death rates.

The Main Causes of Death

Cardiovascular diseases, malignant neoplasms, and accidents are the leading causes of death in all countries with a high degree of social and economic development and, consequently, a high life expectancy. In South America, with a partial degree of development, this is true to some extent. In Temperate South America, heart disease, cancer, and stroke are the three most frequent causes of death; but in Tropical South America, influenza, pneumonia, and diarrheal diseases appear among the three major mortality problems (Table 2).

Table 1. Health Indicators in America, ca. 1985[a]

	Tropical South America	Temperate South America	North America
Life expectancy at birth (years)	63	6.9	75
Infant mortality rate (per 1000 births)	79	28	12
Death rate adjusted by age (per 1000)	6.6	5.7	4.0
Crude death rate (per 1000)	8.5	7.8	8.7

[a]Source: Pan American Health Organization. The Director's Annual Report, 1984.

TABLE 2. Leading Causes of Death in the Americas, ca. 1980[a]

Order	Tropical South America	Temperate South America	North America
1	Heart diseases	Heart diseases	Heart diseases
2	Influenza and pneumonia	Malignant neoplasms	Malignant neoplasms
3	Diarrheal diseases	Stroke	Stroke
4	Accidents	Influenza and pneumonia	Accidents
5	Malignant neoplasms	Accidents	Influenza and pneumonia

[a]Source: Reference 1.

As is shown in Table 3, the leading health problems differ in Tr SA and Te SA. In the first region, one-third of all deaths have an infectious, nutritional, or perinatal origin. The risk of suffering those types of ailments is 4–5 times higher than in North America. Another one-third of deaths are due to chronic diseases with a 3–4 times lower risk. Since 17% of all deaths in Tr SA have "ill-defined causes," lack of exactitude in the conclusions is inevitable. In Temperate South America, maternal and child health problems account for 16% of total deaths; but 61% are the result of a group of chronic diseases, which have become the top causes of death at these countries. In Te SA, the health situation is intermedial between the health problems of Tropical South America and those observed in North America.

COMMUNICABLE DISEASES

In spite of various types of efforts, the communicable diseases are still an important problem in Tropical South America, and are not under control in Temperate South America (Table 4). The death risk is especially high in children under 5 years of age (Table 5). Regarding the diseases with international reporting, no cases of cholera have been notified during the past decade in South America. Sporadic cases and small outbreaks of plague show the persistence of the disease in the western areas of the United States and in such tropical South America countries as Bolivia, Brazil, Ecuador, and Peru, due to plague focuses in selvatic rodents. During the years 1976–1980, 698 cases of yellow fever were reported in Tropical South America, most in Colombia and Peru. Differ-

TABLE 3. Causes of Death in South America and North America, ca. 1980[a]

Causes of death	Tropical South America	Temperate South America	North America
Maternal and child and infectious diseases	202 (35%)	116 (16%)	46 (5%)
Diarrheal diseases	51	13	1
Tuberculosis	13	7	1
Other infectious diseases	38	19	6
Influenza and pneumonia	48	25	26
Malnutrition	11	8	1
Maternal deaths	9	7	1
Perinatal deaths	32	37	10
Chronic diseases	179 (31%)	453 (61%)	613 (70%)
Coronary heart disease	41	126	289
Stroke	33	85	79
Other heart diseases	30	68	42
Malignant neoplasms	53	150	179
Chronic bronchial diseases	14	8	10
Cirrhosis of the liver	5	16	14
Accidents and violence	56 (10%)	65 (9%)	71 (8%)
Accidents	37	42	48
Homicide and suicide	19	23	23
Other causes	34 (7%)	39 (5%)	126 (15%)
Ill-defined causes	99 (17%)	67 (9%)	14 (2%)
Total	570 (100%)	740 (100%)	870 (100%)

[a]Death rates per 100,000 population.

ent vectors convey the disease and monkeys are the reservoirs. Selvatic yellow fever is linked with the progressive invasion of the jungle by man.

Several parasitic diseases are still prominent in Tropical South America. In the case of malaria, a total of 270,579 cases were reported in 1980, in comparison with only 341 in Temperate South America and 2,675 in North America. A matter of concern is the fact that the number of notified cases in 1980 in Tropical South America was 87% higher than in 1970, in spite of the eradication programs. The problem is associated with the mosquito resistance, bad housing conditions, and the migration of people to malaric areas, with increasing numbers at risk. The American trypanosomiasis, or Chagas disease, is an important problem of the rural areas from Mexico to Argentina, in any place where ecologic conditions permit contact with *Trypanosoma cruzi*-infected vectors; most of the notified cases come from Argentina, but antibody studies performed in different countries show that a high proportion of adult populations are

TABLE 4. Reported Cases of Selected Communicable Diseases, 1980[a]

Diseases	Tropical South America	Temperate South America	North America
Measles	74	49	11
Whooping cough	38	74	2
Poliomyelitis	0.9	0.1	0.0
Tetanus	2.7	0.7	0.0
Diphtheria	2.7	0.8	0.0
Tuberculosis	70	61	12
Typhoid fever	21	28	0.2
Viral hepatitis	40	62	24
Gonorrhea	89	112	421
Syphilis	41	46	29
Leprosy	9	4	0.1
Malaria	14	1	1

[a]Rates per 100,000 population.

positive reactors to the infection. The problem of leishmaniasis is frequently reported in Peru, and schistosomiasis in Surinam. The incidence rate of leprosy varies from 0.1 per 100,000 in Chile to 146 in Brazil and 167 in Paraguay. More than half the cases are of the lepromatous type of the disease. The incidence rate has doubled during the last decade as a result of better diagnosis and reporting of cases.

In spite of the existence of good vaccination procedures, the incidence of measles, whooping cough, poliomyelitis, tetanus, and diphthe-

TABLE 5. Acute Respiratory Infection and Diarrheal Mortality in Children under 5 Years of Age, 1980[a]

	Tropical South America	Temperate South America	North America
Acute respiratory infection			
Less than 1 year of age	860	450	50
1–4 years of age	75	22	3
Diarrheal diseases			
Less than 1 year of age	790	404	22
1–4 years of age	123	37	0.5

[a]Rates per 100,000.

ria is still significantly higher in South America in comparison with North America, and the same is true for the incidence of typhoid fever. The knowledge of the venereal diseases problem is incomplete because cases are underreported in many countries.

Maternal and Child Health Problems

Children under 15 years of age and women of child-bearing age represent almost two-thirds of total population of South America. For that reason, and the high death risk, the maternal and child problems have had a high level of priority among the health programs of the region. The death risk of children and mothers is several times higher than that observed in North America (Table 6) as a result of a low standard of living, poor housing and sanitation, inadequate medical care programs, and other limitations linked to the low educational level of many mothers.

The health of infants and preschool children remains at a critical level in the majority of the Latin American and Carribean countries, a problem closely associated with poverty. The problems are greater than the official data convey, since only one-half of the countries have a complete death registry. The main factor is children's death underregistration, especially during the first weeks of life. In spite of this situation, a substantial proportion of infant deaths were due to perinatal causes in 1980 (40% in Temperate South America and 27% in Tropical South America). The most important health problems, beside those associated with pregnancy and birth, are communicable diseases, acute respiratory infections, diarrheal diseases, and malnutrition.

In recent years, 24% of all communicable disease deaths in the 1–4-year-old group were due to illnesses preventable by vaccination: measles,

Table 6. Maternal and Child Risks, ca. 1985[a]

	Tropical South America	Temperate South America	North America
Infant mortality rate (per 1000 births)	79	28	12
1–4-year-old death rate (per 1000 population)	4.5	1.3	0.6
Percentage out of total deaths			
Under 1 year of age	24	12	2
1–4-year-old	11	2	0.4
Maternal death rate (per 1000 births)	1.6	0.6	0.2

[a]Rates per 100,000 population.

whooping cough, poliomyelitis, and tetanus; the proportion was less than 1% in North America during the same period of time.

Children under 5 years and aged people are population groups with the highest mortality risks from influenza and pneumonia. Collaborative studies have shown that the incidence of acute respiratory infections is similar in North and South America, but the rate of complications and the fatality rates are significantly higher in the last region.

Diarrheal diseases continue to be a principal cause of morbidity and mortality of children in many Latin American countries. It is a complex syndrome having different etiologies, mainly viral, shigella and salmonella, amebiasis, and other parasitic infections. The problem is specially serious among infants (Table 5).

Malnutrition in preschool children is a very important problem in the developing countries, probably the main factor associated with death in these children. A close relationship between infection and malnutrition, in a sort of circle, can be observed. The frequency of any degree of malnutrition in children under 5 years of age is less than 10% in Temperate South America, but reaches over 50% in other parts of Latin America.

The Health Problems of the Adult Population

Chronic diseases have become the leading cause of death (61%) in Temperate South America and of a major proportion (31%) of total deaths in Tropical South America. In comparison with North America, chronic diseases in Tr SA have a lower risk, with the exception of chronic bronchitis. In Temperate South America the only difference from North America is a lower coronary heart disease death rate (126 instead of 289 per 100,000 population); all the other main problems have a similar risk in North and Temperate South America: stroke, other heart disease, malignant neoplasms, chronic bronchitis, or cirrhosis of the liver (see Table 3).

Main sites of malignant neoplasms vary in different countries (Table 7). The most important cancer sites in North America (lung, intestine, and breast) are the same in two countries of the Temperate South America (Argentina and Uruguay), both with the most aged population in Latin America. On the other hand, the incidence of gastric cancer is higher in South America; the frequency of cervix uteri neoplasms is similar in both regions.

Among life-style habits, cigarette smoking represents an important health danger. The collaborative studies in the region show that roughly 40% of men and a lesser proportion of women are smokers.[2] A matter of concern is the upward trend of smoking in females, mainly young women. In a country like Chile, the number of deaths attributable to smoking

TABLE 7. Main Sites of Malignant Neoplasms in America[a]

Sites	United States	Temperate Uruguay	South America		Tropical South America
			Argentina	Chile	
Lung	43	33	26	9	3
Intestine	20	18	12	4	3
Breast	16	16	12	5	2
Stomach	7	24	14	25	10
Cervix uteri	5	7	5	6	6

[a]Rates per 100,000 population.

accounts for 7% of total adult deaths and the habit of cigarette smoking makes a contribution of 10% to the infant mortality rate of the country through the lower birth weight of babies (220 g less than babies of non-smoking mothers.[3]

Alcoholic beverage consumption is high in Temperate South America, explaining the great incidence of cirrhosis of the liver, especially observed in Chile, and also linked to high rates of accidents and violence (see Table 3).

In sum, several Latin American countries present a quite complex pattern of mortality. On one hand, infant mortality, malnutrition, and infectious diseases, and on the other, increasing rates of heart disease, malignancies, and other chronic conditions pose different issues for health care.

ASSOCIATED FACTORS OF HEALTH PROBLEMS

Generally speaking, the health situation of a community is the result of the impact of different geographic, ethnic, demographic, social, economic, and cultural conditions, the latter operating through the existence of sanitation facilities, nutritional programs, and medical care and health services organization.[4] In the South America case, all these factors are important for understanding present health conditions.

The geographic location of the region explains the high frequency of different types of tropical diseases, since most of the area is situated in the vicinity of the equatorial line. The exception is the so-called Temperate South America, located between the 25° and the 55° southern parallels and in a temperate zone, south of the Capricorn Tropic line. Geographic and ecologic conditions also explain the unusual frequency of some digestive cancers, especially neoplasms of the stomach, observed in some places of Chile, Colombia, or Venezuela.[5]

The population of the countries in Tropical South America is the result of a mixture of Europeans, Africans, and American Indians in different proportions. In opposition to this situation, Temperate South America has only a white population of European descent, mainly Spanish and Italian, as in Argentina and Uruguay, or a white majority population, as in Chile. It is important to remember that several communicable diseases known for centuries in Europe, such as tuberculosis, where people were acquainted with them, were not known by the American Indians or African people. During the last 400 years there has been no time for a natural selection process with increase of natural antiinfective defenses. The ethnic factors also explain the unusual frequency of some diseases in certain South America groups. This is the situation observed in Chile with the highest world prevalence of gallbladder diseases[6]; the great incidence of intrahepatic cholestasis during pregnancy, linked to the American Indian component of the population[7]; the fragility of Chilean livers to the cirrhotic effects of alcohol, having twice the liver cirrhosis expectable according to the average alcoholic beverage consumption,[8] or the unusual frequency of peptic ulcers located in the upper third part of the stomach, associated significantly to the O blood group.[9]

Tropical South America is an example of a young demographic type of population, while Temperate South America is in an intermedial situation (Table 8). Both sectors of South America have significant health problems, according to the demographic features: Tropical South America faces high maternal and child risks, while Temperate South America has a great amount of chronic diseases, parallel to a higher expectancy of life. The young population structure depends on high fertility rates, which also means an important rate of population increase, making difficult the efforts to obtain total health services for the population. In South America, an increasing migration to urban areas is observed. That implies, initially, difficulties in providing medical care, and greater health risk but, since in the urban areas it is easier to organize health services, ultimately living in urban condition determines a lower health risk for the population, not only for access to medical care, but in relation to the betterment of other components of the standard of living situation.

The gross national product per capita in 1980 was U.S. $1,859 in Temperate South America and U.S. $1,504 in Tropical South America, ranging from U.S. $2,457 in Venezuela, an oil producer country, to U.S. $567 in Bolivia. According to these figures, all South American countries can be classified as developing countries. This explains the problems

TABLE 8. Selected Demographic Features of South America, ca. 1980

	Tropical South America	Temperate South America	North America
Age of the population (percentage)			
Under 15 years	42	29	23
15–64 years	55	63	66
65 years and over	3	8	11
Dependent population ratio (%)	82	59	51
Fertility rate (per 1000 population)	29	23	16
Increase of population (percentage per year during the period 1975–1980)	2.8	1.3	1.0
Geographic distribution of the population (%)			
Urban	66	83	74
Rural	34	17	26

attributable to scarcity in economic resources in the areas of nutrition, sanitation, medical care, or educational services, which are extremely important to improving health conditions. In the field of sanitation, only three of the 12 South American countries (Venezuela, Chile, and Uruguay) have 90% or more of the total urban population with controlled water services in the dwellings, and only three (Ecuador, Colombia, and Chile) have 65% or more of the population with sewage systems in urban areas. This situation explains the high incidence of diarrheal diseases and other water- or food-origin diseases.

Illiteracy has become a rare condition in the South American cities, but still remains a problem in the villages and rural population of some countries. A worse educational level is observed in Tropical South America in comparison with Temperate South America, where a major part of the population has 9 or more school years (Table 9). Illiteracy, as an expression of poverty, has been always associated with higher risk of infectious disease, maternal and child problems, and high fertility rates. The increasing educational levels of the young-generation mothers is an important factor for significant changes in health and family planning behaviors.

THE IMPORTANCE OF MEDICAL CARE

In many South American countries, the factor that plays a major role in health progress is the development, organization, and functioning of

TABLE 9. Quality of Life Indexes in America, ca. 1980

	Tropical South America	Temperate South America	North America
Adult literacy rate (%)	81	90	99
Gross national product per capita (in US$)	1,100	1,900	11,000
Infant mortality rate	42	33	13

health care activities. This arises in those nations that have overcome many of the very serious limitations imposed by the low levels of personal income, education, sanitation, or nutrition. Moreover, the introduction of family planning programs has led to an intermediate demographic condition, without the burden of a great aged population, and with considerably fewer problems of coronary heart disease, malignant neoplasms, and other chronic diseases.[4] Under such conditions, health care acquires special importance and the health resources development appears a milestone in achieving medical care in the required amount and quality.

Table 10 shows some important features of medical care activities. In comparison with North America, South American countries have roughly one-half the hospital beds per 1000 population, a greater proportion of small hospitals, fewer nurses, and fewer medical doctors. The high frequency of maternal and child problems determines an important number of physicians working in the areas of pediatrics, obstetrics, and gynecology.

With less resources, the admission rate to hospitals in South America (100 per 1000 population) is approximately two-thirds that observed in North America. The frequency of medical calls varies from five visits a year in some Argentinian cities to near zero in the rural areas of Tropical South America. A great deal of variation is also observed in the amount of well-baby clinic visits and in other important types of services. The best immunization programs of the region are observed in Chile, with more than 90% of infants receiving BCG as tuberculosis protection, a third dose of DPT (diphtheria–pertussis–tetanus), and poliomyelitis and measles vaccine.[10]

Human Health Resources

Around the world it can be noted that countries have come up with different answers in the process of providing health care to the population. The participation of physicians, nurses, assistant or auxiliary

TABLE 10. Human Resources and Health Services in America, 1980–1985

	South America	North America
Number of hospital beds	722,000	1,573,000
Ratio per 1000 population		
Total beds	3.5	6.5
Beds in short-stay hospitals	2.3	5.1
Property of the hospitals (%)		
Ministry of Health	18	2
Other public agencies	22	44
Private sector	60	54
Hospital size (%)		
Under 100 beds	31	14
100–499 beds	44	60
500 and over	25	26

Human resources (per 10,000 population)	Tropical South America	Temperate South America	North America
Physicians	9	21	19
University nurses	2.3	5.3	6.1
Auxiliary nurses	19	15	33

Physicians (per 10,000 pop.)	Canada	U.S.A.	Chile
Type of practice (%)	18.2	16.7	8.7
General practice	42	15	10
Pediatrics	3	7	14
Obstetrics and gynecology	3	6	10
Other specialties	52	72	66

nurses, or other personnel can be quite different because the diverse solutions are linked to the level of development of the countries. With enough financial resources, health care is usually provided by medical doctors. But in countries with a shortage of physicians, other types of personnel are needed for solving important health problems. In young nations with high proportions of children and many malnutritional or infectious diseases, the contribution of nurses or assistant personnel for health promotion activities, education, or specific preventive measures is very important in a group of activities that in developed countries are usually performed by doctors. In the same way, in the rural areas of the poor countries with a great number of scattered population, the best solution is the deployment of permanent auxiliary personnel, living in the area, instead of resident physicians.

Around the world there is agreement on the fact that the activities that should be done in the secondary and tertiary levels of medical care should be performed by doctors. But no unanimity appears regarding the type of personnel needed for the primary health care level, mainly in well-baby clinics or other types of services in the family planning or the pregnant women services.

The old WHO Expert Committee recommendation for the countries to have or reach a rate of 10 physicians per 10,000 people seems obsolete today. The nations with the best health indexes—expectancy of life at birth, infant mortality rate—now have 14–15 doctors per 10,000 population. The rate of physicians varies widely in the world, from 29 in Israel or the Soviet Union, to 0.1–0.2 per 10,000 population in Ethiopia or Niger, according to data of the last years of the 1970's decade. In Latin America, as a whole, the rate amounts to 9.2 per 10,000, being higher in Temperate South America (21 per 10,000) due to the very high rate in Argentina (26.7), than the observed in Tropical South America (9 per 10,000) as is shown in Table 10. The number of doctors is high in a few countries like Uruguay (19 per 10,000) or Cuba (15 per 10,000), but extremely low in Guyana (1.0) and other Central American or Caribbean countries.

During the last 20 years, the Latin American universities have made an important effort to solve the problem of the lack of medical doctors. In South America, for instance, the rate of physicians increased from 5.6 to 8.9 per 10,000 population between the year 1960 and 1980. Unfortunately, this trend, which seems positive for solving the important health problems of the region, has also generated some important problems in terms of an overproduction of physicians in relation to the economic capacity of the countries, creating increasing numbers of underpaid or unemployed young doctors.

Thus, if it is very difficult to solve health problems efficiently without enough numbers of doctors, it is also true that a surplus of physicians is not the answer, especially if the increase has happened in a short period of time without an upward trend in financial resources, hospital facilities, and professional work incentives. If this trend does not happen, a great concentration of underpaid doctors in the great cities or massive migration to other countries are the costs of such policies.

Obviously, the lack of balance observed in Latin America between the human resources needs, its production at the universities, and the finances of the health system operating in the countries is the result of bad planning systems, due not only to weak links between the health and the educational sectors but also associated with the chronic political instability of the countries and changes in the short- and long-term planning policies.[11,12] Generally speaking, achievements in health resources planning are few in the world, usually due to lack of realism in taking account of the social, economic, and political limitations of the countries.[13]

In almost all nations there is a tendency toward the concentration of health professionals in cities in comparison with the rural areas—the trend historically associated with the existence of a greater number of hospital beds in the cities. For solving the problem of few doctors in small towns and rural areas, which tend to have greater death risks, the Latin American countries have tried different systems. One of them has been compulsive rural work for young doctors or senior medical students during their internship, before getting the professional degree. Chile, for two decades, had a system in which the incentives of significantly higher salaries and a fellowship for specialization after three to five years of general practice in rural areas and small cities, provided enough physicians for all the rural areas and small hospitals of the country.[14]

During the 20th century, a clear trend toward more specialists in medical work has been noticed all over the world, probably associated with the progress in knowledge and the difficulty for doctors to manage efficiently all types of health problems. This trend for working in medical specialties has been different in the countries of North and South America. In Canada, Trinidad, Puerto Rico, or Panama, almost one-half of the doctors are in general practice, and there is an availability of 4.4 to 4.7 general practitioners per 10,000 people. But in the United States, only 15% of the physicians practice medicine in this way and the rate is only 2.5 per 10,000. Other countries are in an intermedial situation. In 1980, 40% of the total number of doctors were general practitioners and in 27 of 42 Latin American or Caribbean nations, the general practice amounted to over 50% of the total number of doctors.

When a country or a region has enough general practitioners it is easier to provide medical services to the rural areas. When the number is limited, there can be noted in such countries high numbers of obstetricians, pediatricians, and internists—indicating a sort of replacement of the general practitioners by two types of specialists, pediatricians and internists, who work as general practitioners for children or adults, respectively.

The lack of medical doctors has led many Latin American countries to the policy of giving nonmedical personnel a great deal of responsibility in the well-baby or pregnant women clinics, the family planning programs, or the chronic disease control. But this policy has been not successful because the lack of doctors is parallel to scarcity in any type of professional or university health workers. The number of registered nurses in Latin America being extremely low (2.7 per 10,000 people in 1972), the Decennial Health Plan for the Region, approved by almost all Latin American countries, established as a goal to obtain a regional average of 4.5 university nurses and 14.5 assistant or auxiliary nurses, through the training of 125,000 new nurses and 360,000 nurse's aides. In 1980, the rates were 4.2 and 10.8 for each type of personnel having a double number of nursing personnel (76,000 in 1972 and 152,000 in 1980). In spite of this effort, the Latin American availability of nurses continues to be low, only one-tenth of that observed in North America. When the number of nurses is low, most of them work in hospitals (70% in Latin America and the Caribbean) making it more difficult to work efficiently in community health and giving entry to the assistant personnel in activities classically performed by professional nurses. But the difficulties and the costs of preparing well-trained auxiliary nurses has led some countries to a trend of preparing community health workers with a very low level of training, in paid or voluntary systems, for doing tasks traditionally performed by nursing personnel. For these reasons, the analysis of the nursing situation has become increasingly complex, with new types of personnel in a wide range of professional capacities.

As was discussed in the cases of the physicians, there also has been noted defective planning in nursing human resources production. It has been observed in several countries that the effort of training nurses has not been linked with increases in financial resources for paying them, appearing in some countries in high rates of unemployed nurses.

Good care during pregnancy and in birth assistance are crucial points to lowering infant mortality, usually very high in many Latin American countries. Only Cuba, Costa Rica, and Chile have infant mortality rates under 20 deaths per 1000 births. In many rural areas of Latin America, one-half the deliveries have no professional assistance, the women being helped by traditional midwives. Efforts have been made to train these midwives in the principles of a nonrisk birth assistance in normal cases and in the decision to send the mothers to the hospital in complicated cases, using short-term courses and supervision of the professional health personnel.

The different types of nurse's aides, or the community health workers, are trained in service, for doing well-defined tasks such as community and family survey, health education, sanitation, maternal and child health, nutrition, vaccines, and other functions. Experience shows that the auxiliary personnel can be effective if: (1) they have good personal conditions for working with communities, getting enough status for their work; (2) they are trained; (3) they receive periodic supervision (2–4 times a month); and (4) they have the possibility for sending patients to higher medical care complexity levels when the problem of the patient oversteps the capacities of the auxiliary personnel. When these conditions are not present, there are few possibilities that this personnel could really solve the health problems with improvement of the local health conditions.[15,16]

In poor countries, like many Latin American nations, there is a great temptation to have low-qualified assistant health personnel, mainly for financial reasons, since the cost of training one medical doctor is about the amount needed for training 8 auxiliary nurses,[17] and, afterwards, the salary costs are lower. The important point is perhaps to know which has the real capacity for solving the common health problems demanding medical care. In Chile, for instance, we know that in our communities the capacity of the auxiliary nurse personnel with 9 months of training is roughly 60% of the primary health care demand; the figure grows to 90% when a medical doctor is present. Both figures show that in any case, but in different proportion, many patients' problems cannot be solved at the primary health level and the patients should be sent to a hospital either for diagnostic or therapeutic reasons.

Probably the idea to have community health workers is viable in some countries when other solutions are not possible. That was proved in China, with their "barefoot doctors." But it is advisable to remember that in this experience the results have been linked to: (1) a very careful appraisal of the personal qualifications of the candidates, especially their IQ; (2) the wish of the workers to improve their condition in the future, perhaps becoming medical doctors; (3) the selection of a few tasks related mainly to health promotion and family planning; and (4) supervision and help from the higher medical care levels. When these conditions are not fulfilled, success is rarely achieved.

In 1980 several Latin American countries had accomplished the goal of having 14.5 auxiliary nurses per 10,000 people (Costa Rica, 21.9; Puerto Rico, 21.3; Venezuela, 21.0; Chile, 20.7; Uruguay, 20.4; Panama, 18.2; Barbados, 17.2). No information is available regarding the number of community voluntary health workers in Latin America. Generally speaking, the "health promoters" or "health auxiliaries" initially concentrated their efforts in health promotion activities in the maternal and child field—greatly needed because of the young demographic condition of the countries—but being the only member of the health team in the villages and rural areas they have been compelled to extend their role to problems of morbidity for which they have not been trained.

Trends and Perspectives

During the last years a clear downward trend in mortality has been observed in South America (Table 11), mainly in children under 5 years of age, which represents an accomplishment of the expected goals of the Decennial Health Plan for the Americas of the 1970's decade. The decline of the death rates is a result of different types of improvement: sanitation, nutrition, women's educational level, and especially the extension of medical care services with a primary health care approach, including immunization programs, child growth and development activities, nutrition, health education, and medical care. The result of such an effort has been a decrease in the main causes of child disease (diarrheal and other communicable illnesses and malnutrition); a lowering of the fatality rates by oral rehydration procedures in diarrheal diseases, or by treatment in acute respiratory conditions. A crucial point has been

Table 11. Trends in Health Indicators and Population Changes in America

	Tropical South America	Temperate South America	North America
Reduction in age-adjusted mortality 1970–1978 (%)	23	22	17
Infant mortality rates			
1960	88	83	26
1970	65	66	20
1980	43	38	12
Accomplishment in infant mortality reduction according to Decennial Health Plan (countries)	3/5	2/3	2/2
Reduction in the 1–4-year-old mortality (%)			
1960–1970	30	40	27
1970–1980	52	44	20
Reduction in maternal mortality rates (1970–1980) (%)	18	40	55
Life expectancy at birth (1980)	61	68	74
Increase in life expectancy comparing 1965–1970 and 1975–1980 (number of years)	4	3.5	2
Fertility rates 1975–1980 (per 1000 population)	36	23	16
Expected rate for 1995–2000	29	18	14
Population (millions)			
1970	154	36	226
1980	204	41	246
1990 (expected)	267	46	270
Population increase 1970–1980 (%)	2.8	1.3	0.9

the increasing outreach to the population of medical services, particularly at birth and during the first years of life.

Analysis of South American health trends leads to the conclusion that at very low levels of development, medical care cannot change the prevalent health conditions because of the restraints posed by housing, sanitation, nutrition, or educational problems. But, in a second phase, when these problems are partially solved, the preventive programs and medical care services appear the most important factors for bettering health conditions. Many South American countries or regions of these countries are in this phase. In a third stage, when virtually all of the population has medical care, new progress in health is linked to the development of mental health activities, changes in life-style, and improvement in the ecologic conditions.[4]

The decrease in the death risk has determined an impressive population increase, Latin America being at the present time the region of the world with the highest rate of growth, since the fertility rates remain at a high level. Nevertheless, during the last decade, the fertility rates of most South American countries have declined, reducing the rate of population increase. The fertility decrease is the consequence of childbearing women attaining a better educational level and cost-free programs of fertility regulation methods.

A downward trend in death risk should not lead to the conclusion that the frequency of disease is now significantly less than in the past and there will be a decrease in medical care needs. Some recent research performed by us[18] shows that the young-generation mothers, with only one or two children per family, make a medical care demand for their children that is several times greater than that observed in the women of the previous generation. In the young women, almost each disease episode represents a medical care demand for the sick child. On the other hand, another source of increasing medical care demand depends on the aging population process in South America, which has determined an increase in chronic disease prevalence. The mass communication media has also changed the perception of chronic disease and the medical behavior of the people.

The final result is that health needs today are greater than ever, and an increasing need has appeared for financial resources to manage this new and demanding situation. There is an interest in new types of medical organization and also a concern for the costs and efficiency of medical care activities, and for better planning and management systems. Medical care and public health in South America are facing changes that have happened in a very short period of time and are challenging the old structures of medical organizations of the countries.

At the root of the situation appears the fact that, in many South American countries, the diseases linked to underdevelopment are not completely controlled, and malnutrition, infectious diseases, and maternal and child problems still appear as priorities; but, on the other hand, such problems as heart disease, malignant neoplasms, the consequence of the population aging process, or accidents appear as the main causes of death for these countries. For the control of these threats, new strategies are needed. To the primary health care strategy, so useful for controlling the maternal and child problems, it is necessary to add other strategies mainly located in the areas of public education for change in life-styles and screening systems of chronic diseases with a more extensive use of the tertiary level of care, meaning greater economic resources than are considered at the present time. It appears that the need is to review all the classic priorities, while giving consideration to the new problems that have appeared in a short period of time as major public health concerns. These changes in the importance of different diseases are compelling the initiation of deep changes in priorities, strategies, services, human resources, and types of training if the goal of Health in 2000 is to be attained for the South American populations.

References

1. Pan American Health Organization: *The Health Situation in America, 1977–1980.* Scientif Publ No. 427, Washington D.C., 1982.
2. Joly D: *The Smoking Habit in Latin America.* Pan Am Health Org Scientif Publ No. 337. Washington D.C., 1977.
3. Medina E, Rojas C, Miranda R et al: Smoking habit in pregnant women and birth weight (in Spanish). *Rev Chil Pediatr* 1984; 55: 279–286.
4. Medina E, Kaempffer AM: An analysis of health progress in Chile. *Pan Am Health Org Bull* 1983; 17: 22–30.
5. Armijo R, Orellana M, Medina E et al: Epidemiology of gastric cancer in Chile: a case-control study. *Internat J Epidemiol* 1981; 10: 53–57.
6. Medina E, Kaempffer AM, Irarrazaval M et al: Epidemiological features of gallbladder diseases in Chile (in Spanish). *Bol Ofic Sanit Panam* 1976; 80: 220–227.
7. Reyes H, González M, Ribalta J et al: Prevalence of intrahepatic cholestasis of pregnancy in Chile. *Ann Int Med* 1978; 88: 487–493.
8. Medina E, Kaempffer AM: Epidemiology of liver cirrhosis. (in Spanish.) *Rev Med Chile* 1974; 102: 466–476.
9. Csendes A, Medina E, Obaid E: Blood groups ABO and Rh in peptic ulcer, gastric cancer and control groups (in Spanish). *Rev Med Chile* 1975; 103: 470–476.
10. Carrasco R, Dintrans E, Montalto I et al: The cold chain and the expanded program on immunization in Chile: an evaluation exercise. *Bull Pan Am Health Org* 1982; 16: 261–267.
11. Vidal C: The human resources development in America (in Spanish). *Educ Med Salud* 1984; 18: 9–24.

12. Mejia A. World trends in health manpower development: a review. *World Health Statist Quart* 1980; 33: 112–115.
13. Hall TL, Mejia A: *Health Personnel Planning* (in Spanish). Geneva, WHO Publications, 1979.
14. Medina E: Health: a social need of the world (in Spanish). *Rev Med Chile* 1975; 103: 451–461.
15. Skeet M: The community health agent: An impellant or a restraint to primary health care (in Spanish). *Foro Mundial Salud* 1984; 5: 333–338.
16. Ratnaike RN, O'Neil P, Chynoweth R: The rural health agent and the malnutrition: a project that failed (in Spanish). *Foro Mundial Salud* 1984; 5: 361–363.
17. Gruber FJ: Primary health care given by health teams: Principles, strategies and methods (in Spanish). *Bol Ofic Sanit Panam* 1981; 90: 304–310.

II

Problem Areas in International Health

7

International Scientific Cooperation for Maternal and Child Health

ELENA O. NIGHTINGALE, DAVID A. HAMBURG, AND ALLYN M. MORTIMER

INTRODUCTION

Most of the world's people still cannot take for granted their ability to meet basic needs for food, water, shelter, and other factors essential for survival. The problems that face industrialized nations are related to sociotechnical conditions that have appeared very recently in the evolution of the human species. In developing countries, the shift from old to new ways is occurring even more rapidly. Many of the developing nations are undergoing rapid social change. These social changes are having important effects on the physical and mental health of the population. Such changes involve urbanization, industrialization, and large-scale migration, as well as unemployment, vast increases in scale of the community of reference, and greater cultural heterogeneity. Taken together, these factors tend to weaken or even rupture the fabric of traditional cultures and attenuate their socializing, orienting, and supportive functions. This weakening of traditional family and community roles may have a critical impact on maternal and child health, including adolescent outcomes.

Across much of Africa—especially in sub-Saharan Africa—Asia, and Latin America, population growth and abject poverty have contrib-

ELENA O. NIGHTINGALE • Special Advisor to the President, Carnegie Corporation of New York, Washington, D.C. 20036. DAVID A. HAMBURG • President, Carnegie Corporation of New York, New York, New York 10022. ALLYN M. MORTIMER • Program Associate, Carnegie Corporation of New York, Washington, D.C. 20036.

uted to extremely severe health problems that stand as an enormous obstacle to continued development and social progress. Malnutrition and infectious diseases take the lives of a great many infants before they reach one year of age, and handicap for life many of those who survive. Fourteen to seventeen million children die each year worldwide from the combined effects of poor nutrition, diarrhea, malaria, pneumonia, measles, whooping cough, and tetanus. Susceptibility to a wide variety of diseases is heightened by the marginal character of subsistence in many regions.

In industrialized countries, such as the United States, attention to the needs of children is complicated by the fact that a major shift in allocation of resources has occurred from the younger to the older end of the population.[1] In the past 20 years, the economic status of children in the United States has worsened while the proportion of older age groups in poverty has greatly diminished. Nearly 40 percent of all poor people in America are children. Of these children, only about half are immunized against preventable diseases; only 39.9 percent of the non-white preschool children are fully immunized against polio, and only 51.3 percent against diphtheria, whooping cough, and tetanus.[2] Similar problems occur in other countries.

A useful estimate of the well-being of a society is provided by the infant mortality rate, measured by the number of babies that will die before the age of 12 months per 1000 babies born. For example, in Mali in 1985, the infant mortality rate was 175 per 1000; other African countries had rates ranging from about 63 to 175 deaths per 1000 live births. Remote rural areas reach rates of 200 to 250 per 1000. By comparison, the overall infant mortality rate in the United States in 1985 was 11, and in Japan, Finland, and Sweden it was 6.[3] The worst record for infant mortality in the United States is held by the nation's capital. Despite major improvements in recent years, infant mortality remains over 20 per thousand for the District of Columbia, where many births are to very young black women, who are impoverished and receive little or poor prenatal care—a situation comparable to but not as grave as that of the vast majority of women in Africa.

But why, when problems of hunger, poverty, health care, and survival are so pervasive in the less developed nations, should we focus on the improvement of the health of mothers and children, including adolescents? First, mothers, children, and adolescents make up three-quarters of the population of the less developed countries; therefore, reaching out to them directly reaches the largest and most vulnerable segment of the population—the segment with the least power. Second, by reaching mothers with primary health care—including family planning, literacy, nutrition, and health education—the mother, as the primary caretaker, improves the status of the entire family. Finally, but of critical importance, most of the causes of death and severe disability among mothers and children are interrelated, and are preventable at low cost and without the need of sophisticated technologies.

During the past 10 years, biomedical and behavioral scientific inquiry has made it possible to learn a great deal about preventing damage to mothers, children, and adolescents. Among some of the modern scientific and technical interventions that have made a powerful contribution to improving human welfare are antibiotics, oral rehydration therapy, and immunization. Improvements in the delivery of services for women and children have also been made. Alternative approaches to service delivery, such as the "risk approach," have been used as a managerial tool in reallocating resources to improve coverage and efficiency of maternal and child health care.[4] Scientific research, including a number of longitudinal studies, has helped to clarify the relationship between risk factors and later outcomes. Sufficient and early prenatal care, breastfeeding, adequate nutrition, early education, and social support networks for health and education are a few interventions that are proven or plausible.

There is a growing interest in cooperative efforts among nations to assess worldwide problems and increasing concern for helping developing countries adapt and apply technology to their own circumstances. Since science provides a powerful problem-solving tool, it is essential that its strengths are brought to bear on the problems of maternal and child health to the maximum extent possible. The success of cooperative efforts, however, will depend in large part on the interaction between behavior and technology. The existence of technologies to deal with a particular problem has frequently not been sufficient to solve the problem; in order to be effective, methods for using and maintaining these technologies must be taught correctly, understood adequately, and distributed widely. To translate an interest in promoting greater cooperative efforts to improve the conditions of life for mothers and children, it is important to link technical expertise to the behavioral and social sciences.

Selected Health Problems of Women and Children

Since a large proportion of the population of developing and newly industrialized countries is young, maternal and child health is a prime preoccupation and a way of tackling major health problems. Development of the human infant begins at conception, although the nature and extent of a child's vulnerability to environmental influences stems in part from factors present prior to conception: the mother's age, general health and nutritional status, education, life-style and habits, and the socioeconomic circumstances of both father and mother. A combination of low birth weight, malnutrition, and care by a very young, poor mother may retard the growth and development of some children by the age of two. Large cohorts of children reach school far behind their contemporaries on a variety of cognitive and social measures. During adolescence, a significant number of young people in developing countries have no access to or drop out of school, commit a crime, become pregnant, succumb to mental illness, abuse alcohol or drugs, become disabled, attempt suicide, or die from injuries.[5]

There are many causes underlying the developmental problems of the young. The most profound and pervasive exacerbating factor, however, is poverty. Almost every form of childhood damage is more prevalent among the poor—from increased infant mortality, gross malnutrition, recurrent and untreated health problems, and child abuse to educational disability, low achievement, early pregnancy, alcohol and drug abuse, and failure to become economically self-sufficient. Health problems occur not only more frequently, but they are more serious among the poor. For example, poor children are more likely to suffer from middle-ear infections, to receive no or incomplete treatment, and to suffer permanent hearing loss that can retard learning in school.

Women of childbearing age and children are especially at risk of ill health and premature death in poor areas because of the particular vulnerability of certain stages in growth and development—those related to childbearing in women and the very rapid development and growth in prenatal life and early childhood. During adolescence people often adopt self-damaging behavior patterns that can sometimes shorten life. These behaviors of adolescence include poor health practices (poor nutrition, exercise, hygiene); alienation from school; reckless driving; assaultive behaviors; and the use of tobacco, alcohol, and illicit drugs. These behaviors can occur in all communities.[6]

If family health is to be attained, the health needs of mothers and children, including adolescents, are a first priority. The basic principle underlying maternal and child health is that there are specific biological and psychosocial needs inherent in the process of human growth that must be met in order to ensure the survival and healthy development of the child and future adult.

MALNUTRITION

Malnutrition of the mother and the newborn constitutes the single most important cause of health problems carried through to adult life.

Whether it is chronic or acute, associated with famines or undramatic, the fetus and the newborn are particularly vulnerable to it. Malnutrition before birth and during the first 5 years is early protein-energy malnutrition. It is the most extensive and serious public health problem affecting the human species. In Africa, more than a quarter of children under four—more than 20 million children—are affected, and several million die each year.[7] Although it is very difficult to disentangle early protein-energy malnutrition per se from interrelated cultural, familial, and institutional influences, the available evidence suggests that it has a negative effect on intellectual, physical, and social development. A high incidence of the conditions may entail a heavy economic burden and be a serious obstacle to development in many countries.

Nutritional deficiencies, such as insufficiency of vitamins A and D, adversely affect thousands of children worldwide. Each year about one-quarter of a million children are blinded by xerophthalmia induced by severe vitamin A deficiency. In general, a well-nourished child with a vitamin A deficiency is at greater risk of infection than is a generally malnourished child without vitamin A deficiency. Most commonly occurring in the rice-eating areas of Southeast Asia and India, vitamin A deficiency in children is also found in the Middle East, in part of the Caribbean, in northeast Brazil, and in Central America.[8] The most vulnerable age for vitamin A deficiency is between 6 months and 5 years; this debilitating disease affects the poor predominantly.

Maternal malnutrition not only represents a drain on the woman herself, but also increases the risk that her baby will have a low birth weight, a significant factor negatively influencing the chances of the child's survival. A woman's nutritional requirements during pregnancy and lactation increase considerably; there is a dramatic increase in vitamin, mineral, and energy requirements. It has been estimated that 100,000 calories are expended per pregnancy, about 1800 calories per day during lactation.[9] Malnutrition during pregnancy is particularly severe in developing countries, where it has been estimated that about two-thirds of all pregnant women are anemic.[10]

Diarrheal Diseases and Acute Respiratory Infections

Diarrheal diseases and acute respiratory infections are major causes of illness and death among young children in developing countries. In India, more than 500,000 young children die from acute respiratory infection each year, while in Bolivia, over 100,000 children have been dying each year from diarrheal dehydration. Both of these conditions constitute a group of diseases with multiple etiologies—bacterial, viral, or parasitic—and both may predispose children to malnutrition. Children under 5 years of age are especially susceptible. In poor communities, children may contract a diarrheal infection six or more times a year, with each episode lasting for more than one day, while episodes of pneumonia, bronchiolitis, acute laryngitis, and epiglottitis frequently are fatal.[11,12] As many as 9 million children under 5 years of age die annually from acute diarrheal disease and pneumonia. There is an age-specific vulnerability to diarrhea that is closely associated with the introduction of weaning foods or the cessation of breast-feeding. The earlier the bottle is introduced, the higher the risk of diarrheal disease and death.[13] Acute respiratory infections are also less likely to be problematic to infants when a strategy of breast-feeding is implemented.[14]

In addition to improvements in socioeconomic conditions, advances in knowledge have allowed for improvements in the treatment and prevention of diarrheal disease and acute respiratory infections. Such measures include immunizations, appropriate use of antimicrobial drugs, application of oral rehydration therapy in the case of diarrhea, and correct identification of the severity of the diseases and informed referral to hospital care for infants and children most severely affected. In the case of diarrheal disease, where studies of use and impact of oral rehydration therapy have been done, the results have given inadequate consideration to sociocultural factors. The ultimate health benefit depends upon the actual use of the intervention. A mother may be introduced to the technique, but her decision to use it and her ability to use it effectively are influenced strongly by her social support system. The main thrust of research indicates that the most effective interventions for diarrheal disease are those that interrupt the transmission of infectious agents in the home. There are well-documented findings concerning the fundamental importance of fecal contamination of food and water in the home and controlled studies showing the effectiveness of such simple actions as handwashing in preventing infection, but the international research literature on diarrheal diseases is unfortunately lacking in field studies designed to learn how to make household hygiene effective in poor countries. Such studies could have great practical benefit in a relatively short time, and could help to instill health habits with long-term gains.

A 1986 report by the Institute of Medicine of the National Academy of Sciences (U.S.A.) identified 19 diseases (with global distribution) of the less developed countries for which vaccines could probably be developed in the next 10 years, given sufficient resources.[15] Top priority was given to development of a vaccine for pneumonia, middle ear infections, and meningitis caused by *Streptococcus pneumoniae*. The incidence of these diseases is particularly high in the very young, and the available vaccine is not effective in this age group.

Rotavirus diarrhea is ranked second for vaccine development. Nearly 900,000 children under the age of five die every year from dehydration that accompanies rotavirus diarrhea. Immunization of women of childbearing age could provide protection through breast milk; that, plus immunization of infants could provide protection to the population at highest risk.

New vaccines will require investments in research and production that most developing countries cannot afford. New approaches for international cooperation in research, development, and funding of vaccine production, availability, and delivery could markedly reduce the burden of death and disability borne by the children of the developing world.

Low Birth Weight

Babies born too soon or too small are at high risk of death or, if they survive, of disability. These babies are disadvantaged from birth. Female infants of low birth weight have an increased chance of becoming mothers of such infants themselves. Prevention of low birth weight is of crucial importance to child survival.

A 1985 Institute of Medicine-National Academy of Sciences (U.S.A.) report assessed the impact of the frequency, periodicity, and content of prenatal care of prevention of low birth weight in the United States.[16] As in less developed countries, babies born too small for their gestational age are concentrated among minorities, the poor, and the young teenage mothers. Here as elsewhere, low birth weight is a major determinant of infant mortality and increases the risk of lifelong problems, physical and mental, in the survivors. Very little is known about the specific biological mechanisms of low birth weight, but factors that increase its chance of occurrence have been identified. These include low socioeconomic status, low level of education, nonwhite race, childbearing at extremes of the reproductive age span, and being unmarried; medical risks that can be identified before pregnancy, such as a poor obstetric history, selected diseases and conditions, and poor nutritional status; medical risks that are detected during pregnancy, such as poor weight gain, urinary infections, preeclampsia and toxemia, short interpregnancy interval, and multiple pregnancy; behavioral and environmental risks, such as smoking, alcohol, and other substance abuse, and exposure to various toxic substances; and the health care risks of absent or inadequate prenatal care. Many of the established risk factors are amenable to prevention or therapy, especially those recognized before pregnancy occurs. Smoking is the best example of a preventable risk. Teenage girls in the United States and many European countries now smoke more than boys of the same age. Other risks include poor nutritional status, certain chronic illnesses, and susceptibility to infections such as German measles (rubella). Even demographic risk factors, such as age, can be managed—e.g., by avoiding pregnancy at extremes of the reproductive age span. The risks posed by high parity and brief intervals between pregnancies can be decreased through family planning.

The risk of low birth weight declines sharply among mothers with at least 12 years of education. The relationship between education and low birth weight is independent of maternal age and race. The risk of low birth weight is reduced among mothers who initiate prenatal care during the first three months of pregnancy. Moreover, the Institute of Medicine analysis suggests that the content of care may have an important influence on the risk of low birth weight.

While this report focuses on prevention of low birth weight in the United States, the risk approach taken is applicable to prevention of low birth weight and other aspects of maternal and child health care in less developed countries. By identifying risk factors and how they cluster in people, relative risk can be used to target prevention programs and allocate resources. Further, the obstacles to prenatal care are basically similar in many different countries—lack of money, lack of providers and services, attitudes that further impede seeking help, lack of transportation and child care, and lack of systems to recruit hard-to-reach women. This is an area of maternal and child health care in which experience in technically advanced and less developed countries can be exchanged to mutual advantage. It is an area requiring education, but also the collaboration of the behavioral and biomedical sciences, particularly for the design of efficient delivery systems in rural, poor areas.

Maternal Mortality

About half a million women die each year in developing countries from fertility-related causes—pregnancy, abortion attempts, and childbirth.[17] In sub-Saharan Africa, the maternal mortality rate is 2 to 6 per 1000 births—some 100 to 300 times the Western European rates.[18] In rural Bangladesh, maternal mortality rate was found to be 570 per 100,000 live births. Maternal mortality accounted for 57 percent of deaths of women aged 15 to 19 years old in this area and 43 percent of deaths of women aged 20 to 29. In Afghanistan, maternal mortality has been estimated to be about 700 per 100,000 live births. Thus, high population growth results from high fertility and relatively high mortality and is achieved at the very high price of the lives and health of women and infants.

Among the most important causes of these deaths are postpartum hemorrhage (often with anemia as an underlying cause), sepsis (infections), and hypertensive disorders of pregnancy, such as toxemia. Although there is widespread underreporting, illegally induced abortions are a significant cause of maternal deaths. This problem is particularly notable in Latin America, where in some cities as many as one maternal death in three was the result of abortion; nearly all these deaths were sepsis-related. In hospital studies in India and Papua New Guinea more than one-tenth of all maternal deaths were due to abortion.[10,17] High fertility rates thus affect the health status of both women and their children. Too many or too closely spaced pregnancies give rise to health risks both for the mothers and the infants. The health needs of other children in the family, especially very young ones still dependent on maternal feeding, may consequently not be met. Pregnancies that are too closely spaced also leave little time for a woman to build up her nutritional reserves. For African women, childbearing is usually started as soon as it is biologically possible, and stops at the menopause. On average, the African woman spends 18 to 20 years of her adult life in childbearing—that is, 18 to 20 years elapse between the first birth and the last, compared to 3 to 5 years for women in most developed countries. Not only is the African woman's potential for other pursuits exceedingly limited by her reproductive functions, but in some poor rural areas of Africa, by the time women complete their families, they have had 6 to 8 children without health care. The prevention of maternal deaths and improvement in maternal care is an area that will require a shift in the priorities of developing countries and a cooperative effort on the part of the international medical and scientific community.

Vaccine-Preventable Diseases

In 1983, 5 million children died from six diseases that can be prevented by immunization: diphtheria, whooping cough, tetanus, measles, poliomyelitis, and tuberculosis.[19] An equal number were disabled physically or mentally. In 1985, 3 million children died from measles, neonatal tetanus, and whooping cough.[12] In the developing world, up to one-third of childhood deaths are associated with vaccine-preventable diseases. These diseases tend to be severe, since the resistance of many of the children is already compromised by multiple infections and, mostly, by severe malnutrition. Neonatal tetanus results mainly from unsanitary handling of the umbilical cord, and could be controlled by immunizing women twice before the birth of the baby. In many areas, tetanus accounts for up to 10 percent of all neonatal mortality. In India, for example, 288,000 neonates die from tetanus annually.[20]

Measles is a surprisingly important and problematic disease worldwide. In general, the complications of measles are much more severe in developing countries, chiefly because the disease occurs in malnourished children, and malnutrition is an important factor in determining outcome. In Mexico, there are several million children in absolute poverty who are chronically hungry. Mexico had 54,000 deaths from measles in 1983. There were also thousands of children left with mental impairment from encephalitis associated with measles. Thus, prevention is very important and requires further effort. The measles vaccine in the United States is not recommended for children under one year, yet the mortality (especially in developing countries) is highest in that age group. Recent trials with inhalation vaccine by aerosol in babies nine months old could help in this regard, but the data are not complete.

Acquired Immune Deficiency Syndrome (AIDS)

AIDS has become widespread in many parts of the world, although patterns of transmission vary. For example, the pattern in Africa is notably different from that in the United States, where male homosexuals account for the highest percentage of AIDS victims. In Africa, heterosexual contact is the dominant mode of transmission.

In Central Africa, the AIDS problem has reached critical proportions. For example, in Zaire the incidence of infection with the AIDS virus has been estimated to be more than 1 percent of the population; in the U. S. the prevalence of infection is less than 1 percent overall, but can exceed 50 percent in intravenous drug users and in promiscuous male homosexuals.[21] Women suffering from AIDS can transmit the infection to their unborn or newborn baby, although the mechanism is not clear. In the United States, about three-quarters of the more than 1,000 children under 13 years of age who have AIDS are from families where one or both parents are AIDS victims. Other risk factors for childhood AIDS include being a hemophiliac or receiving repeated blood transfusions for other reasons. AIDS in children is more difficult to diagnose than adult AIDS. Infants with AIDS may lack the characteristic clinical and laboratory indicators. The AIDS epidemic has potentially tragic consequences for the health and well-being of mothers and children worldwide. Although the pace of AIDS research has been rapid, so has the advance of the disease. A concerted global research and surveillance effort is required.[22]

Risk-Taking Behaviors in Adolescence

Adolescence has been neglected because in most societies adolescents are perceived as relatively healthy, although such perceptions are often wrong. It is during adolescence that people adopt self-damaging behavior patterns that often shorten life. Rapid biological and psychological changes take place in adolescence. In many countries in Africa, for example, menarche in girls coincides with the beginning of childbearing. In developing nations and under conditions of poor health and nutrition, menarche may not occur until 15 or 16 years of age, compared to an average of 12 years in more developed nations. Nonetheless, the trend is to earlier maturity. Problems related to pregnancy in early adolescence are frequent and serious. Adolescent pregnancy is a worldwide problem, although many variations exist.

Statistics on the health problems of adolescents are scarce and often unreliable, but the data that exist indicate that in many developing countries, adolescents are a significant proportion of the population, and for them the leading cause of death is from injuries. Abuse of tobacco, alcohol, and other drugs strongly affects health, injuries, and violence.[6] The rates of abuse are increasing. In more developed countries, death and disability are primarily the result of motor vehicle accidents, while in developing countries death occurs most often from falls, fires, poisoning, and drowning. Murder and suicide are also major causes of death among young people, particularly in urban areas.

Smoking in developing countries is increasing. In Uganda, for example, 31 percent of university students smoke; in Lagos, 17 percent of boys and 2 percent of the girls smoke.[23] In the United Kingdom, there was a sharp increase in the number of girls taking up cigarette smoking, from 15 percent in 1982 to 24 percent in 1984.[24] Many young people experiment with alcohol and other drugs (including cigarette smoking) in an attempt to work through the usual difficulties of adolescence. Some risk factors and antecedents of risk-taking behaviors, such as low self-esteem, social depreciation, poverty, low expectations and achievement, negative peer pressure, and tenuous human relations are related to long-term emotional deprivation.

Young people are apt to engage in unplanned and unprotected sexual activity, especially after drinking. The sexual behavior of adolescents is undergoing changes in many parts of the world, moving toward more and earlier sexual activity. In many industrialized countries and in many parts of Africa, the incidence of sexually transmitted diseases among adolescents is twice as high as it is among those in their late 20s.[25] Information about teen pregnancies in developing countries is limited, although it is known that in some countries 50 percent of the first births occur to mothers under the age of 20 years. Early teenage pregnancies pose serious health risks for the mother and the child. For female adolescents, early childbearing also has serious consequences for future options, limiting educational, employment, and social opportunities. In some cultures where pregnancy in young adolescents is outside of the social norm, the young girls may be ostracized and resort to prostitution, or die from attempts at abortion.

The experience of industrialized nations suggest that rapid social changes, the breakdown of family supports and prolongation of adolescence are associated with an increase in these behavior-related problems. Adolescents need to be motivated to participate in prevention programs, most of which are essentially educational in nature.

Mechanisms for Promoting Maternal and Child Health

The 1978 declaration of Alma-Ata, supported by 134 governments and representatives of 67 organizations of the United Nations or in official relations with the World Health Organization (WHO) and the United Nations Children's Fund (UNICEF) reaffirmed that the existing gross inequality in the health status of people between developed and developing countries is unacceptable and of common concern to all countries.[26] Primary health care was viewed as the key to attaining a level of health that permits a socially and economically productive life.

Primary health care is defined to include education about prevention and control of health problems, promotion of food supply and proper nutrition, adequate safe water, basic sanitation, maternal and child health care that includes family planning, immunization against the major infectious diseases, prevention and control of locally prevalent diseases and injuries, promotion of mental health and provision of essential drugs. Primary health care is one of the basic underlying principles behind the global strategy for health for all by the year 2000.[27]

Female Literacy

The success of primary care for mothers and children depends on an effective linkage of health, family planning, nutrition, and education. Health interventions are ineffective if the people are not educated for health. Mothers are uniquely motivated for education for health. Further, health interventions can serve as an entering wedge for the general education of girls and women, including basic literacy. Health is affected by what happens in other sectors, and cannot be promoted adequately by specific health activities alone. The most effective and efficient approach is to promote health and prevent disease by involving individuals, families, and communities and viewing them as resources in themselves and not only as recipients of health care.

The link of health to education is illustrated in the United States by the high rate of low birth weight babies born to women with less than a high school education. In developing countries, infant mortality is clearly related to maternal education. Over 24 separate studies in 15 nations have established that the level of the mother's education—even within the same economic class—is a key determinant of her children's health. In Pakistan and Indonesia, the infant mortality rate among children whose mother had four years of schooling was 50 percent lower than among children of women who were illiterate. In Bolivia, the infant mortality rate was 209 per 1000 live births for infants of mothers with one to three years of school, but 110 for those with ten years. And in Kenya, it is estimated that female education has accounted for 86 percent of the decline in infant mortality in the past 20 years.[28] In 1985, infant mortality rates were consistently high in countries with low literacy rates. For example, Afghanistan, with a female literacy rate of 8 percent, had an infant mortality rate of 189; Nigeria had an infant mortality rate of 110 and a female literacy rate of 31 percent.[3]

Literacy of women is not a simple determinant of infant mortality. Female literacy is a surrogate for many social and economic variables that influence nurturing of the infant and child as well as ability to understand instructions and make health-promoting decisions. According to UNICEF's 1984 report, *The State of the World's Children,* it is

> usually the mother's level of education and access to information which will decide whether or not she will go for a tetanus shot; whether a trained person will be present at birth; whether she knows about the advantage of breastfeeding; whether her child will be weaned at the right time; whether the best available foods will be cooked in the best possible way; whether water will be boiled and hands washed; whether bouts of diarrhea will be treated by administering food and fluids; whether a child will be weighed and vaccinated; and whether there will be adequate interval between births.[29]

The leverage of education of the mother on the well-being of the child is powerful even in very poor environments and empowering women by education—even as little as four years of education—can have a remarkable impact. It is encouraging that since 1960 the proportion of 6- to 11-year-old girls who are enrolled in school in the poorest half of the world has jumped from 34 percent to 80 percent. This is a breakthrough that must be sustained. Mothers who are literate tend to have more opportunity to learn about new ideas and more confidence to put them into practice.

Family Planning

Family planning is in fact a primary care measure of great value in preventing disease and improving public health, but there are pressures to keep the size of poor families large. When wages are low, income lost by the mother during a child's infancy may often be recovered by the child later on. Parents in poor communities may have fewer children if they perceive that this will open up educational and hence occupational opportunities. But if schooling opportunities for children are lacking altogether, this incentive disappears. Poor parents worry about who will take care of them in their old age or when they are ill, and for many the need for support in old age outweighs the immediate costs of children. Since many children die young—for example, in some parts of Africa one out of five children die before reaching the age of one and again as many die before their fifth birthday—the incentive to have many babies to ensure that a few survive is very great. Limited information about, and access to, cheap, safe, and effective means of contraception also contributes to high fertility among the poor.

However, parents and children often do not gain where there are many children. Inadequate access to land, or the poor health of both mothers and children (often as a result of closely spaced births), can confound the parents' expectations. In a sense, the persistence of high fertility in developing countries is a symptom of lack of access to services that the industrial world more or less takes for granted. This is particularly true of health services, which reduce the need for many births to ensure against infant and child mortality; and of education, which raises parents' hopes for their children, and broadens a woman's outlook and life options.

Thus, rapid population growth in poor countries contributes to a large burden of illness for mothers and children; and a large burden of illness and death among infants and children is a stimulus for a woman to have too many children over too long a period of time and too closely spaced, thereby jeopardizing her health and that of her children, and leaving little time for other life pursuits.

Interventions to prevent this high burden of illness and death include promotion of family planning services with dispensing of contraceptives that are safe, easy to deliver and explain, inexpensive, and acceptable. Family planning services are widely in demand in developing countries. Family planning efforts to prevent untimely pregnancies, pregnancy before age 18 and after 35, after four births, or less than two years apart are necessary to save lives and improve health in less developed countries. Family planning is one approach; other important approaches center on improving the status of women—educational, social, and economic—and increasing the healthy survival of children and adolescents.

COMMUNITY-BASED EFFORTS

Community-based efforts to change behavior for health are rapidly eliciting worldwide interest, and more attention is being paid to building a scientific basis to enhance their effectiveness. How is it possible to change behavior for health without coercion? This involves analyzing cultural values, and determining the specific knowledge deficits in a community with respect to health. It involves social learning, including the skills necessary to maintain health-promoting behavior. It involves learning how to use constructive motivations, for example, those of pregnant women to provide the best protection and care for their babies. It involves finding the channels through which members of a particular population may understand and take seriously information pertinent to their own health. These community-based initiatives to promote lifestyle changes are difficult to achieve, and research is necessary to clarify the conditions under which the changes actually occur—for example, in preventing heavy smoking or heavy alcohol use, and in improving nutritional, family planning, and sanitation practices.

Several key elements have been identified in research into major behavioral changes affecting health:

- Getting the facts straight: accurate biomedical and behavioral information about risk factors in a community.
- Clarifying the psychosocial obstacles to health-promoting behavior change in order to cope with them.
- Using modern behavioral and social sciences, including communications research, to learn how to study a given population in such a way that opportunities for promoting health may be fully understood by the population. A useful line of inquiry in developing countries would be to assess which principles and techniques of conveying health information in the developed world are applicable to their own conditions, and how they can be adapted to specific cultures.

If preventive action is taken in pregnancy and early childhood, its effectiveness and impact on health are great. Preventing illness and promoting health involve concrete measures that form part of a forward-looking orientation to life. Yet it is only in the past few decades that the necessary scientific and operational foundations have been laid that have allowed families throughout the world to plan for their own future or for that of their children with any degree of certainty. The concepts involved in taking action now for a better life tomorrow are becoming more widely understood. The remarkable progress achieved in recent decades in the prevention of childhood diseases has unfortunately benefited only a small proportion of the world's children. To establish a link between health and education sectors, it is necessary to foster connections between health and education ministries, and to increase the role of universities and other institutions of higher education in improving the health of their communities.

Global Strategies and Approaches for Scientific Cooperation

In the decades following World War II, there was a gradual, though irregular, decline of interest in the United States' scientific and technical community in developing-country problems and a concomitant decline of funding for cooperative research on such problems. Recently, however, the scientific community has realized that the issues of globalization and the interdependence of the human species offer opportunities to become involved in greater cooperative efforts aimed at promoting science and technology for health and development.[30] Maternal and child health is a logical focus for international scientific cooperation since it is the backbone of primary care and a cutting edge for improving health and quality of life in developing countries.

Two general strategies of promoting science and technology have emerged. One involves efforts to establish, support, or strengthen a central organization in a country or region that can develop an infrastructure to address needs which that country or region has identified as critical. The second is to build a mutual interest network of scientific and technological colleagues working in many countries, both industrialized and developing, to solve a problem or set of problems concerning developing nations.

The international center model focuses on an institution established within a single developing country. This institution may draw upon scientists from various nations who will work together on a specific research problem of major importance to that region. There are both virtues and drawbacks to the international center model. On one hand, a center run by an international board and funded by external sources can protect participating scientists from the political pressures of the host country. On the other hand, the reliance on outside support carries with it considerable vulnerability. Too often institutions have been built only to decay and crumble after the external support used to create them has been terminated.

An interesting model of a second approach to the problem is offered by a program for protection of the world's children sponsored by the World Health Organization, UNICEF, the World Bank, the United Nations Development Programme (UNDP), and the Rockefeller Foundation. The mission of the program is to accelerate immunizations as an entering wedge for primary care and to address the constraints, especially managerial, in the way of full immunization of children. The Task Force for Child Survival is developing country-based plans for accelerated immunization program proposals using primary health care. The plans will be presented to bilateral and multilateral donor agencies for funding. They will also review present research needs in biotechnology, management, and operations, and identify resources for the research. Initially, three countries—Colombia, India, and Senegal—were included. The program now involves approximately 25 additional countries and is still developing and expanding. A newsletter, published every two months in English, Spanish, and French reaches 10,000 people throughout the world with information on progress and issues about immunization of children (personal communication from William Watson, the Task Force on Child Survival, to Elena Nightingale, on December 17, 1986).

There are also programs aimed at classes of diseases with a high burden of illness for children and mothers. An outstanding example is UNDP–World Bank–WHO special program for research and training in tropical diseases. This program was built on careful planning and brought the best minds to bear on the problem, selected the best research opportunities, and enlisted the support of world leaders in their work. Similarly, the World Health Organization's Advisory Committee on Medical Research laid the foundation for an expanded program of research in the biobehavioral sciences and health. The strengthening of knowledge in this area is viewed as a fundamental underpinning for maternal and child health—physical and mental.[31]

Similar programs, if carefully designed and evaluated, could serve as models to stimulate interest in education for healthy child development in other settings. Likewise, their principles and techniques have value for their potential application to other problems. Building a network of scientists working in developing and industrialized countries toward a common end has many positive outcomes, such as strengthening the research capability of the developing countries by engaging scientists in those nations directly in significant research projects, and linking scientists and their institutions in developing countries with counterparts in the industrialized nations. Three elements are crucial to the success of this approach to international cooperative efforts:

- Identification and recruitment of outstanding individual researchers to work on a targeted problem.
- The necessary infrastructure.
- The general environment—social, economic, and political—that will permit research activities to begin and be sustained over time.

Another facet of the network model is the role of universities in strategies for improving world health.[32] Through research, universities can diminish heavy burdens of illness by extending the spectrum of the health sciences to its full length—from the community to the patient's bedside to the laboratory bench. Thus, the health sciences extend beyond the biomedical to include those epidemiological, biostatistical, social, and behavioral sciences needed to get accurate data on crucial interventions affecting health, in this context the health of women and children.

Universities can bring together novel conjunctions of talent to clarify complex issues in human resource development and provide continuously improving answers to health-related problems. They can involve the scientific and scholarly community more deeply in these issues than it is now engaged. They can foster the dissemination of intelligible, credible syntheses of state-of-the-art information on maternal and child health questions.

The scientific and technical community of more developed countries represents a strong potential asset for developing countries—if ways can be found to educate that community more deeply about the problems and opportunities that exist in the developing world, and if present mechanisms can be strengthened or new ones devised for ensuring effective technical cooperation over the long term. Universities can play a useful role in bringing decision makers together across disciplines, sectors, and national boundaries to focus on these problems and to follow with ways to study, test, and disseminate ideas. Universities can also explore ways to encourage the scientific and technical community to exercise more leadership in moving technically advanced nations toward solutions of human development problems.

Some developing and newly industrializing countries have made much progress in education, health, family planning, and nutrition. Other countries have accomplished much less. It is extremely important to sort out these experiences and to learn about the underlying factors and general principles that contributed to their success or lack of it. Universities can seek effective ways to get the nature and sources of such progress better understood, to identify particular models that have potential application elsewhere and on a larger scale, and to develop clearer understanding of how such lessons might be absorbed and applied by other countries.

In recent decades, most technically advanced nations have given little attention in research, education, and practice to some of the most important disease problems in the world today—those concentrated heavily in developing countries. In light of major recent advances in the life sciences, there are remarkable opportunities for such research—including capacity building in developing countries so that they can tackle their own problems. Priority areas include: (1) epidemiological assessment of specific needs; (2) studies of efficacy, organization, and cost of health services; (3) applying molecular biology to parasitic diseases, with a view toward prevention; (4) devising a wider array of birth spacing methods with special reference to cultural acceptability and feasibility of use; and (5) clarifying relations of health and behavior, with special reference to breast-feeding, nutrition, child care, sanitation, water use, and family planning. What is fundamentally needed is a heightened awareness within the scientific community of the opportunities that exist, since even a modest shift of attention to such problems could yield major benefits.

The scientific community could have a greater influence than it currently does on political decisions bearing directly on health throughout the world. It is the closest entity the world has to a genuinely international community, one with shared standards, values, curiosities, and interests. Cooperative efforts to meet the health needs of mothers and children on a global basis will require creative, multidisciplinary approaches that draw on the life sciences broadly defined—behavioral, social, biological, and biomedical. Ideally, the scientific community can provide not only a deeper understanding of the problems of humanity everywhere—and the tools to address those problems—but also a model for human relations across national boundaries and historic barriers.

References

1. Richman HA, Stagner MW: Children: Treasured resource or forgotten minority? in Pifer A, Bronte L (eds): *Our Aging Society: Paradox and Promise.* New York, WW Norton & Co, 1986, p 161.

2. National Center for Health Statistics: *Health, United States*. 1985, DHHS Publication No. (PHS) 86–1232, Washington, D.C., U.S. Government Printing Office, 1985.
3. *UNICEF: The State of the World's Children 1987*. New York, Oxford University Press, 1986.
4. World Health Organization: *New Trends and Approaches in the Delivery of Maternal and Child Health Care in Health Service*. Geneva, WHO, 1976.
5. Liskin L: *Youth in the 1980s: Social and Health Concerns*. Population Reports, Series M, No. 9, November–December 1985.
6. Hamburg DA: *Reducing the Casualties of Early Life: A Preventive Orientation*. New York, Carnegie Corporation of New York, 1985.
7. Chandler WU: *Investing in Children*. Worldwatch Paper 64. Washington, D.C., Worldwatch Institute, 1985.
8. *UNICEF: The State of the World's Children 1986*. New York, Oxford University Press, 1985.
9. Sivard RL: *Women . . . A World Survey*. Washington, D.C., World Priorities, Inc., 1985.
10. Division of Family Health: *Health and the Status of Women*. Geneva, World Health Organization, 1980.
11. Acute respiratory infections in third world children. *Lancet* 1986, 2:1049.
12. *The Task Force for Child Survival: Protecting the World's Children*, "Bellagio II" at Cartagena, Colombia, October 1985. Decatur, Georgia, The Task Force for Child Survival, 1986.
13. Rohde JE: Acute diarrhea, in Walsh JA, Warren KS (eds): *Strategies for Primary Health Care: Technologies Appropriate for the Control of Disease in the Developing World*. Chicago, University of Chicago Press, 1986, p 14.
14. Berman S, McIntosh K: Acute respiratory infections, in Walsh JA, Warren KS (eds): *Strategies for Primary Health Care: Technologies Appropriate for the Control of Disease in the Developing World*. Chicago, University of Chicago Press, 1986, p 29.
15. Institute of Medicine: *New Vaccine Development: Establishing Priorities*, Vol. II—*Diseases of Importance in Developing Countries*. Washington, D.C., National Academy Press, 1986.
16. Institute of Medicine: *Preventing Low Birth Weight*. Washington, D.C., National Academy Press, 1985.
17. Rosenfield A, Maine D: Maternal mortality—A neglected tragedy. *Lancet* 1985; 2:83–85.
18. Sai FT: *The Population Factor in Africa's Development Dilemma*. Paper presented at the annual meeting of the American Academy for the Advancement of Science in New York, 28 May 1984.
19. Protecting the World's Children: *Vaccines and Immunization within Primary Health Care*, A Bellagio Conference, March 13–14, 1984. New York, The Rockefeller Foundation, 1984.
20. Joseph SC: Toward universal child immunization: Lessons learned and questions raised since the Bellagio Conference of 1984, in: *The Task Force for Child Survival: Protecting the World's Children*. "Bellagio II" at Cartagena, Colombia, October, 1985. Decatur, Georgia, The Task Force for Child Survival, 1986, p 45.
21. Nichols EK: *Mobilizing against AIDS: Revised and Enlarged Edition.*. Cambridge, MA, Harvard University Press, 1989.
22. AIDS: Be Informed. *World Health*, November 1985, p 6.
23. Nath UR: Smoking in the Third World. *World Health*, June 1986, p 6.
24. Player DA: The big killer. *World Health*, June 1986, p 4.
25. World Health Organization: *Towards a Better Future: Maternal and Child Health*. Geneva, WHO, 1980.

26. World Health Organization: *Primary Health Care,* Report of the International Health Conference on Primary Health Care, Alma-Ata, USSR. Geneva, WHO, 1978.
27. World Health Organization: *Global Strategy for Health for All by the Year 2000.* Geneva, WHO, 1981.
28. *UNICEF: The State of the World's Children 1985.* New York, Oxford University Press, 1984.
29. *UNICEF: The State of the World's Children 1984.* New York, Oxford University Press, 1983, p 57.
30. Salvatore G, Schachman HK (eds): Proceedings of the international symposium on the role and significance of international cooperation in the biomedical sciences. *Perspectives in Biol and Med* 1986; 29 (part 2):1–229.
31. Hamburg D, Sartorius, N (eds): *Health and Behavior: Selected Perspectives.* Cambridge, Cambridge University Press, 1989.
32. World Health Organization: *The Role of Universities in the Strategies for Health for All.* Geneva, WHO, 1984.

8

Mental Health Programs
An International Perspective

THOMAS A. LAMBO AND NORMAN SARTORIUS

BACKGROUND

The past 20 years have seen a significant increase in priority assigned to mental health programs in many countries. This is particularly true for developing countries and could be due to four partly independent factors:

- First, to the awareness that mental disorders, as well as problems related to substance abuse, are increasing in numbers and are of a frightening magnitude in developed and developing countries, east and west, north and south;*
- Second, to the demonstration that prevention and treatment of mental disorders are possible and can be done using effective low-cost technology;
- Third, to the recognition that the hopes that were placed in technological solutions to problems caused by diseases in general did not come true and that it will be necessary to rely on behavioral and mental health approaches in preventing many such diseases and coping with their consequences; and that there are no obvious solutions to the almost universal growth of psychosocial problems, such as juvenile delinquency, problems of adaptation in migrants to towns, disintegration of families; and

*In many developed countries this awareness was heightened by the closure of mental hospitals and consequent increase of chronic mentally ill people in the community.

THOMAS A. LAMBO • Deputy Director General (Retired), World Health Organization, Geneva, Switzerland. NORMAN SARTORIUS • Director, Division of Mental Health, World Health Organization, Geneva, Switzerland.

- Fourth, to the emergence of a new mental health doctrine which stresses the need for a wide scope of mental health programs, the links of mental health efforts with primary health care, and the need and possibilities for an active involvement of different social sectors.

This chapter will first examine these developments, then present a possible set of recommendations for the future, and end with a brief description of WHO's program.

The Pandemic of Mental and Neurological Disorders and the Menace of Substance Abuse

Mental and neurological disorders are widespread in all populations and cultures and continue to be a source of distress, impaired productivity, and diminished quality of life for significant numbers of people and families.

In most populations the lifetime incidence of mental disorders can be estimated at no less than 15%; and at any point in time a significant proportion of the population suffers from disability due to mental illness or impairment. In developed countries, the main causes of such disability today are chronic psychoses such as schizophrenia, dementia, and other organic brain syndromes of mid- and late life, epilepsy, consequences of cerebrovascular disorders, neurosis, and psychosomatic disorders; there is a clear tendency of increase in the prevalence of senile dementia and other diseases occurring in middle and late age in many countries, and in Europe and North America there is an increase in the incidence of depressive illnesses in younger age groups. In developing countries, the principal causes of chronic mental and social impairment are similar to those found in developed countries, but in addition, there is an excess of psychological reactions associated with different types of severe environmental stress, and of organic brain syndromes due to a variety of causes including trauma and infectious and parasitic diseases.

Recent studies carried out in different countries showed that neurological disorders such as epilepsy, stroke and its sequelae, parkinsonism, and peripheral neuropathies, previously believed to be of little relevance to developing countries, are important contributors to disability and excess mortality all over the world. While the incidence of stroke shows a tendency to stabilize or even decline in some developed countries, there is an alarming increase of this disorder in parts of the developing world, notably Africa. High rates of exposure to toxic substances are significant causes of brain damage, while parasitic and tropical diseases are among causes of high rates of epilepsy in certain areas of the Third World. Insufficiently developed general health care and, in particular, poor postnatal care lead to damage to the central nervous system before, during, or after birth and to motor and learning disability. Nutritional deficiency such as iodine deficiency is among the other significant causes of mental retardation and disorder in spite of the fact that many of these deficiencies are amenable to correction even in countries where health systems operate under severe financial constraints.

There is a growing recognition throughout the world that alcohol and drug abuse are creating major social and health problems. These can be seen as the consequence of complex interactions involving a wide range of factors including the pharmacological and toxicological properties of the substance or combinations of substances used, the poor accessibility of appropriate health care, the nutritional habits and status of those dependent on alcohol or drugs, and their level of social integration.

The analysis of trends in the frequency and severity of health problems related to drug abuse reveals their continuing increase in most countries, particularly in the developing world. Although different drugs are predominant in particular cultures, there is a general trend towards wider diffusion of drug use across national boundaries. There is an increasing tendency to multiple drug use and to drug use in conjunction with consumption of alcohol. At the same time, expressions of concern over alcohol abuse are no longer confined to countries that have traditionally recognized its presence; reports have been received from countries all over the world, including those with long traditions of abstinence from alcohol, indicating sharp increases in health damage, family problems, crimes, and accidents in which alcohol has played a part.

The social and individual problems related to substance abuse show significant similarities in many countries. Besides their direct effects on health and life expectancy, alcohol and drug abuse are also associated with suicide, accidents, absenteeism, negative impact on family life and offspring, prostitution, and delinquency. Changes that occur in individuals as a result of alcohol or drug abuse are linked to increasing neglect of their professional and personal affairs, of social responsibilities and to health-damaging life-styles. Although the social implications of this process are less well quantified and documented than the health consequences, they present an even more serious problem to communities and societies at large. Where psychoactive substance abuse is a frequent phenomenon in a given population, substance abuse problems are compounded and have an even more serious impact on the overall development and on the economy of the community.

An issue that has grown in importance over the past few years is the route of administration of drugs. Injecting drugs intravenously multiplies health risks, because needles and syringes are often contaminated and adulterated substances are added to heroin, amphetamines, or cocaine. The spread of AIDS through the use of contaminated needles is an especially vivid example of this phenomenon. Increases in mortality are also seen in a number of countries in which cocaine is now inhaled or smoked rather than sniffed, since the rapid action and the difficulty of controlling the dosage impose additional risks.

The changing patterns of alcohol consumption around the world are another cause for concern. Although some countries in Western Europe and North America are now reporting a leveling off and even a moderate decline in alcohol consumption, the global trend is still that of continuing growth, with particularly sharp rises in commercial production of alcoholic beverages in some developing countries in Africa, Latin America, and the Western Pacific. The rapid growth of alcohol consumption in developing countries is likely to be followed by increases in related problems which will put a severe strain on scarce economic and social resources.

Prevention and Treatment Possibilities

The last decade witnessed significant advances in basic neurosciences, clinical research, and epidemiology, or ingenious combinations of these different approaches. Examples are the identification of a deoxyribonucleic acid (DNA) marker for Huntington's disease as a result of epidemiological, clinical, and laboratory studies; the discovery of endogenous ligands for receptors in the brain which bind psychoactive substances; the development of immensely powerful investigative techniques (e.g., neuroimagery); new leads to the origin of transmissible dementias; the development of refined, specific diagnostic criteria for the major mental disorders and of instruments for their identification in community surveys and clinical settings; major developments in artificial intelligence; and increased knowledge about the structure and functions of protective social networks. WHO-coordinated research has contributed new data on the age- and sex-specific incidence of schizo-

TABLE 1. Measures That Could Prevent a Significant Proportion of Mental Retardation

Prenatal and perinatal care
Immunization
Family planning
Epilepsy control
Nutrition
Day care
Accident prevention
Provision of family support
Teaching of parenting skills
Improvement of conditions in institutions providing long-term care or shelter (e.g., orphanages)
Recognition and correction of sensory and motor handicaps

phrenia in different cultures, on the effects of psychotropic drugs in various populations, and on the prediction of impairments of social functioning in severe psychiatric illness. Reliable estimates of the prevalence of neurological disorders in a variety of countries are now available.

The technology for the treatment of many mental and neurological disorders has also developed over the past few decades. Most significant progress in recent years has been achieved in the adaptation of the available techniques for use in general care and although the number of mental health personnel in developing countries remains insufficient, it is now evident that services to the mentally and neurologically ill can be provided through general health and other social service workers. This is already happening in many countries; in others, there is still a need to change attitudes of specialists and general health workers, the general population, and governments to ensure the wide application and use of the well-proven training approaches now in existence.

Prevention of a significant number of mental and neurological disorders is also possible: a recent paper submitted to the World Health Assembly presented preventive measures of demonstrated effectiveness and of a price affordable even by poor countries. So, for example, the measures proposed to prevent mental retardation included those in Table 1.

Similar lists of measures were proposed for other mental, neurological, and psychosocial disorders, and it was estimated that a wide and systematic application of the measures proposed would lead to the prevention of at least half of all such disorders in the world.[95]

Psychosocial Perspectives of Health and Development

Recent research showed that, all over the world, a significant proportion of the people who present themselves to health workers do so because they have psychological and social problems. Even when they present with a physical complaint or disease, there may be psychological or social factors that have caused or precipitated the physical problem, or that may affect its course and outcome. Survey of health workers' education in many countries showed that health workers are being introduced only to techniques and language for dealing with physical problems. Psychological and social problems are dismissed as "not real" or as being outside the competence of the health worker. The necessity to organize health care in a way that enables health workers to deal with psychosocial problems and see their patients as people functioning in a specific way within their community rarely receives sufficient emphasis even when an awareness of needs in the psychosocial area exists.

On a larger scale, the role of psychosocial factors is also neglected. Rapid social change resulting from economic development, industrialization, and urbanization is reported from countries all over the world and has profound effects on the structure of communities, the functioning of families, and on the psychological well-being of individuals. Social disorganization often linked to social change exacerbates problems such as juvenile delinquency, violence, and accidents at work and in traffic.

Social stresses exert their most serious pathogenic effects on mental health in the absence of the protective and buffering mechanisms that have evolved in human groups in all societies.[88] The deprivations and stresses of an unpredictable and generally hostile environment can be less pathogenic if a supportive social network (family, friends, neighbors) is available. Social networks and other features of community life, which have until recently played an important protective role in many countries, are disappearing. Recent trends of community disintegration and breakdown leave the population more vulnerable and make it a prey to health damage due to a variety of psychosocial factors.

Technological solutions for disease problems that were to result from advances of science failed to materialize. This is true for both communicable and noncommunicable diseases. Insecticides can reduce the population of vectors but pollute the environment; even such evidently useful measures as immunization against frequent infectious diseases do not get applied because of psychological resistances and bureaucratic and financial constraints; diseases make their appearance and spread in spite of the fact that health services have technologically correct measures available to them. As a result of the perception of failure of technological solutions, increased reliance on techniques that will result in changes in human behavior (which in turn could lead to lesser disease incidence, better outcomes, and less expensive solutions) has become (rationally) accepted in many settings. In some countries this has led to a significant increase in research on behavioral aspects of health and a wide-ranging change in the population's behavior without any support or leadership by the medical profession. In other settings the awareness of the importance of psychosocial factors and of the benefits of appropriate application of knowledge from the behavioral sciences has not yet been translated into higher priority for funding and support.

Changes in Scope of Mental Health Programs

The awareness of the developments sketched out above among governments, top level health administrators, and decision makers in developed and developing countries has led, in many settings, to the recognition that classical "mental health" programs—which in reality deal only with psychiatric and neurological disorders—cannot be accepted to respond to these challenges in an effective way. Numerous countries have therefore formulated mental health programs of much broader scope, using public health approaches in defining problems and in seeking ways to their solution. The value of mental health for individual, community, and national well-being has been recognized and specific promotive activities as well as program components focusing on psychosocial aspects of health and health care have been added to the program. New ways of handling alcohol and drug abuse and their health consequences have been proposed and often used with success. Care for mental and neurological diseases changed emphasis from predominant attention to specialist care to the incorporation of mental health program components in primary health care, and the development of community support systems that permit patients—even if they suffer chronic impairment—to live a socially and economically productive life. Medical disciplines other than psychiatry and social sectors other than health are increasingly often involved in mental health programs.

A variety of managerial issues still remain unresolved. Coordination between different social sectors often presents formidable problems. Linkage with those involved in developing primary health care and their understanding of the essential public health nature of mental health programs remains insufficient. The multidisciplinary and multisectoral nature of programs also means that there are few professionals with the knowledge, skills, and attitudes necessary to lead and manage such programs.

The evaluation and monitoring of programs are still hampered by the lack of agreement about indicators suitable for these purposes and by the weakness of mental health information support services and systems, which could generate the necessary data.

The position of mental health and psychosocial development is still low on the scale of values of most individuals, communities, and nations, and the motivation essential for a vigorous individual action and national program development is often missing.

The Next 20 Years

The size and severity of mental health problems now present in the world will not diminish in the next two decades. Even if it were possible to introduce all the preventive measures described above in all countries—and thus halve the incidence of mental and neurological disorders—the challenge confronting mental health programs and societies at large would hardly diminish. It is likely to consist of three components.

First, the burden of care for the impaired and chronically ill will increase because of growing life expectancy of those disabled; because of the increase of population in age groups at higher risk for mental disorders; and because of decreases in family size and capacity to support its disabled members.

Second, psychosocial problems will increase because of the growing dissonance between human capacity for adaptation and the rate of changes linked to technological progress, depletion of natural resources, and related processes.

Third, the low value that individuals, communities, and nations give to mental life and development will, unless resolute measures are taken now, continue to decrease motivation for activities that could lead to adequate program development.

To meet these challenges, mental health programs must change.

First, they have to become multisectoral, not only in name but in reality. Coordinating mechanisms bringing together social welfare, health education, judiciary, and other allied sectors are already coming into existence at national level in a number of countries; they should be established also at provincial and district level. The redefinition of the scope for mental health programs and multisectoral action in their implementation is inevitable for economic as well as ideological reasons. If psychiatrists refuse to accept a leadership role in bringing about this change, their position will become even less enviable tomorrow than it is today in many countries.

Second, mental health programs will have to give up making detailed long-term plans and utilize "rolling horizon planning" in which decisions on what should be done are made only for the immediate future, keeping in mind a few well-defined major and long-term policy goals. These goals are likely to include the increase of value attached to mental health and functioning; an intensive input into general health care and development programs; an advocacy of rehumanization of both medicine and economic growth; a better and continuing translation of knowledge into a form that can be offered for broad application to different social sectors; and an effort to bring together and involve the different disciplines relevant to mental health programs.

Third, the mental health programs, while uniform in policy, will have to be decentralized in responsibility and authority for action. This will require attitude change, as well as procedural backing, on an unprecedented scale.

Fourth, mental health programs will have to utilize radically new arrangements concerning funding of activities. Not only is the distribution of funds the single most powerful determinant of health system orientation: it also has delayed and remote effects on psychiatric training, on the image of psychiatry, and on other disciplines involved in the program.

Fifth, the field of action of mental health programs has to be split into recognizable, well-defined tasks. The replacement of the description of roles of members of professions by the definition of mental health tasks, regardless of who will do them, has already had revolutionary effects on service organizations in the best programs of Third World countries. It is clearly a managerial strategy of central importance in a field so depleted of personnel resources as are the mental health programs in most countries.

Sixth, changes in the methods and contents of training for health and other social services workers are needed now. There are new themes that have emerged and that make this revision urgent. They include the need to harmonize training of various social agents—doctors, teachers, lawyers, administrators, and others—in matters concerning mental health; the need to ensure that the training of health personnel in general fosters positive attitudes to mental illness; the need to ensure that the humane requirements of health care remain foremost in the minds of future graduates; and the need to contribute, through training, to efforts to maintain (or place) human well-being in the center of overall development efforts.

Seventh, the research components of future mental health programs must respond to a number of needs that are emerging; there is a need for a new paradigm of research in mental health; a need for more knowledge about normal functioning; a need to test multicausal etiological hypotheses that may require considerable inventiveness and new skills. The new century's programs in mental health will have to create better opportunities for longitudinal, long-term research; foster and facilitate multicentric studies, both within and across countries; and make arrangements for sharing of the incredibly expensive equipment currently lying idle for much of the time and becoming obsolete at a frightening pace.

Eighth, the search for the best way to provide services for the mentally ill must continue. Today, there is no universally applicable model that could be recommended to all countries, or even to all provinces within a country: it is unlikely that it will ever be possible to construct such a model. There are, however, two elements common to many models, and likely to extend into the next century. The first is that people can and should participate in maintaining their health, in surviving their disease, and in living with their own and other people's impairments. The second is that in the absence of a model valid for all settings, the primary goal in improving services should be to reach consensus on principles that may be helpful in developing the structure of services. Among these is the need for equal emphasis on quality of care and on its efficiency, the need for diversity in congruence with cultural and socioeconomic norms; responsiveness to new opportunities; and precedence of humanism and common sense over rigid plans and over-adherence to theory in service development.

Reflections on the Mental Health Program of the World Health Organization

Global reviews cannot do justice to the wealth of innovations and experience that have become available in mental health programs of many countries. Many of the trends visible when viewing the broad canvas of development of mental health programs in different countries will therefore be neither observable nor obviously relevant to a specific country or province.

Nevertheless, a global analysis can often help in thinking of how best to proceed in making a program as useful and as harmonious with other programs and with national development in general. With this in mind, the last part of this chapter will therefore present a selective review of results of the research and technology development activity of the mental health program of WHO.[75]

The mental health program of WHO has been formulated through a process of consultation within WHO, with other United Nations bodies, with governments, with the scientific community, and with various nongovernmental organizations.[49,56,90]

The program's objectives are broad and cover three main areas: prevention and control of mental, neurological, and psychosocial disorders, such as those related to the abuse of alcohol and drugs; mental health aspects of general health care; and psychosocial aspects of overall health and development. These three areas of concern were identified in the review of the situation in the countries and are often reflected in national programs. They also open possibilities for collaboration with a variety of other programs within WHO and with various agencies within the United Nations' system.

For its implementation the program relies on a network of collaborating centers in more than 60 countries, expert advisory panels, nongovernmental organizations, and governments of WHO member states. The main types of activity are collaboration with countries in mental health policy and program formulation; transfer of information involving the collection, assessment, and distribution of experience and data relevant to mental health programs from a variety of sources; participation in training activities; publication of material necessary for national programs; development of consensus statements of key issues; and an extensive effort to stimulate and coordinate research activities.

The themes for WHO research are selected from proposals consonant with the medium-term program of the organization. The criteria for selection of topics include the social relevance of the subject of research (e.g., research on prevalent disorders leading to serious disability would have higher priority), the likelihood that such research could not be carried out without WHO's involvement, and that useful results will become available in the foreseeable future, the interest of institutions and individuals to collaborate with WHO on the topic, and ethical acceptability. Projects promoting cooperation with and between developing countries and bringing together scientists from different regions, political and economic spheres, and language areas are given higher priority than those involving a single institution or country.

WHO is an international organization which carries out its functions in cooperation with member states. It has a unique position in the field of health care and represents a neutral platform that can be used to bring about international collaboration in research. Over the years the organization has gained experience in the management of international collaborative projects and obtained access to leading institutes and scientists in most countries of the world. In the following pages the results of WHO's efforts in coordinating and stimulating research will be briefly described to illustrate the potential that WHO has in the global effort to improve health.

Research activities included in the program fall in five groups: (1) those concerned with the development of a common language; (2) those concerned with specific clinical, biological, and social characteristics of widespread mental and neurological disorders and psychosocial problems; (3) those concerned with the development of methods of treatment and prevention; (4) those concerned with the provision of care; (5) and those dealing with psychosocial aspects of general health care.*

Development of a Common Language

An essential prerequisite for collaboration in the field of mental health is agreement on a language that can be understood and will be used by all concerned. Such an agreement must cover terms used in the description of mental and neurological functioning and pathology (including diagnosis); indicators of mental, neurological, and psychosocial problems (e.g., those related to alcohol and drug dependence) and of the success of measures undertaken for their solution; terms referring to environmental factors or situations relevant in mental health investigations; and methods of investigation, e.g., how biological samples are obtained, sent to other centers, and so on.

After some 10 years of work, WHO produced a classification of mental disorders, now included in the ninth revision of the *International Classification of Diseases*.[76] The methods used to achieve this included a series of case-history exercises, reviews of the literature and diagnostic practices in many countries, and intensive discussions between mental health experts and statisticians from some 30 countries on the most acceptable categorization of mental disorder.[4,5,25,29,45,48,58,59,60,69,70]

To ensure agreement on the content of categories included in the classification, a glossary with definitions of categories of mental disor-

*References for the work described in this chapter are given at the end of the chapter. A list of documents and publications of the Mental Health Programme is available on request.[76]

ders listed in the classification was developed in collaboration with experts in 61 countries.[73,78] In addition, work has been undertaken on standardization of terms in relation to epilepsy and cerebrovascular disorders, in collaboration with experts from different countries and centers collaborating in neuroscience projects.[70,77]

The work of the chapters dealing with mental and neurological disorders became even more intensive in the preparation for the tenth revision of the *International Classification of Diseases* (ICD). More than 170 centers in some 50 countries are involved in extensive tests of the applicability and usefulness of the new proposals, this time accompanied by detailed guidelines for classification.

A whole "family" of classificatory instruments is being developed simultaneously. These include guidelines for diagnosis and classification in research, lexical definitions of terms used in the *ICD*, a classification of impairments and disabilities, classifications for use at the primary health care level and various "crosswalks" facilitating the translation of terms between different classifications and their revisions.[56]

In a series of projects undertaken over the years and still continuing, instruments have been adapted or developed for a standardized description of mental states and other characteristics of a patient's condition. The most widely used of these instruments, the Present State Examination (PSE), is a description of the patient's present mental state.[67] This instrument, first developed in English by J. K. Wing and his colleagues, has been extensively tested in some 20 countries and now exists in more than 30 languages; the fact that its application closely resembles a clinical interview is an important feature because it allows the acquisition of reliable data about the mental state in a manner familiar and acceptable to both the research worker and the patient.

The instrument was initially used to assess functional psychoses; subsequent testing proved its applicability in less severe conditions and most recent work indicates that, with appropriate modifications, it can be used for the assessment of mental disorders of varied etiology and severity.

A shortened version of the PSE has been used with success as a screening instrument in nonpatient populations by Wing et al.,[68] Cooper et al.,[11] and by investigators in WHO coordinated studies on the extension of mental health care[22] in Colombia, India, Senegal, and Sudan, and on the psychosomatic sequelae of female sterilization in Colombia, India, Nigeria, the Philippines, and the UK.[89]

The PSE has more recently been incorporated into a system for the comprehensive assessment in neuropsychiatry (SCAN),[100] which is being tested in the framework of a major project carried out jointly by

WHO and the Institute for Alcohol and Drug Abuse, and Mental Health of the United States of America.[33] The same project is also engaged in testing two other instruments: the Combined International Diagnostic Instrument, which will be used mainly in epidemiological research,[44] and the International Personality Disorder Examination.[36]

The PSE was also used in a major international study on schizophrenia. In this investigation some 1200 patients were examined to establish whether similar cases of schizophrenia exist in different cultures and to develop instruments needed to obtain comparable clinical and social data that would allow transcultural mental health studies.[71,74,84] Several other instruments standardizing the assessment of relevant facts have been developed in the course of this and subsequent studies.[30,46] These include screening methods to identify patients with functional psychoses, instruments to assess the psychiatric history and social condition of the patient, and others. More recently, the centers involved in the schizophrenia study examined reasons for differences in outcome of schizophrenia between developing and developed countries and a set of new instruments was developed in this work: they deal with the assessment of impairment and disabilities; the perception of mental illness by families in different cultures; and the recording of life events, of follow-up information, and of other facts relevant to the investigation of the origin, course, and outcome of mental disorders.

Instruments for the assessment of specific conditions have also been developed. So, for example, an instrument for the assessment of depressive disorder resulted from a multinational study of depression.[54] This instrument was originally tested in five countries and is by now available in some 15 languages. It covers the clinical state, psychiatric history, and sociodemographic data and was found to be applicable and acceptable in the populations studied. Instruments for the assessment of alcohol- and drug-related problems have been developed in the framework of the projects on community response to alcohol-related problems and in the research and reporting program on drug dependence.

Instruments for the assessment of impairments, handicaps, and associated disabilities in psychiatric patients have been developed in a collaborative study involving eight countries in Europe and Sudan.[98] The present versions of the Psychological Impairments Rating Schedule (PIRS) and the Disability Assessment Schedule (DAS) are designed for use in conjunction with the PSE.

In addition to developing instruments for the assessment of mental states of individuals, the organization has also undertaken to develop methods for evaluating the mental health needs and resources of communities and countries. These include a first-stage screening procedure for the detection of psychiatric cases in primary health care settings (for both adults and children), an interview schedule for use with key informants, to assess their attitudes and obtain help in case identification, and a method for the assessment of the effects of psychiatric illness on his immediate family.[23,63] These instruments have been shown to be applicable and acceptable in a number of developing countries. Equivalent versions of the whole set of instruments exist in Arabic, English, French, Hindi, Tagalog, Portuguese, and Spanish.

A project coordinated by the European Regional Office brought together investigators from most European countries aiming to define methods for the description of needs and resources for mental health care in defined catchment areas. In each of these areas teams of research workers have carried out a census of patients and facilities providing care and proceeded to study pathways of patients in the services.[97] Routinely available data were used in this investigation, which has resulted in several publications. In another study, data available at national level are being examined to define a minimal set of information necessary to monitor mental health needs for purposes of planning and evaluation of national programs concerned with mental health.[85]

The response of communities to major psychosocial problems—such as those related to alcohol consumption—needs careful assessment prior to intervention programs. A study on community responses to alcohol-related problems has been carried out in Mexico, Scotland, and Zambia, and its report indicated ways of collecting data and problems likely to arise in assembling and interpreting such data.[24] Instruments for the assessment of drug-dependence problems have also been developed in collaborative projects.[21,27]

Instruments and protocols for the epidemiological assessment of neurological problems constitute another area in which there is a need to achieve agreement, and studies have been carried out in a variety of countries.[13,41,61]

Finally, there is another area of standardization which has been given attention—biological investigations in psychiatry. Centers collaborating in the WHO projects in biological psychiatry have agreed on several such methods and use them in investigations of biological factors possibly involved in the pathogenesis or treatment of mental disorders.[79,80] Standardization of this kind of work covers details of techniques for taking samples of blood, urine, cerebrospinal fluid (CSF), and other biological material and transporting them from laboratory to laboratory, often in different countries. Similar work has been initiated in the program concerned with the research on and control of neurological disorders.

Characteristics of Mental and Neurological Disorders and of Psychosocial Problems of Major Public Health Importance

WHO's first major research effort was concerned with schizophrenia; the International Pilot Study of Schizophrenia[72] was launched to establish whether it is feasible to carry out collaborative projects in psychiatry using a commonly agreed protocol with the active involvement of investigators from different countries. Centers in Denmark, Colombia, China, India, Nigeria, Czechoslovakia, the UK, U.S.A., and USSR participated in a study in which a series of patients consecutively admitted to psychiatric facilities were examined by means of standardized research instruments. The study proved that international collaboration in psychiatric research is feasible. It also produced instruments for standardized assessment of patients in different cultures and contributed to our knowledge about schizophrenia by demonstrating that: (1) similar schizophrenic syndromes exist in all of the cultural settings included in the study; but that (2) the course and outcome of schizophrenia show significant differences between countries—patients in developing countries having on the whole a more favorable course and outcome than their counterparts in the developed world.[84]

The centers participating in this program were then engaged in a series of studies aiming to explore some of the possible reasons for the differences in outcome. To exclude errors in sampling as an explanation of differences, an incidence study has been launched in geographically defined areas involving all agencies that are likely to be contacted by patients and their families.[53] Other studies to test hypotheses explaining differences in outcome include an investigation of emotional interaction in families in different cultures[35,64,65]; a project exploring the frequency and type of stressful life events in different settings;[15] and a study of social and individual factors likely to contribute to the development of impairments and disabilities in patients with schizophrenia.[31] In another study the frequency of specific physical disorders—such as cancer, cardiovascular disease, and congenital anomalies—in schizophrenic patients was examined using a record linkage technique.[16]

Immunological and other biological studies of schizophrenia have also been undertaken. A network of centers located in Basle, Gröningen, Munich, Washington, Moscow, Epsom, and Copenhagen has been established and collaborates in this work. The blood sera from schizophrenic patients and normal controls have been examined to establish whether there are differences in the antithymic activity (ATA) between the two groups. The study showed that, although there were many schizophrenic patients with high levels of serum ATA, the ATA values did not discriminate between patients with schizophrenia and normal persons. In view of high ATA values in relatives of schizophrenics, high ATA was considered by the investigators as an indication of high risk for schizophrenia.[28]

Acute Psychoses

Acute psychoses, often described as the most frequent reason for admission to hospitals in developing countries, are being investigated in Ibadan, Agra, Chandigarh, Cali, and Aarhus to obtain information that will lead to a better psychopathological delineation of the syndrome and facilitate sociological, clinical, and biological studies of this condition. Methods developed in the study of Determinants of Outcome of Severe Mental Disorders and other WHO projects have been used in this investigation, with appropriate additional parts developed on the basis of an analysis of case histories of patients with acute psychoses seen in the centers collaborating in the study.

Alcohol-Related Problems

The growing realization that alcohol dependence syndromes represent only a part of alcohol-related problems ranging from cirrhosis to traffic accidents, as well as recent developments pointing the way to effective intervention in the field, revived WHO's commitment to action in this area. First, a research project to explore the response of communities to alcohol-related problems was carried out in Mexico, Scotland, and Zambia; it developed instruments for the acquisition of data relevant to the assessment of the size and nature of problems and responses in geographically defined communities. In another part of this project, the cross-cultural applicability of prevention and treatment techniques has been explored.

Arising from this work, a number of more recent studies have examined the effectiveness of particular interventions in a variety of cultural settings. Of these, the most complex has been concerned with the identification and management of individuals who experience alcohol-related health problems but without necessarily being sincerely dependent upon alcohol. The first phase of this study involved centers in Australia, Bulgaria, Kenya, Mexico, Norway, and the U.S.A.; it has led to the development of a simple screening instrument.[57] In the second phase, these six centers have been joined by four more (Costa Rica, UK, USSR, and Zimbabwe) and testing is now taking place of a range of simple treatment interventions suitable for delivery in primary health care settings.

A parallel study examines the effectiveness of health promotion approaches to the prevention of alcohol-related problems. Centers in Botswana, Costa Rica, Fiji, and Sri Lanka are collaborating in the preparation of assessment guidelines based upon the results of the research undertaken at national level in these four countries. Linked to this study has been an evaluation of the relative effectiveness of peer-led and teacher-led approaches to alcohol education for young people in Chile, Norway, Swaziland, and Western Australia. The analysis of the results of this study[42] is particularly encouraging, in that peer-led education, well-suited to the needs of developing countries, appears to produce rather positive changes, not only in terms of increase in knowledge, but also in stimulating more health-oriented attitudes and behavior.

In collaboration with researchers from 15 countries, WHO is involved in the reanalysis of data from some 40 longitudinal studies on drinking behavior and alcohol-related problems.[18] The impetus for this work came from a 1984 task force meeting of the Advisory Committee on Medical Research's subcommittee on biobehavioral science and mental health. Utilizing a research methodology based upon techniques of meta-analysis, this project explores the interrelationships between alcohol use and abuse, chronological age, culture, and history.

Through a series of small pilot studies in a range of countries in the Americas, Africa, and the Western Pacific, WHO is examining the role of alcohol as a causative factor in admissions to emergency rooms for accidental injuries. This work is supported by a constant effort to improve the collection and dissemination of health and other (e.g., trade) statistics concerning alcohol-related problems.[66] This work will greatly benefit from earlier studies carried out jointly with the Finnish Alcohol Foundation[9] and a major review of approaches to the prevention of alcohol-related problems in some 70 countries.[39] The European WHO Regional Office also collaborated in an International Study of Alcohol Control experiences carried out jointly by centers in Europe, the UK, and Canada.[19] More recently the organization has also initiated biological investigations of alcohol problems. A first study examined characteristics of alcohol in different populations;[99] plans for a multicentric study of biological predictions of relapse after treatment have been developed, and it is expected that work in this area will start soon.

Depressive Disorders

A program of investigation of depressive disorders was started in 1972. This program contains studies with an epidemiological orientation, biological studies, and operational research.[47,50,51]

Among projects with an epidemiological orientation, the largest was a prospective 10-year follow-up study of depressive patients in four different countries.

Some 550 patients with depressive conditions were included in the study. All of them were assessed by means of a standardized method of assessment developed by the centers in Basle, Montreal, Nagasaki, Teheran, and Tokyo, in collaboration with WHO.[91] It was shown that psychiatrists in the different centers used the same diagnostic criteria to distinguish between endogenous and nonendogenous depressive conditions, and that the clinical characteristics of the patients within those groups did not differ among centers. Before it can be said that depression in different countries shows the same characteristics, it is clearly important to prove that its course and outcome do not show major differences from country to country. A 10-year follow-up study has therefore been carried out and its results will be published shortly.

Another set of studies explored the biological characteristics of depressive disorders. In a collaborative study genetic linkage of bipolar manic–depressive illness and red–green color blindness was examined. Sixteen pedigrees were identified and analyzed in four centers—Basle, Bethesda, Brussels, and Copenhagen—leading to the conclusion that bipolar illnesses are significantly heterogeneous. This study illustrated one of the advantages of collaborative studies that can help to speed up the accumulation of data relating to those rare cases in which an important issue can be examined (such as those in which bipolar illness and color blindness coincide).[20] In another biological study human lymphocyte antigens in patients with affective disorders were studied in four centers: the study failed to show any consistent results.[79,80] In the same direction of enquiry, possibilities for developing a biological classification of depression are being explored in a study on differences between endogenous and nonendogenous depressive patients in responses to the clonidine growth stimulation test.[79,80] Another study has dealt with the treatment of depressive conditions in patients living in different geographical locations (see below).

The trends in suicide prevalence have been examined periodically and these reviews are published at regular intervals.[8,89]

Drug Dependence

An important component of projects dealing with the implementation of drug demand reduction programs is evaluative research.*

*These projects are undertaken in cooperation with countries and often involve the United Nations Division on Narcotic Drugs and the United Nations Fund for Drug Abuse Control, as well as UN specialized agencies such as WHO, International Labour Office, United Nations Educational, Social and Cultural Organization, and Food and Agriculture Organization.

To be able to undertake it, a project was launched in 1972, aiming to develop instruments and techniques necessary to enable countries to report on changes in drug-dependence problems and learn about trends in other parts of the world. In carrying out this work, WHO has collaborated with centers in Burma, Indonesia, India, Malaysia, Pakistan, Thailand, Canada, Mexico, the U.S.A., and others. This work has so far resulted in an internationally tested instrument for surveys of drug use in student populations; in a reporting card that can be used in treatment facilities for drug-dependent people; in the definition of a "core" data set for surveys and case reporting; and in protocols for the evaluation of results of treatment in different settings.

Other studies examined the dependence liability of thebaine[81]; the pharmacological and clinical effects of khat[87]; the clinical and social consequences of long-term use of cannabis[62]; the coca leaf chewing/coca paste effects[2]; and the effectiveness of antidepressants in the pharmacological treatment of drug (opium) dependence. Instruments and methods necessary to assess public health and social problems associated with the use of psychotropic substances have been developed.[34] These methods will be used in studies undertaken to help WHO fulfill its responsibilities under the Convention on psychotropic substances which require WHO to make recommendations to the United Nations Economic and Social Council concerning international control of these medicaments.

The use of methadone in the treatment of opiate dependence has been subject to international review.[3] In addition, centers in a number of American and European countries are collaborating in an assessment of the relative importance of a variety of risk factors for the development of drug dependence. This work has been given renewed impetus by the emergence of the AIDS epidemic, which raises important questions for research on the nature of HIV infection through the use of contaminated needles and syringes. Equally, the epidemiology of intravenous drug use, which is of importance to WHO's programs on the prevention and control of drug abuse and of AIDS, is now being taken forward through a series of pilot studies in major cities where HIV infection rates are thought to be linked to rates of drug abuse.

Neurological Disorders

A program concerned with the control of neurological disorders was started in the early 1970s and involves leading neuroscience centers in Canada, France, Mexico, Nigeria, Senegal, Switzerland, the U.S.A., and USSR.[6,7] The centers were engaged in several WHO-coordinated research activities, including a study on peripheral neuropathy and a study on transient ischemic cerebrovascular attacks. Following a meeting of a study group on applications of neurosciences in the control of neurological disorders,[82] epidemiological surveys of neurological disorders in African and other developing countries have been carried out.[40]

Development and Improvement of Treatment Methods

A study of the effectiveness of antidepressant medication has been undertaken by a network of centers in Basle, Gröningen, Munich, Epsom, Moscow, Bethesda, and Copenhagen. In this study, plasma levels of amitriptyline have been measured and correlated with clinical responses assessed with standardized instruments.[12]

A new set of studies dealing with the effectiveness of medicaments has been undertaken. The largest of these were the WHO-coordinated studies of the effects of psychotropic drugs in different populations.[83,96]

Anecdotal accounts and occasional reports in the literature seem to indicate that populations living in settings differing in climatic, nutritional, and sociocultural conditions require significantly different dosages of common psychotropic drugs. The importance of this finding is obvious and WHO carried out double-blind collaborative studies on dose effectiveness of the frequently used antidepressants and neuroleptic medicaments in several countries. A set of instruments for the assessment of the clinical conditions and their changes was produced using some of the schedules mentioned above and some newly developed techniques. Antidepressants have been examined in centers in Basle, Bombay, Cali, Nagasaki, Lucknow, Sapporo, and Nashville. Three striking findings emerged: first, that antidepressant treatment is effective in a vast majority of cases; second, that there are few if any differences in treatment effects between the low and high dose of antidepressant drugs; and third, that most of the differences in dosage across countries can be explained by diagnostic and therapeutic habits of psychiatrists. The effectiveness of benzodiazepines was also examined in some of the centers participating in these investigations. It clearly demonstrated the value of counseling and the superiority of the combined use of counseling and medicament use over the use of medicaments alone. It also produced instruments that can be used in the assessment of effects of treatment of mild mental disorder in different cultures. Other studies in this area include the investigation of the therapeutic "window" of neuroleptics, the effects of naloxone on schizophrenic and manic syndromes,[43] and regular surveys of the use of psychotropic drugs in different populations.

Organization of Mental Health Services: Assessment and Development of New Models

A major focus of WHO's cooperation with countries is the improvement of provision of mental health care. To ensure that appropriate advice is provided to governments wishing to improve mental health care, several studies have been initiated.

The most important among these is a multinational study aimed at developing new strategies for the provision of essential mental health care in developing countries. Teams in Colombia, India, Sudan, and Senegal were the first to join in this study; Brazil, Egypt, and the Philippines have joined the study soon afterward. In each country an area was selected, and the extent and nature of mental health problems in the communities were assessed in a standardized and comparable manner. On the basis of this information "priority" conditions were selected using as criteria frequency, harmful consequences, community concern, and availability of effective, simple, and inexpensive treatment. Specific, short training courses were designed to instruct health workers already working in the area on how to detect these "priority" mental health disorders and how to deal with them effectively.[93] These studies demonstrated that decentralized, nonspecialist mental health care provided largely by auxiliary health care workers can function well and be acceptable to both health workers and the community.

In conjunction with this study the usefulness of algorithmic approaches was examined in a study dealing with methods of management of mental disorder in primary care. A set of flowcharts were produced[17] and evaluated in Lesotho in 1986.[37] The study showed that the use of flowcharts can enable nurses to deal competently with a number of mental disorders after only 13 hours of training.

Parallel to studies of the pilot study areas (see above) WHO and its European Regional Office have made a continuous effort to define roles of different types of health workers in the provision of mental health care.[86]

An investigation of the understanding and use of the concept of dangerousness by psychiatrists, jurists, and law enforcement personnel was carried out in six countries (Brazil, Denmark, Egypt, Swaziland, Switzerland, and Thailand). The three main components of this study are (1) a review of legal provisions; (2) a description of the processes used to arrive at a conclusion about the dangerousness of a mentally ill person[38]; and (3) an assessment of the degree of reliability (i.e., interrater agreements) that experts can achieve in their assessments. This study was initiated after a thorough review of mental health legislation in some 40 countries, which pointed to the assessment of dangerousness as a key element in mental health legislation.[14]

Another set of investigations aiming at facilitating care provision dealt with the improvement of information about the functioning of mental health services. These studies helped to develop an internationally acceptable and applicable method of collecting and presenting useful data about mental health needs and resources at national level. Teams of investigators in Bulgaria, Thailand, Panama, Ghana, the U.S.A., Papua New Guinea, and Kuwait were involved in this study.[21]

Psychosocial Aspects of General Health Care and High-Risk Group Research

One of the mental health program objectives deals with psychosocial aspects of general health and development. This objective is being pursued by several means. One of them is the organization of workshops that involve health planners and behavioral scientists and in which specific health service delivery issues are being examined to establish possible contributions from a psychosocial point of view.[88] Another approach is the establishment of multidisciplinary groups and centers at national level; there are, however, also specific studies dealing with specific problems in this area.

One such study dealt with psychosomatic consequences and perceptions of tubal ligation, a widely used fertility regulation intervention.[94] Another study in several European countries is underway to examine the nature and frequency of problems in children of transnational and intranational migrants. The investigations on high-risk groups also include studies on the emotional interaction in families in which one or more members are suffering from a severe disease.

The frequency and impact of life events on patients with mental disorders were studied to obtain information on differences among cultural settings in the frequency of life events and on coping strategies employed to overcome their negative effects.[15]

The reasons for contacts of patients with health care agents were examined in a multicentric study carried out in seven countries. The results of this study served as a basis for the development of a classification of psychological and social problems encountered in primary health care and for the formulation of a triaxial recording procedure.[10,52]

A series of other projects have been initiated recently. These deal with various aspects of disease prevention and control as well as with the promotion of health.[55] In this effort the potential contributions of behavioral sciences are being systematically examined.[26]

Concluding Remarks

The tale about Achilles and the tortoise exemplifies the difficulty of catching up with a point in a progression regardless of the amount of effort: descriptions of problems (and programs) are outdated even before they are finalized. The review presented here is no exception: it must therefore be seen as a snapshot taken at a randomly selected point in a process, a snapshot that reminds us of the past and of the future and makes us aware of the imperfections of the apparatus that we are using to capture the wealth of events and features contained in a moment of time.

Acknowledgment

This chapter was prepared by the authors but the work described in its second part has been carried out by many individuals in countries and in WHO over the years. Among them are the members of WHO staff currently responsible for coordinating WHO activities in the field of Mental Health, at Headquarters, the Regional Offices, and in the field, namely the following: R. Diekstra, G. Ernberg, M. Grant, W. Gulbinat, J. Henderson, A. Jablensky, C. D. Jenkins, R. Johnson, I. Khan, I. Levav, J. Orley, L. Prilipko, J. Sampaio Faria, H. Sell, N. Shinfuku, A. Uznansky, and N. Wig. Yet their achievements are also based on the work of many others who have had the privilege of coordinating WHO mental health program activities over the years.

References

1. Arif A, Hughes PH, Khan I, Khant U, Klett CJ, Navaratnam V, Shafique M: *Drug Dependence: A Methodology for Evaluating Treatment and Rehabilitation.* WHO offset publication, No. 98, Geneva, 1987.
2. Arif A: *Adverse Health Consequences of Consequences of Cocaine Abuse.* Geneva, World Health Organization, 1987.
3. Arif A, Westermeyer J: The role of methadone in the management of opioid dependence: An international analysis (submitted for publication).
4. Astrup C, Oedegaard O: Continued experiments in psychiatric diagnosis. *Acta Psychiatr Scand* 1970; 46: 180–210.
5. Averbuch ES, Malnik EM, Serebrjakova ZN, Sternberg EA: *Diagnostika i klassifikatsiya psihiceskih zabolevanii pozdnego vozrasta* (Diagnosis and Classification of Psychiatric Disorders in Old Age). Leningrad, 1968.
6. Bolis CL: WHO Neurosciences Programme for Control of Neurological Disorders. *Trends in Neurosci* 1978; 1(4): 1–2.
7. Bolis CL: The WHO approach to neurological disorders. *Trends in Neurosci* 1978; 1(4): 8.

8. Brooke EM (ed): *Suicide and Attempted Suicide.* Public health paper, 58. Geneva, WHO, 1974.
9. Bruun K, Edwards G, Lumio M, Mäkelä K, Pan L, Popham RE, Room R, Schmidt W, Skog O-J, Sulkunen P, Osterberg E: Alcohol control policies in public health perspect. *The Finnish Foundation for Alcohol Studies* (Helsinki) 1975; 25: 1–106.
10. Clare A, Gulbinat W, Sartorius N: A triaxial classification of health problems presenting in primary care: Results of a WHO multicentric study. *Soc Psychia* (in press).
11. Cooper JE, Copeland JRM, Brown GW, Harris T, Gourlay AJ: Further studies on interviewer training and interrater reliability of the Present State Examination. *Psych Med* 1977; 7: 517–523.
12. Coppen A, Ghose K, Montgomery S, Rama Rao VA, Bailey J, Christiansen J, Mikkleson P, van Praag HM, van de Poel F, Jorgensen A: Amitriptyline plasma—Concentration and clinical effect: a World Health Organization Collaborative Study. *Lancet* 1978; i: 63–66.
13. Cruz ME, Tapia D, Proano J, Sevilla F, Carrera L, Barberis P, Bossano F, Schoenberg BS, Bolis CL: Prevalencía de Desordenes Neurologicos en Quiroga (Prov. Imbabura). *Revista Ecuatoriana de Medicina* 1984; Vol. XX, No. 2: 77–91.
14. Curran WJ, Harding TW: *The Law and Mental Health: Harmonizing Objectives.* Geneva, WHO, 1978.
15. Day R, Nielsen JA, Korten A, Ernberg G, Dube KC, Gebhart J, Jablensky A, Leon C, Marsella A, Olatawura M, Sartorius N, Strömgren E, Takahashi R, Wig N, Wynne LC: Stressful life events preceding the acute onset of schizophrenia: A cross-national study from the World Health Organization. *Cult, Med Psychia* 1987; 11: 123–205.
16. Dupont A, Möller Jensen O, Strömgren E, Jablensky A: Incidence of cancer in patients diagnosed as schizophrenic in Denmark, in GHMM ten Horn, Giel R, Gulbinat WH, Henderson JH (eds): *Psychiatric Case Registers in Public Health.* Elsevier, Amsterdam, 1986, pp 229–239.
17. Essex B, Gosling H: Programme for Identification and Management of Mental Health Problems. *Tropical Health Series.* Churchill Livingstone, Longman Group Limited, Essex, U. K., 1982.
18. Fillmore KM, Grant M, Hartka E, Johnstone BM, Swayer SM, Speiglman R, Temple MT: Collaborative longitudinal research on alcohol problems. *Br J Psychia* (in press).
19. Finnish Foundation for Alcohol Studies and WHO Regional Office for Europe: *International Statistics on Alcoholic Beverages: Production, Trace and Consumption, 1950–1972.* The Finnish Foundation for Alcohol Studies (Helsinki), 27, 1977.
20. Gershon ES, Mendlewicz J, Gastpar M, Bech P, Goldin LR, Kielholz P, Raphaelson OJ, Vartanian F, Bunney WE Jr: A collaborative study on genetic linkage of bipolar manic-depressive illness and red-green colour-blindness. *Acta Psychiatr Scand* 1980; 61: 319–338.
21. Gulbinat W: *Monitoring of Mental Health Needs.* Report of a WHO-coordinated study in seven countries. WHO document MNH/NAT/84.3, Geneva, WHO, 1984.
22. Harding TW: Psychiatry in rural agrarian societies. *Psychiatr Ann* 1978; 8: 74–84.
23. Harding TW, de Arango MV, Baltazar J, Climent CE, Ibrahim HHA, Ladrido-Ignacio L, Srinivasa Murthy R, Wig NN: Mental disorders in primary health care—A study of their frequency in four developing countries. *Psych Med* 1980; 10: 231–241.
24. Hawks DV: Improving community response to alcohol-related problems: An interim report. Proc 24th International Institute on the Prevention and Treatment of Alcoholism, Tongue EJ (ed). Zurich, 1978; pp 27–39. ICAA: Lausanne, 1978.
25. Helmchen H, Kielholz P, Brooke E, Sartorius N: Zur Klassifikation neurotischer und psychosomatischer Störungen. *Nervenartz* 1973; 44: 292–299.

26. Holtzman WH, Evans RI, Kennedy S, Iscoe I: Psychology and Health: Contributions of Psychology to the Improvement of Health and Health Care. *WHO Bulletin* 1987; 65 (6): 913–935, Geneva. WHO.
27. Hughes PH, Venulet J, Khant U, Medina Mora ME, Navaratnam V, Poshyachinda V, Rootman I, Salan R, Wadud KA: *Core Data for Epidemiological Studies of Nonmedical Drug Use*. WHO offset publication, No. 56, WHO, Geneva, 1980.
28. Koliaskina G, Kielholz P, Bunney WG, Rafaelson O, Coppen A, Nippius H, Vartanian F: Antithymic immune factors in schizophrenia: a World Health Organization collaborative study. *Neuropsychobiology* 1980; 6: 349–355.
29. Kramer M, Sartorius N, Jablensky A, Gulbinat W: The ICD-9 classification of mental disorder: A review of its development and contents. *Acta Psychiatr Scand* 1979; 59: 241–262.
30. Jablensky A: The need for standardization of psychiatric assessment: An epidemiological point of view. *Acta Psychiatr Belg* 1978; 78: 549–558.
31. Jablensky A, Schwartz R, Tomov T: WHO collaborative study on impairment and disabilities associated with schizophrenic disorders: A preliminary communication: Objectives and methods. *Acta Psychiatr Scand* 1980; Suppl 285, 62: 152–163.
32. Jablensky A, Sartorius N, Gulbinat W, Ernberg G: Characteristics of depressive patients contacting psychiatric services in four cultures: A report from a WHO collaborative study on the assessment of depressive disorders. *Acta Psychiatr Scand* 1981; 63: 367–383.
33. Jablensky A, Sartorius N, Hirschfeld R, Pardes H: Diagnosis and classification of mental disorders and alcohol- and drug-related problems: A research agenda for the 1980's. *Psych Med* 1983; 13: 907–921.
34. Jdänpään-Heikkilä J, Ghodse H, Khan I: Psychoactive drugs and health problems: A report of a meeting by the World Health Organization with the collaboration of the government of Finland, the government of Thailand and the United Nations Fund for Drug Abuse Control. The National Board of Health, The Government of Finland, 1987.
35. Leff J, Wig NN, Ghosh A, Bedi H, Menon DK, Kuipers L, Korten A, Ernberg G, Day R, Sartorius N, Jablensky A: Expressed emotion and schizophrenia in North India. III: Influence of relatives' expressed emotion on the course of schizophrenia in Chandigarh. *Br J Psychiatr* 1987; 151: 166–173.
36. Loranger AW, Hirschfeld RMA, Sartorius N, Regier DA: The international personality disorder examination: A semistructured clinical interview for use with DSM-III-R and ICD-10 in different cultures. *Arch Gen Psychiatry* (submitted for publication).
37. Meursing K, Wankiiri V: The use of flow charts in mental health by mid-level general health workers. *WHO Bull* 1988; 66, No. 4: 507–514.
38. Montandon C, Harding TW: The reliability of dangerousness assessments: A decision-making exercise. *Br J Psychiatry* 1984; 144: 149–155.
39. Moser J: *Prevention of Alcohol Related Problems: An International Review of Preventive Measures, Policies and Programmes*, Geneva, WHO; and Toronto, Canada, Drug Addiction Research Foundation, 1980.
40. Osuntokum BO, Schoenberg BS, Nottidge V, Adeuja A, Kale O, Adeyefa A, Bademosi O, Bolis C.L: Migraine headache in a rural community in Nigeria: Results of a pilot study. *Neuroepidemiol 1982;* 1, No. 1: 31–39.
41. Osuntokun BO, Schoenberg BS, Noddidge V, Adeuja A, Kale O, Adeyefa A, Bademosi O, Olumide A, Oyediran ABO, Pearson CA, Bolis CL: Research protocol for measuring the prevalence of neurologic disorders in developing countries: Results of a pilot study in Nigeria. *Neuroepidemiol* 1982; 1, No. 3: 143–153.

42. Perry, CL, Grant M: Comparing peer-led to teacher-led youth alcohol education in four countries. *Alcohol, Health & Research World* 12(4): 322–326.
43. Pickar D, Bunney WE Jr, Douillet P, Sethi BB, Sharma M, Vartanian ME, Lideman RR, Hippius H, Naber D, Leibl K, Yamashita I, Koyama T, van Praag HM, Verhoeven WMA: Repeated naloxone administration in schizophrenia: A Phase II World Health Organization Study. *Biol Psychiatr*, 1987.
44. Robins LN, Wing J, Wittchen HU, Helzer JE, Babor TF, Burke J, Farmer A, Jablensky A, Pickens R, Regier DA, Towle LH: The composite international diagnostic interview. *Arch Gen Psychiatry* 1988; 45: 1069–1077.
45. Rutter M, Shaffer D, Shepherd M: *A Multi-axial Classification of Child Psychiatric Disorders*. Geneva, WHO, 1975.
46. Sartorius N: The programme for the World Health Organization on the epidemiology of mental disorders. In *Proc Vth World Congress of Psychiatry*, Mexico, 1971 de la Fuente R, Wiseman MN (eds). p 13. Excerpta Medica: Amsterdam, 1973.
47. Sartorius N: Epidemiology of depression. *WHO Chron* 1975; 29: 423–427.
48. Sartorius N: Classification: An international perspective. *Psychiatr Ann* 1976; 4: 359–367.
49. Sartorius N: The new mental health programme of WHO. *Interdiscipl Sci Rev* 1978; 3: 202–206.
50. Sartorius N: Research on affective disorders within the framework of the WHO programme. In Schou M, Strömgren E (eds) *Aarhus Symposia: Origin, Prevention and Treatment of Affective Disorders*. pp 207–213. Academic Press: London, 1979.
51. Sartorius N, Jablensky A: Collaborating research for the development of guidelines for treatment and rehabilitation of depressed patients in developing countries. In *Proc Third World Congress of International Rehabilitation Association*. Basle 1978, Huber: Bern, 1980.
52. Sartorius N, Gulbinat W: *Recording Health Problems Triaxially*. World Health Organization/National Institute of Mental Health, Rockville, 1983.
53. Sartorius N, Jablensky A, Korten A, Ernberg G, Anker M, Cooper JE, Day R: Early manifestations and first-contact incidence of schizophrenia in different cultures: A preliminary report on the initial evaluation phase of the WHO Collaborative Study on Determinants of Outcome of Severe Mental Disorders. *Psych Med* 1986; 16: 909–928.
54. Sartorius N, Ban TA: *Assessment of Depression*. Springer-Verlag, Heidelberg, New York, Tokyo, 1986.
55. Sartorius N, Diekstra R: Psychosocial approaches to health: Outline of a long-term research programme undertaken by WHO, 1989.
56. Sartorius N: International perspectives of psychiatric classifications. *Br J Psychiatr* 152 (suppl.): 9–14.
57. Saunders JB, Aasland OG: *WHO Collaborative Project on Identification and Treatment of Persons with Harmful Alcohol Consumption*. Report on Phase I: Development of a Screening Instrument. WHO document WHO/MNH/DAT/86.3, 1987.
58. Shepherd M, Sartorius N: Personality disorder and the International Classification of Diseases. *Psych Med* 1974; 4: 141–146.
59. Shepherd M, Brooke E, Cooper JE, Lin T-Y: An experimental approach to psychiatric diagnosis: An international study. *Acta Psychiatr Scand* 1968; 44(suppl. 201).
60. Tarjan G, Tizard J, Rutter M, Begab M, Brooke EM, de la Cruz F, Lin T-Y, Montenegro H, Strotzka H, Sartorius N: Classification and mental retardation: Issues arising in the fifth WHO seminar on psychiatric diagnosis, classification and statistics. *Am J Psychiatr* 1972; 128(suppl. 11): 34–45.

61. Wang Chung-Cheng, Cheng Xue-Ming, Li Shi-Chuo, Bolis CL, Schoenberg BS: Epidemiology of cerebrovascular disease in an urban community of Beijing, People's Republic of China. *Neuroepidemiol* 1983; 2, No. 3–4: 121–134.
62. Wig NN, Varma VK: Patterns of long-term heavy cannabis use in North India, and its effects on cognitive functions: A preliminary report. *Drug Alcohol Depend* 1977; 2: 211–219.
63. Wig NN, Suleiman M, Srinivasa Murthy R, Routeledge R, Ladrido-Ignacio L, Ibrahim HHA, Harding TW: Community reactions to mental disorders—A study in three developing countries. *Acta Psychiatr Scand* 1980; 61: 111–126.
64. Wig NN, Menon DK, Bedi H, Ghosh A, Kuipers L, Leff J, Korten A, Day R, Sartorius N, Ernberg G, Jablensky A: Expressed emotion and schizophrenia in North India. I: Cross-cultural transfer of ratings of relatives' expressed emotion. *Br J Psychiatr* 1987; 151: 156–160.
65. Wig NN, Menon DK, Bedi H, Leff J, Nielsen JA, Thestrup G, Kuipers L, Ghosh A, Day R, Korten A, Ernberg G, Sartorius N, Jablensky A: Expressed emotion and schizophrenia in North India. II: Distribution of expressed emotion components among relatives of schizophrenic patients in Aarhus and Chandigarh. *Br J Psychiatr* 1987; 151: 160–165.
66. Walsh B, Grant M: *Public Health Implications of Alcohol Production and Trade.* WHO offset publication, 88, WHO, Geneva, 1985.
67. Wing JK, Cooper JE, Sartorius N: *The Measurement and Classification of Psychiatric Symptoms.* London, Cambridge University Press, 1974.
68. Wing JK, Nixon JM, Mann SA, Leff JP: Reliability of the PSE (ed 9) used in a population survey. *Psych Med* 1977; 7: 505–516.
69. World Health Organization: *Report of the Fifth Seminar on Psychiatric Diagnosis. Classification and Statistics.* Mental Retardation (Washington, 1969). (offset) Geneva, WHO, 1970.
70. World Health Organization: *Report of the Eighth Seminar on Standardization of Psychiatric Diagnosis, Classification and Statistics, 1972.* Geneva, WHO, 1973.
71. World Health Organization: *Dictionary of Epilepsy.* Part I, *Definitions* (H. Gastaut). Geneva, WHO, 1973.
72. World Health Organization: *The International Pilot Study of Schizophrenia,* Vol. L. Geneva, WHO, 1973.
73. World Health Organization: *Glossary of Mental Disorders and Guide to Their Classification.* Geneva, WHO, 1974.
74. World Health Organization: *Schizophrenia: A Multinational Study.* Public Health Papers no. 63. Geneva, WHO, 1975.
75. World Health Organization: *Selected Documents and Publications of the Mental Health Programme,* 1947–1988. (MNH/POL/89.4) Geneva, WHO, 1978.
76. World Health Organization: *International Classification of Diseases* (rev 9). Chapter V. Mental disorders. Geneva, WHO, 1978.
77. World Health Organization: *Cerebrovascular Disorders: A Clinical and Research Classification.* WHO offset publication No. 43. Geneva, WHO, 1978.
78. World Health Organization: *Mental Disorders: Glossary and Guide to Their Classification in Accordance with the Ninth Revision of the International Classification of Diseases.* Geneva, WHO, 1978.
79. World Health Organization: *Report on the Third Exchange of Visits of Investigators in Biological Psychiatry* (WHO/MNH/78.2). Geneva, WHO, 1978.
80. World Health Organization: *Report on the Fourth Exchange of Visits of Investigators in Biological Psychiatry* (WHO/MNH/78.26). Geneva, WHO, 1978.

81. World Health Organization: *Research on Dependence Liability of Thebaine and Its Derivatives: Interim Progress Report* (WHO/MNH/78.28). Geneva, WHO, 1978.
82. World Health Organization: *The Application of Advances in Neurosciences for the Control of Neurological Disorders: A Report of a WHO Study Group*. Technical Report Series, 629, Geneva, WHO, 1978.
83. World Health Organization: *Report on the Second Meeting of Investigators of the WHO Project on the Effects of Psychotropic Drugs in Different Populations.* (WHO/MNH/78.16) Geneva, WHO, 1978.
84. World Health Organization: *Schizophrenia: An International Follow-up Study*. Chichester, John Wiley & Sons, 1979.
85. World Health Organization: *Report of Third Meeting of Investigators Collaborating in the Project on Monitoring of Mental Health Needs*. New Delhi, 1978. Unpublished document: Geneva, WHO, 1979.
86. World Health Organization: Regional Office for Europe Report of a Conference on Mental Health Services. In Pilot Study Areas, Lysebu (ICP/MNH/007) 1977. Copenhagen, 1977.
87. World Health Organization: Review of the pharmacology of khat: Report of a WHO Advisory Group. *Bull Narc* 1980; Vol. XXXII, No. 3: 83–93.
88. World Health Organization: *Stress, Lifestyle and the Prevention of Disease*. Report of a WHO Scientific Working Group, Sofia, Bulgaria, 5–12 October 1981, Geneva, WHO, 1982.
89. World Health Organization: Validity and reliability of trends in suicide statistics. *World Health Quarterly* 1983; 36, No. 3/4, pp 339–348.
90. World Health Organization: *Global Medium-Term Programme (1984–1989). Protection and Promotion of Mental Health.* (MNH/MTP/83.19). Geneva, WHO, 1983.
91. World Health Organization: *Depressive Disorders in Different Cultures*. Geneva, WHO, 1983.
92. World Health Organization: *Global Medium-Term Programme (1990–1995). Protection and Promotion of Mental Health* (MNH/MTP/88.1). Geneva, WHO (in press).
93. World Health Organization: *Mental Health Care in Developing Countries: A Critical Appraisal of Research Findings.* Report of a WHO Study Group. Technical Report Series, 698, Geneva, WHO, 1984.
94. World Health Organization: Mental health and female sterilization. Report of a WHO collaborative prospective study. *J Biosoc Sci* 1984; 16: 1–21.
95. World Health Organization: *Prevention of Mental, Neurological and Psychosocial Disorders* (WHO document A39/9). Geneva, WHO, 1986.
96. World Health Organization: Collaborative study on dose effects of antidepressant medication in different populations. *J Affec Dis* (suppl 2), 1986.
97. World Health Organization: *Pathways of Patients with Mental Disorders* (WHO/MNH/NAT/87.1). Geneva, WHO, 1987.
98. World Health Organization: *WHO Psychiatric Disability Assessment Schedule* (WHO/DAS). Geneva, WHO, 1988.
99. Yamashita I, Ohmori T, Koyama T, Mori H: WHO Collaborative study of alcoholism with reference to ethnic differences. *Clin Neuropharmacol* 1986; 9: 442–449.
100. Wing JK, Babor T, Brugha T, et al: SCAN: Schedules for clincial assessment in psychiatry. *Arch Gen Psychiatr* (submitted for publication).

9

International Cancer Care

H. VAINIO, D. M. PARKIN, AND L. TOMATIS

INTRODUCTION

Cancer is a major source of morbidity and mortality in developed countries, and both are rapidly increasing in developing countries, so that prevention and control have a high priority in public health. Time trends and worldwide incidence and mortality figures provide clues to the multiple causative factors involved in human cancers. Such data are supplemented by observations on changes in risk of cancer in migrant populations who in time acquire the cancer pattern of the host country. Ad hoc epidemiological studies and analysis of data obtained under controlled conditions in animal models have defined specific carcinogenic factors. Considerable progress has been made during the last decade in the understanding of the mechanisms of cancer and the mode of action of carcinogenic agents, including, recently, the biological processes triggering uncontrolled division of cells. In this review we describe briefly the worldwide cancer burden and the principal known causative factors, and discuss the potential for cancer prevention.

THE WORLD CANCER BURDEN

The importance of a disease in a population is measured by its impact in terms of mortality and morbidity. Death rates are convenient and widely used for comparative purposes (geographic, time trends, etc.) although, as an (inverse) measure of health status, they are not entirely satisfactory. Even for a disease such as cancer, with a relatively poor prognosis, many persons affected do not die of the disease; thus mortality rates can

H. VAINIO, D. M. PARKIN, AND L. TOMATIS • International Agency for Research on Cancer, 69372 Lyon, Cedex 8, France.

only represent one dimension of the impact of illness and are only a proxy indicator of disease occurrence. Incidence is a more useful measure for epidemiological purposes. It provides an estimate for the risk of disease for the individual and the community. For most diseases, incidence rates are difficult to obtain, although reasonable data for cancer are available, thanks to systems of cancer registration.

Prevalence of different cancers in the community is sometimes advanced as a useful indicator of cancer burden, although the meaning of "prevalence" in this context is unclear; it should cover everyone alive who has ever in the past been diagnosed as having had a cancer, but would then clearly include many "cured" cases who no longer require medical services. On the other hand, limiting the term "prevalence" to cancer cases who are still receiving treatment or medical supervision measures the availability of services to the same extent as the level of disease in the community.

Measures of incidence or mortality provide little information on the level of disability or quality of life in persons affected by cancer. Unfortunately, there are no standard international definitions of disability, so that comparative studies are not possible, and even within different countries estimation of disability in the population usually requires special surveys.

Mortality

Figure 1 shows the distribution of estimated mortality according to certain broad cause groupings for the six regions of the World Health Organization in 1980. Overall, it is estimated that there were 4.2 million deaths due to cancer that year, but the percentage of deaths due to this cause varies considerably between regions and countries; in the developing world, cancer causes 8–9% of deaths, compared with 20–25% in the developed world.[1] Much of this difference can be accounted for quite simply by the age structure of the population. Mortality rates for the major cancers increase logarithmically with age (for most epithelial cancers, rates are proportional to the fourth or fifth power of age[2]). Thus the most important overall determinant of the number of cancer cases in the population and the number of deaths will be the age structure of the population. In the less developed regions of Africa, Latin America, and South Asia, about 40–50% of the population are children under 15 years of age and only 3–4% are aged over 65, whereas in Europe and North America only one-quarter of the population are children and 10–12% are aged 65 or more.

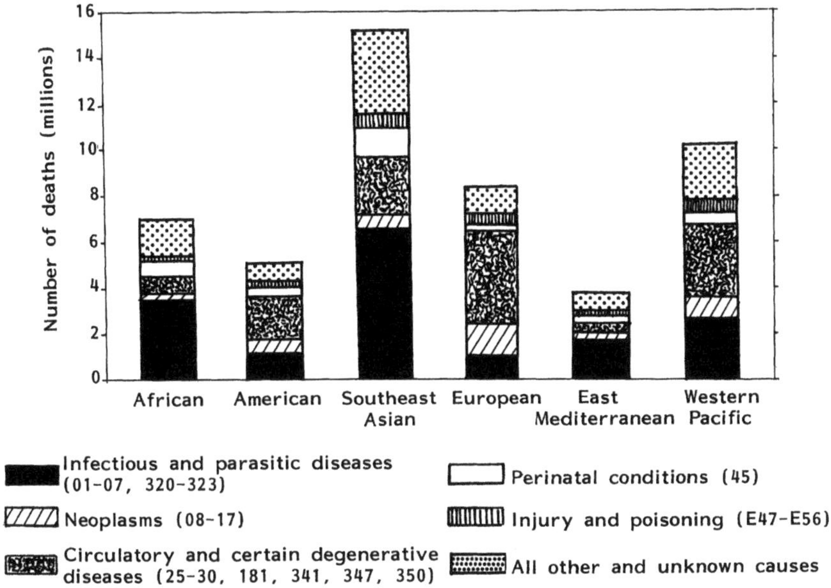

FIGURE 1. Estimated number of deaths by cause, WHO regions, 1980.

Table 1 shows that there are correspondingly wide differences in crude death rates from cancer (i.e., for all ages combined); for example, in males, the ratio of death rates in Africa to those in Europe is 1 : 4.3. However, for the individual age groups, the differences are much smaller, so that the ratio of rates (Africa : Europe) at age 65+ is only 1 : 1.7. Some of the remaining difference is due to the fact that, within these broad age bands, the actual distribution of ages will tend to be younger in developing countries.

Of course, age differences do not explain all of the variation in cancer mortality; the geographic and temporal distribution of individual cancers is related to the presence of causative factors in the environment, and the acquisition of knowledge about such risk factors and the means to control them form the goal of epidemiological studies. Nevertheless, it is undoubtedly true that cancer emerges as an increasingly important public health problem as nations undergo the so-called demographic transition away from the pattern of high fertility and high overall mortality that characterizes most developing countries where infec-

TABLE 1. Estimated Death Rates from Neoplasms, 1980[a] (per 100,000)

Area	All ages	Age groups			
		0–14	15–44	45–64	65–
Males, world	101	5	20	266	1029
Developed regions	196	7	22	314	1356
Developing regions	70	5	20	241	770
Africa	56	3	15	230	879
Latin America	61	5	13	177	792
North America	201	5	18	344	1395
East Asia	99	5	25	290	783
South Asia	59	5	18	210	811
Europe	241	8	24	345	1458
Oceania	157	6	19	302	1365
USSR	122	8	23	241	1030
Females, world	89	4	23	219	667
Developed regions	169	6	24	232	792
Developing regions	60	4	22	211	525
Africa	59	3	26	237	610
Latin America	55	4	17	166	551
North America	160	4	20	265	803
East Asia	73	4	20	197	506
South Asia	57	4	24	224	554
Europe	187	6	24	232	818
Oceania	124	5	23	234	798
USSR	167	6	28	236	773

[a]From WHO (unpublished data).

tious and parasitic diseases and respiratory infections are frequent causes of mortality, especially at young ages, and where expectation of life at birth is low.

CANCER INCIDENCE

The existence of an extensive network of cancer registries throughout the world permits estimates to be prepared of the number of new cancer cases, by site of cancer, in different countries. Where incidence rates are not available, mortality by cause can be used to estimate likely patterns of incidence. Cancer incidence (like mortality) is strongly related to age, so that the incidence rate for the whole population (crude incidence) is related to its age structure, and the actual *number* of cases to the population size. Table 2 shows the estimated rates of incidence in 24 world areas (for around 1975) and Table 3 summarizes the numbers of cases estimated for different sites in developed compared with developing countries.[3] Overall, there were estimated to be 5.9 million new cases of cancer in 1975, almost equally divided between males and females, and slightly more cases in the developing than in the developed world. In 1975, stomach cancer was thought to be the most common tumor, followed closely by lung cancer, but by now this pattern has almost certainly reversed. The importance of the two specifically female cancers—breast cancer and cervix cancer—is emphasized in Table 3, but comparison of their incidence rates in Table 2 shows that their relative importance varies considerably, with cervix cancer being more common in the developing world and breast cancer in developed regions.

Potential Years of Life Lost

An additional dimension of the burden presented by cancer for the purpose of defining health priorities, especially for prevention, is given by potential years of life lost (PYLL). The calculation of PYLL gives each death a weighting that may be equal to the normal expectation of life remaining at the age of death (derived from a life table), or up to a maximum age of 65 to 70 (sometimes considered as the remaining "productive" years of life under the (usually implicit) assumption that retirement age marks a cessation of productivity. Deaths under one year of age are sometimes excluded, as they are often due to ill-defined causes ("prematurity," etc.) and, because of their large weighting, come to constitute an important component of PYLL. PYLL depends upon the number of deaths occurring and their distribution by age, the latter depending upon the age-specific rates that are present and the age structure of the population. Young populations, such as those in developing countries, will have a larger proportion of deaths at young ages, so that causes of death that predominate in the young will produce a PYLL that is relatively large in relation to the size of the population. Table 4 compares the percentage of total PYLL from different causes for nine very different populations around 1980. In males, the extent of injury and poisoning (an important cause of death in the young) means that cancer is rarely the major cause of PYLL—however, in females, it is only in certain developing countries that cancer is not the major cause of PYLL.

TABLE 2. Estimated Crude Rates of Incidence

Area	Buccal cavity/ pharynx (140–149)[b]		Esophagus (150)		Stomach (151)		Colon and rectum (153, 154)		Liver (155)	
	M	F	M	F	M	F	M	F	M	F
East Africa	7	6	5	1	4.5	3.5	2.5	2	22	6
Middle Africa	5	3	0.9	0.6	3.5	2	4	3	18	6.5
Northern Africa	11.5	5.5	2	1.5	4.5	1.5	5.5	3.5	3	2
Southern Africa	8.5	4	13	3	13	8	4.5	7.5	13	2.5
Western Africa	2	1.5	0.4	0.2	2.5	2	1.5	1.5	9	3
Caribbean	12	3.5	7.5	3	15.5	7.5	10	11	4.5	3
Middle America	2.5	2	2	1	9	6.5	4.5	6	2	1.5
Temperate South America	18	6.5	11.5	3.5	27	17	23	27	5.5	3.5
Tropical South America	9	4	4	1	19	11	7	7.5	3	3
North America	16	6.5	5	2	12	7	48	46	3	1.5
China	8	4.5	23	13	29	15	8.5	8	17	6.5
Japan	3.5	2	8	2.5	85	50	17	15	14	7
Other East Asia	7	3.5	3.5	0.8	28	14	8	6	18	4
Eastern South Asia	9	4.5	3.5	1.5	8	4.5	6.5	5.5	15	4
Middle South Asia	18	9.5	6	4.5	4.5	2.5	3.5	2.5	1.5	1
Western South Asia	4	2	2.5	2	6	3.5	5	4	2	1
Eastern Europe	12	3	3.5	1	41	25	22	22	7	5.5
Northern Europe	9	5	7	5	31	21	43	46	2.5	1.5
Southern Europe	14.5	3	8	2.5	44	30	30	30	11	5
Western Europe	20	4	10	1.5	34	22	43	45	4.5	2.5
Australia/New Zealand	15.5	4	5	2.5	16	10	38	39	1.5	0.8
Melanesia	19	14	2	0.3	4	2.5	5	2.5	14	5
Micronesia/Polynesia	4	1.5	3	0.4	7	3	6.5	5	5	2.5
USSR	13	4	8	5.5	47	36	11	15	7	5.5

[a]From Parkin et al.[3]

[b]Numbers in parentheses indicate the *ICD* codes according to the Eighth Revision of the *International Classification of Diseases*. Values >10 rounded to nearest whole number; values <10 rounded to nearest 0.5; values <1 rounded to nearest 0.1.

CANCER CAUSATION

CULTURAL HABITS

TOBACCO USE Tobacco consumption is a worldwide problem. Although, until recently, attention was directed primarily towards the carcinogenic effects of tobacco smoking, the recent increase in North America and northern Europe in the use of so-called "smokeless" tobacco products (chewing tobacco and snuff used orally) has stimulated (per 100,000) by Sex, Site, and Area[a]

Bronchus/ lung (162)		Breast (174)	Cervix (180)	Prostate (185)	Bladder (188)		Lymphatic tissue (200–203)		Leukemia (204–207)		All sites (140–207) (excl. 173)	
M	F	F	F	M	M	F	M	F	M	F	M	F
2	0.4	9	21	5.5	3.5	1	10	5.5	1.5	1	86	83
2.5	1	12	21	6	3	1.5	12	7.5	1	0.6	90	100
2.5	0.6	25	19	2	16	6	11	5.5	5	3.5	100	110
19	3	20	27	8	3.5	1.5	6	3.5	3.5	2.5	121	116
0.9	0.5	7	11	3	2	1	9	5.5	2	1.5	42	52
35	12	30	20	19	7.5	2	8	5	5	3.5	146	123
7.5	3	14	21	7.5	3.5	1	4	3.5	2.5	2.5	73	94
39	7	79	24	22	16	6	6	4.5	7	5	232	256
11	3	27	32	10	5	1	7	4.5	4.5	3.5	104	135
68	21	87	13	55	22	7.5	16.5	14	11	8	323	315
11	5	12	29	2	2	0.6	3	25	4.5	3.5	138	123
24	9	20	17	4	4.5	2	5.5	4	4.5	4	199	171
13	5	16	26	3	3.5	1	4	2	4	3	128	144
17	6	14	21	2.5	2	0.6	3.5	2	4.5	3	91	89
6	1.5	15	24	1.5	1.5	0.4	4.5	2	3	2	72	79
11	2.5	15	4.5	3.5	5	0.9	6.5	4	4	3	82	72
59	8.5	36	24	17	11	2.5	11	8.5	7.5	5.5	234	216
93	23	82	17	37	22	7.5	14	11	9	7.5	334	313
62	13	61	13	26	21	3.5	12	9.5	10	6.5	310	253
87	11	84	23	42	25	5.5	12	9.5	9.5	7.5	365	325
57	12	66	13	34	18	5.5	15	12	9	6.5	273	254
4	1	13	20	1	1	0.3	8	2.5	4	1.5	107	114
8	2	7	20	12	0.8	0.9	6	2.5	3.5	1.5	80	90
43	10	23	23	7	9	3	4	3	5.5	4.5	175	168

investigations into the carcinogenic effects of these forms of tobacco use also. In large areas of the world, tobacco is consumed orally, either alone or in betel quids containing lime or other ingredients. In many of these areas, tobacco smoking is also prevalent.

Chewing of tobacco or the placing of a quid of tobacco next to the gingiva has been practiced throughout the world since the introduction of tobacco from the Americas. In Southeast Asia, and particularly in India, the habit of betel quid chewing existed long before the introduction of tobacco. The betel quid consists traditionally of a leaf of the *Piper betle* bush wrapped around a piece of areca nut (the fruit of the *Areca* palm) to which lime and various flavoring ingredients are added.[4] The

TABLE 3. Numbers (and Percentages) of All Cancer at Different Sites: Developed versus Developing Countries (in Thousands)[a]

Site	Developed countries[b]		Developing countries	
	Male	Female	Male	Female
Mouth/pharynx	70.7 (4.9)	23.7 (1.7)	162.2 (10.6)	82.9 (5.6)
Esophagus	37.3 (2.6)	17.1 (1.2)	156.7 (10.2)	85.2 (5.7)
Stomach	204.3 (14.2)	147.4 (10.5)	217.4 (14.2)	113.2 (7.6)
Colon/rectum	160.3 (11.2)	175.6 (12.5)	90.9 (5.9)	80.0 (5.4)
Liver	34.4 (2.4)	19.4 (1.4)	148.1 (9.7)	57.3 (3.8)
Bronchus/lung	318.6 (22.2)	77.3 (5.5)	145.7 (9.5)	49.4 (3.3)
Breast	—	315.8 (22.4)	—	225.4 (15.1)
Cervix	—	105.1 (7.5)	—	354.3 (23.7)
Prostate	148.1 (10.3)	—	49.6 (3.2)	—
Bladder	86.5 (6.0)	26.1 (1.9)	44.2 (2.9)	13.3 (0.9)
Lymphatic	55.9 (3.9)	47.6 (3.4)	73.6 (4.8)	43.7 (2.9)
Leukemia	43.4 (3.0)	35.1 (2.5)	56.9 (3.7)	40.3 (2.7)
All sites	1433.8 (100)	1408.5 (100)	1534.7 (100)	1493.3 (100)

[a]From Parkin et al.[3]
[b]Europe, North America, Japan, Australia/New Zealand, USSR.

addition of a piece of local, sun-dried tobacco augments the feeling of well-being derived from this combination. The habit of chewing tobacco alone is also widespread, particularly in the tobacco-growing states of India.

The oral use of smokeless tobacco is carcinogenic to humans, giving rise to cancers of the oral cavity, pharynx, and esophagus.[4]

There is overwhelming evidence that tobacco smoking is the major cause of lung cancer and is responsible for the rapid increase in mortality from lung cancer in developed countries over the last four decades.[5]

With regard to the type of tobacco product, the smoking of not only cigarettes but also bidis (small cigarettes smoked in India), cigars, and pipes results in an increased risk for lung cancer. With long duration and heavy intensity of cigarette usage, the proportion of lung cancer attributable to smoking is approximately 90%. This figure applies to men in most Western populations; in populations in which more and more women smoke cigarettes, the proportion is approaching the same level.

A large number of case-control and cohort studies have shown that tobacco smoking, particularly in relation to cigarettes, is an important cause of bladder cancer and cancer of the renal pelvis. The proportion of these diseases attributable to smoking in most countries where there has

TABLE 4. Potential Years of Life Lost, to Age 70, as a Percentage of the Total, 1980

	Cancer	Infectious/ parasitic	Cerebrovascular	Other circulatory diseases	Respiratory diseases	Injury/ poisoning	Senility/ ill-defined
Males							
Chile	6.7	8.0	21	4.8	9.5	28.4	6.6
USA	13.3	1.3	2.2	19.1	3.5	34.7	3.8
Japan	21.1	2.1	9.2	11.2	3.9	28.1	0.5
Hong Kong	23.7	4.0	5.1	7.4	10.9	21.0	3.0
Kuwait	5.0	10.8	1.5	12.3	9.9	22.0	1.3
Hungary	15.1	1.4	5.9	20.3	5.4	23.5	0.1
Sweden	17.2	0.9	3.5	23.7	3.2	28.3	1.7
Spain	15.7	5.2	4.0	13.5	6.9	21.3	2.5
Australia	15.5	1.3	2.8	19.8	5.7	30.3	5.9
Females							
Chile	10.7	9.2	3.0	4.7	11.2	13.0	8.0
USA	21.7	1.8	3.6	13.9	4.1	20.1	4.3
Japan	29.0	2.2	9.2	9.5	4.7	17.1	0.6
Hong Kong	21.8	3.7	6.3	7.6	9.9	15.4	1.4
Kuwait	5.5	17.1	1.2	9.0	12.3	11.5	1.2
Hungary	21.5	1.1	7.4	15.3	5.2	12.8	0.2
Sweden	32.8	1.5	4.8	11.5	3.8	18.5	2.0
Spain	20.6	6.2	5.1	11.0	6.9	10.6	2.6
Australia	23.5	1.4	5.0	12.3	4.3	19.8	4.2

been a long history of cigarette usage is approximately 50% for men and 25% for women.

Tobacco smoking is also causally associated with cancers of the oral cavity, upper respiratory and digestive tracts, and pancreas.[5]

ALCOHOL Alcohol is the oldest and most widely diffused intoxicating substance known to man. Although present in very early history, recent decades have witnessed a steady increase in the production and consumption of alcoholic beverages in virtually all regions of the world. Between 1965 and 1980, the total commercial production of alcohol rose by almost 50%, while production per capita rose by just under 15%. Two-thirds of the world's production at both dates occurred in Europe and North America.[6]

The relationship between alcohol intake and cancer has been convincingly documented in several investigations (for review, see Tuyns[7]). Most of them have been retrospective, starting from a series of cancer patients. These studies provide consistent evidence that the consumption of alcoholic beverages entails an increased risk of developing cancer of the oral cavity, pharynx, esophagus, and larynx. Beverages with high alcohol content carry a higher risk for cancer of the above-mentioned sites than those that contain less alcohol. In these cancers, the role of tobacco is also important, and the effects of these two factors, drinking and smoking, are usually combined in an additive or even multiplicative manner.[8]

OCCUPATIONAL EXPOSURES

Occupational exposures normally affect relatively small groups of individuals and tend to exceed those of the general population by one or more orders of magnitude.[9] This is perhaps why epidemiological research has demonstrated a causal association between a number of occupational exposures and increased risk of cancer in various organs (Table 5). The fact that occupationally associated cancers are caused by exposure to agents such as chemicals or ionizing radiation implies that they can be prevented.

About 4% of all cases of cancer in industrialized countries have been attributed to occupational exposures.[10–12] The risk attributable to occupation is a function of the relative risk associated with a given set of exposures, and of the proportion of people exposed; it represents the proportion of cases that would not have occurred in the absence of the exposure.

Some epidemiological studies have estimated the contribution of

TABLE 5. Occupations Involving Exposure to Chemicals, Groups of Chemicals, Industrial Processes of Complex Mixtures for Which There Is Sufficient Evidence of Carcinogenicity to Humans[a]

Industry	Occupation	Cancer site	Substance reported or suspected to be the causative agent	*IARC Monographs* reference
Agriculture, forestry, and fishing	Arsenical insecticide application in vineyards	Lung, skin	Arsenic	23[82]
Mining	Arsenic mining	Lung, skin	Arsenic	23[82]
	Asbestos mining	Lung, pleural and peritoneal mesothelioma	Asbestos	*14*[83]
	Uranium and hematite mining	Lung	Radon daughters	—
Asbestos production	Insulating material production (pipes, sheeting, textile, clothes, masks, asbestos cement products)	Lung, pleural and peritoneal mesothelioma	Asbestos	*14*[83]
Petroleum industry	Shale-oil production	Skin, scrotum	Polynuclear aromatic hydrocarbons	35[84]
Metal industry	Copper smelting	Lung	Arsenic	23[82]
	Chromate production	Lung	Chromium	23[82]
	Chromium plating	Lung	Chromium	23[82]
	Ferrochromium production	Lung	Chromium	23[82]
	Nickel refining	Nasal sinuses, lung	Nickel[a]	*11*[85]
	Metal machining	Skin	Mineral oils (containing various additives and impurities)	33[86]

(continued)

TABLE 5. (*Continued*)

Industry	Occupation	Cancer site	Substance reported or suspected to be the causative agent	*IARC Monographs* reference
Shipbuilding, motor vehicle and transport	Shipyard and dockyard	Lung, pleural and peritoneal mesothelioma	Asbestos	*14*[83]
Chemical industry	Bis(chloromethyl)ether (BCME) and chloromethyl methyl ether (CMME) production and use	Lung (oat-cell carcinoma)	BCME, CCME	*4*[87]
	Vinyl chloride producers	Liver angiosarcoma	Vinyl chloride monomer	*19*[88]
	Isopropyl alcohol manufacture (strong-acid process)	Paranasal sinuses	Not identified	*15*[89]
	Pigment chromate production	Lung	Chromium	*23*[82]
	Dye manufacture and use	Bladder	Benzidine, β-naphthylamine, 4-aminobiphenyl	*29*[90], *4*[87], *1*[91]
	Auramine manufacture	Bladder	Auramine (and other aromatic amines used in the process)	*1*[91]
Pesticides and herbicides production industry	Arsenical insecticides production and packaging	Lung	Arsenic	*23*[82]
Gas industry	Coke plant work	Lung	Polycyclic aromatic hydrocarbons	*34*[92]
	Gas work	Lung, bladder, scrotum	Coal carbonization products, β-naphthylamine	*34*[92]
	Gas retort-house work	Bladder	β-naphthylamine	*34*[92]

Rubber industry	Rubber manufacture	Lymphatic and hematopoietic system (leukemia)	Benzene	29[90]
		Bladder	Aromatic amines	1[91], 4[87]
	Calendering, tire curing, tire building	Lymphatic and hematopoietic system (leukemia)	Benzene	29[90]
	Milling, mixing	Bladder	Aromatic amines	1[91]
	Synthetic latex production, tire curing, calender operating, reclaim, cable making	Bladder	Aromatic amines	4[87]
Construction industry	Insulating and pipe covering, demolition work	Lung, pleural and peritoneal mesothelioma	Asbestos	14[83]
Leather industry	Boot and shoe manufacture, repair	Nose, bone marrow (leukemia)	Leather dust, benzene	25[93]
Wood pulp and paper industry	Furniture and cabinet making	Nose (adenocarcinoma)	Wood dust	25[93]
Textile industry	Mule-spinning	Skin	Mineral oils (containing various additives and impurities)	33[86]
Other	Roofing, asphalt work	Lung	Polycyclic aromatic hydrocarbons	35[84]
	Jute processing	Skin	Mineral oils (containing various additives and impurities)	33[86]
	Chimney sweeping and other exposures to soot	Scrotum	Polycyclic aromatic hydrocarbons	35[84]

[a]The specific compound(s) responsible for a carcinogenic effect cannot be precisely specified.

occupational exposures to cancers of specific sites. The proportion of lung cancer in men in Norway, the U.S.A., and Italy ranged from 13 to 33%.[13–16] Similarly, the risk of bladder cancer attributable to occupational factors ranged between 1 and 19% for men in the U.S.A., England, and Italy.[17–19]

Diet and Nutrition

There is a widespread consensus that the proportion of all cancer cases attributable to diet is relatively high, even though the percentages proposed by different authors vary considerably.[10–12] In spite of the presumed importance attributed to the role of diet, however, none of the risk factors causally associated with cancer in humans appears to be directly related to dietary exposure, with the exception of alcohol. This may be due to the difficulties in carrying out analytical epidemiological studies in populations that have heavily contrasting dietary habits. Most dietary customs that have been incriminated—excess intake of fat, excess calorie intake, and deficit of fiber—are characteristic of the so-called "Western diet."

There is a strong positive correlation between per capita fat consumption and the incidence of colorectal, breast, endometrial, and prostatic cancer internationally.[20–21] A number of case-control studies have shown an association between high fat intake or fat-containing foods and the risk of colorectal, breast, or prostatic cancer (for references, see IARC[22]). Most of these studies showed relatively weak associations with relative risks for high versus low consumption of the order of two.

The epidemiological evidence that high total calorie intake increases the risk of cancer is weak. In studies of breast or colon and rectal cancers, a weaker association was found with high calorie intake than with high fat intake.[23,24] Total calorie intake was associated with risk of colorectal cancer in South Australia, but dietary protein was a more consistent risk factor.[25]

Although obesity and excess body weight is associated with breast and endometrial cancer, it does not seem to be associated with colorectal cancer. In addition, there is no direct relationship between obesity and calorie intake.[26]

Some studies suggest excess risk of breast or colorectal cancer from excess protein intake (e.g., Potter and McMichael[25]; Haenszel et al.[27]; Lubin et al.[28]); however, there has been little experimental evidence that protein per se is a carcinogenic risk factor.

An IARC study in areas with large variations in colon cancer incidence revealed a significant inverse relationship between dietary fiber intake and large-bowel cancer frequency.[29] Dietary fiber intake was significantly higher in a low-risk area (Kuopio, Finland) than in Copenhagen (Denmark). In a second IARC-coordinated study,[30] a significant inverse trend between large-bowel cancer incidence and cereal consumption and total dietary fiber intake was observed.

Viruses and Other Biological Agents

Viruses Many animal tumors can be transmitted by DNA viruses (whose genetic material becomes integrated with that of the host) or retroviruses (RNA viruses capable of transcribing genetic material in reverse from viral RNA to host DNA). In both cases, the resulting integrated viral DNA is replicated together with that of the host, and this process of integration of viral DNA is associated with malignant transformation.

Associations can be demonstrated between several human tumors and viruses. Evans[31] has suggested criteria that can be used to establish whether such associations represent a causal link:

- Antibodies to the virus should occur more frequently and at higher titers in cases of disease than in controls, and, preferably, *before* the onset of the disease;
- A viral genome should be found in tumor tissue, but should be absent in normal tissue;
- The virus should be able to induce malignant transformation of cells in vitro;
- Experimental data on tumor induction and viral integration in animals are also important.

Convincing evidence will be provided by the demonstration that prevention of infection by a given virus (by vaccination) reduces the incidence of a tumor in the setting (geographical or environmental) in which their association has been shown to exist.

The first human retrovirus to be isolated, now referred to as HTLV I, was discovered in patients with a distinct clinicopathological entity called adult T-cell leukemia/lymphoma (ATLL). Clusters of this disease have been identified in Japan, in the West Indies, in the southern U.S.A. among blacks, and in certain African nations. The virus appears to be capable of transmitting cancer in vitro and the epidemiological features of the disease in endemic areas suggest that this also occurs in human populations.[32]

The Epstein-Barr virus (EBV) has been implicated in the causation of

Burkitt's lymphoma and has also been associated with nasopharyngeal cancer. Burkitt's lymphoma occurs in high incidence in children in many parts of sub-Saharan Africa, between 10° North and 10° South of the equator, and in Papuà-New Guinea—areas where malaria is holoendemic—and at a much lower frequency elsewhere.[33] In high incidence areas, antibody titers to EBV are high and present at a young age, and EBV DNA and EBV nuclear antigen are present in tumor cells in over 95% of cases.[34] EBV has been shown to be oncogenic in experimentally infected New World primates,[35] although the lymphoma induced has important dissimilarities (e.g., polyclonal versus monoclonal) from Burkitt's lymphoma.[36] The role of EBV in endemic areas appears to occur through early and massive infection leading to a large population of infected B lymphocytes that secrete vast amounts of immunoglobulins and antibodies, while repeated malarial attacks reduce the T-cell control of such populations.[37] This B-cell subpopulation may subsequently be the target of chromosomal translocations that are particularly relevant to neoplastic transformation of these cells. Of more than 100 Burkitt's lymphoma cell lines that have been analyzed, all showed one of three translocations—t(8;14), t(8;22), or t(2;8)—which appear to be relevant to the activation of the *c-myc* protooncogene.[38]

EBV is also associated with nasopharyngeal carcinoma (NPC). Like Burkitt's lymphoma, this tumor has a distinctive geographical distribution, affecting principally populations living in or originating from southern China, with a zone of intermediate risk in northern Africa.[39] The evidence linking EBV with NPC is similar to that for Burkitt's lymphoma, except that elevated titers of viral-capsid-antigen and early-antigen antibodies to EBV are found in the IgA fraction of serum. The presence of these antibodies in the early stages of the disease has suggested that they may provide a useful means of early detection on a mass scale in high-risk areas.[40]

There is considerable epidemiological and experimental evidence linking hepatitis B virus (HBV) with hepatocellular carcinoma (HCC). A close correlation exists between the geographical distribution of the incidence or mortality from HCC and the prevalence of carriers of hepatitis B surface antigen (HBsAg) in the population.[41] Numerous case-control studies suggest that the relative risk of HCC associated with chronic carriage of HBsAg is 10–20,[42] while prospective studies of carriers suggest that their excess risk of HCC may be up to 200-fold that of HBsAg-negative individuals.[43] This strong association between HBV and HCC is also very specific, since there is no risk for other cancers associated with chronic carriage of HBsAg. Experimentally, hybridization studies using cloned purified HBV DNA have shown that it is integrated into the genome of malignant cells from patients with HCC as well as liver cells of long-term HBsAg carriers.[44] Viruses that closely resemble HBV have been found in several animal species—in particular, the American woodchuck (*Marmota menax*) is susceptible to chronic infection by a hepatitis virus, the DNA of which integrates with the host genome, which is associated with the development of chronic active hepatitis and HCC.[45] The evidence that HBV is an important causal factor for HCC is thus very strong, although it is neither a necessary nor sufficient cause, and aflatoxin, a powerful hepatic carcinogen in animals, may also play a role in humans.[46] The ultimate proof of causality will be provided by demonstration that elimination of HBV infection with newly available vaccines is able to prevent the development of HCC.

The human papilloma virus (HPV) causes several benign papillomas, and also flat areas (condylomata) of the uterine cervix which have the histological features of dysplasia, long-known to be a precursor of carcinomatous change in the cervical epithelium. The availability of cloned specific DNA from HPV has allowed the search for HPV DNA in human tissue. DNA specific to types 16 and 18 has been found in some 80% of cell or tissue specimens from patients with dysplasia, and carcinoma in situ and invasive cancer of the cervix, but not in normal tissue. In contrast, types 6 and 11 are more often associated with benign genital warts or mild dysplasia.[47] There is some evidence that women with evidence of asymptomatic HPV infection are at a higher risk of the subsequent development of in situ cancer.[48,49] To date, these studies have lacked a satisfactory design, and the excess risk associated with infection by different HPV subtypes is hard to determine. The lack of a suitable serological test for HPV infection has also made such studies difficult.

PARASITES The link between the malaria parasite (*Plasmodium falciparum*) and Burkitt's lymphoma has been referred to above. The most important link between parasitic disease and human cancer is that between infection with *Schistosoma haematobium* and squamous cell carcinoma of the bladder in Egypt, Southeast Africa, and other areas of the Middle East. Several possible mechanisms have been postulated: chronic irritation due to the presence of schistosome eggs in the bladder, production of carcinogenic toxins by mirecidia or worms, alteration of liver function by hepatic schistosomiasis with consequent urinary excretion, and secondary bacterial infections that may complicate urinary schistosomiasis.[50] There is a close correlation between infection with liver flukes (*Clonorchis sinensis* and *Opisthorchis viverrini*) and the occurrence of cholangiocarcinoma in southern China and other parts of the

Southeast Area.[51] The mechanism of action is obscure, but probably depends not only on the length and severity of infection and the immune response to it, but also upon interaction with other carcinogens, possibly dietary of origin.

Radiation

IONIZING RADIATION The carcinogenic effects of ionizing radiation have been investigated more thoroughly than those of any other environmental agent. Far-reaching developments in atomic energy, notably the production of nuclear weapons and the expanding use of atomic energy for electric power, have created a climate of concern about the potential risks of low-level irradiation.

Ionizing radiation includes electromagnetic radiation (such as X rays and gamma rays) and particulate radiation of varying masses and charges (such as protons, electrons, and alpha particles). When such radiations penetrate matter, they have the capacity of producing ions and reactive radicals from atoms and molecules in their paths by adding or removing electrons. Radiation is thought to induce cancer by the absorption of energy within the cells, leading to the formation of free radicals (OH) that damage DNA; this is followed by an increase in the frequency of mutations and chromosomal aberrations. The molecular mechanisms of radiation carcinogenesis, however, remain to be determined precisely.

The incidence of all major forms of leukemia, except the chronic lymphocytic form, has been seen to increase in humans after irradiation of the whole body or a major part of the hemopoietic bone marrow. The increase can be detected within years after irradiation and is dose-dependent.[52]

Epidemiological studies have also revealed that the thyroid gland is highly susceptible to radiation carcinogenesis. The incidence of thyroid tumors is increased in atomic-bomb survivors,[53,54] in patients given radiation therapy on the neck region during infancy,[55,56] in patients given x-ray therapy on the scalp in childhood for treatment of tinea capitis,[57,58] and in other populations with a history of thyroid irradiation.[59,60]

An increased incidence in lung cancer has been observed in atomic-bomb survivors,[61] in patients treated with spinal irradiation for ankylosing spondylitis,[62,63] and in hard-rock miners exposed to radon.[64–66]

The female breast has been found to be one of the organs most susceptible to radiation carcinogenesis.[52] This is based on epidemiological data on women surviving atomic-bomb irradiation,[67,68] and on women given radiation therapy to the breast for acute postpartum mastitis or other benign diseases.[69,70]

There is also evidence that many other organs, such as the stomach, colon and rectum, liver, pancreas, skin, and bladder, show an increased incidence of cancer (see, e.g., National Institutes of Health[52]; National Research Council[71,72]).

NONIONIZING RADIATION Two forms of nonionizing radiation have been suspected of increasing the risk of cancer: ultraviolet radiation and electromagnetic fields.

Ultraviolet radiation in the form of sunlight: The evidence that sunlight, and therefore presumably ultraviolet radiation, increases the risk of nonmelanocytic skin cancer is quite convincing. Occupational groups of nonpigmented races exposed to sunlight have a substantially increased risk of both basal cell and squamous carcinoma of the lip, face, and arms (cf. IARC[73]; Scott[74]).

Exposure to electromagnetic fields has only recently been suspected of increasing the risk of cancer, particularly acute myeloid leukemia (for references, see Marino and Morris[75]). The evidence is so far inconclusive, especially that from attempts to relate cases of leukemia to assumed exposure to electromagnetic fields through varying voltage patterns in household electricity,[76,77] although there is some evidence that persons occupationally exposed to electromagnetic radiation may have an increased risk of leukemia.[78–81]

POTENTIAL FOR CANCER PREVENTION

PRIMARY PREVENTION

Primary prevention implies avoidance of the occurrence of cancer, either by reducing exposure of individuals to causative agents in the environment or by enhancing resistance to them. The absolute maximum reduction in cancer that could be so achieved can be seen from estimates of the proportion of cancer cases in a given population that can be ascribed to external, environmental causes (as opposed to the component of risk which is endogenous or genetically determined). There have been several exercises designed to estimate this proportion (e.g., Doll and Peto[10]; Higginson and Muir[11]; Wynder and Gori[12]) which use essentially the same methodologies.

Particularly important is the difference in incidence rates between various communities, differences that vary greatly depending on the type of cancer; for example, rates for esophageal cancer and liver cancer may vary as much as 100-fold in different parts of the world. The data recorded in *Cancer Incidence in Five Continents*[94,95] have been widely used to illustrate international variations (see Table 6).

The difference in incidence observed between genetically similar populations has been taken to illustrate the excess risk that might reasonably be ascribed to environmental differences. Table 6 shows the ratio of highest : lowest rates for "European" populations (Europe, North America, Australia/New Zealand). Comparisons of incidence rates *within* countries may also show very large differences in risk, which can only plausibly be ascribed to differential environmental exposure—in China, for example, mortality rates from esophageal cancer vary as much as 25-fold[96] and even for a relatively nonvariable tumor such as colon cancer (Table 6), incidence rates in a small country such as Scotland can show threefold differences.[97] Communities may be defined other than by geography, and information on specific religious, ethnic, or socioeconomic groups may show similar differences in rates. Religious groups that eschew tobacco smoking, for example, have incidence rates for lung cancer that are considerably below the community

TABLE 6. Highest and Lowest Age-Standardized Incidence Rates (per 10^5) for 12 Cancers, Comparing All Registries, and "European" Registries[a]

	Highest		Lowest		Ratio
	World	European	European	World	(European)
Males					
Mouth	13.0	13.0	0.6	0.5	21.7
Nasopharynx	32.9	1.8	0.3	0.3	6.0
Esophagus	24.7	18.9	1.1	1.1	17.2
Stomach	100.2	43.6	5.7	3.7	7.6
Colon	32.3	32.3	5.2	3.1	6.2
Liver	34.4	11.8	0.6	0.6	19.7
Pancreas	18.3	11.4	3.3	1.0	3.4
Lung	107.2	96.8	18.6	1.1[b]	5.2
Prostate	100.2	59.7	6.6	0.8	9.0
Bladder	30.2	30.2	3.1	2.4	9.7
Females					
Breast	87.5	85.6	16.2	8.9	5.3
Cervix	52.9	30.1	3.8	2.1	7.9

[a]From Waterhouse et al.[95]
[b]Rate for Senegal, next lowest in New Mexico Indians, 8.1.

average as recorded by cancer registries, so that the size of the environmental component of risk is greater than that implied in Table 6.

Migrant studies have been particularly useful in illustrating how much the incidence of a particular cancer can be changed by differences in environment. The studies of Haenszel and Kurihara[98] on Japanese migrants to the U.S.A. showed how the mortality experience of this group begins to approach that of the host country, although the speed with which this occurs varies for different cancers, implying differences in the age at which environmental factors are important and demonstrating the rapidity with which certain important life-style elements (e.g., diet) are modified in migrant groups. Similarly, time-trend studies within the same community indicate that the risk of individual cancers can change quite rapidly with time. Although the possibility of artifacts of diagnosis or recording must be considered, there are many instances of quite dramatic change that are only explicable in terms of changes in environmental exposure (see next section).

The generalized approach described above allows an estimate of the overall potential for prevention by indicating the proportion of the risk due to "environment." However, the identification of the environmental exposures that are relevant to causation depends upon both experimental and epidemiological data. Quantitation of the possible preventive effect of eliminating exposure to a risk factor requires that data on the size of the risk posed by defined hazards be available. This is usually expressed as the relative risk (see above). If the proportion of the population that is exposed to the risk factor is also known, then it is possible to calculate the proportion of the disease that would be removed by eliminating exposure. This is known as the *population attributable risk* of a particular exposure, which represents the potential benefit that might be obtained from intervention measures and is usually relatively time or population specific. However, it should be remembered that some causative agents interact with others to produce effects that are greater than the sum of the effects of the agents separately (e.g., alcohol and tobacco in cancer of the esophagus[8]). Thus, eliminating *either* factor may prevent a substantial percentage of the cancer in question, and eliminating both together may not produce much more benefit. This rather complicates calculations of attribution of risk, since it may well be that addition of estimates of population attributable risk for different factors will sum to more than 100%.

Two other factors must be considered when estimating the possible effects of intervention against risk factors in the environment. First, it is generally an oversimplification to consider risk factors as a dichotomy (exposed versus not)—in many cases a quantitative reduction in exposure is more likely. In such cases, the relationship between dose and response in exposure is important—for cigarette smoking and lung cancer this is approximately linear, but this may not always be so, and for some agents (e.g., perhaps dietary fat), there may be a threshold above which additional exposure adds little to risk. Second, exogenous agents act at different stages of the carcinogenic process, so that some interventions may produce relatively rapid reductions in risk (e.g., removing exposure to exogenous estrogen produces a rapid decline in risk of endometrial cancer), whereas with others (e.g., smoking and lung cancer) the decline in relative risk is much slower.

Oral cancer (mouth, tongue, oropharynx) is in theory largely preventable: the major risk factors are alcohol plus tobacco smoking in Western countries and the chewing of tobacco (with or without betel) in many countries of southern and Southeast Asia. Cancer of the nasopharynx appears to be related to infection with EBV virus (as earlier noted) and possibly also to consumption of salted fish in Chinese populations[99]—the advent of a vaccine effective against the former may indicate more clearly the potential for prevention. Both esophageal cancer and larynx cancer are closely related to alcohol–tobacco consumption in western countries, where the population attributable risk from these agents may be up to 80%. In other areas of the world with very high risk of esophageal cancer (parts of China, central Asia, Southeast Africa), the causative agents are less clear; however, poor overall nutrition is a feature of such areas, so that general dietary improvement may be a valuable preventive measure.

Stomach cancer is showing a general decline in incidence everywhere. This is generally ascribed to changes in nutrition, in particular greater availability of fresh food, and a reduction in traditional methods of storage and preservation (smoking, pickling, salting). This trend will almost certainly continue, since it seems from migrant studies which provide data on age at migration (e.g., Japanese to the U.S.A.) that the level of risk is determined at quite an early age. For colorectal cancer, the major associations appear to be with diet—a low fat/high fiber diet decreasing the risk, with a possible protective effect from dietary calcium. It is not clear how effective changes in dietary habits would be in reducing risk, however, and there are no observations available on sufficiently large populations to indicate whether this is likely to be successful.

In high-risk areas (Africa, South and East Asia), the great majority of liver cancer is attributable to chronic infection with hepatitis B virus (as noted in the previous section). Current programs of vaccination will clearly demonstrate the effectiveness of preventive measures. The role of aflatoxin is less certain, but may well by synergistic with HBV infection, so that its effect in noncarriers of HBsAg may be relatively small. However, it will take many years before programs of neonatal vaccination substantially reduce population prevalence of HBsAg, so, in the interim, measures to reduce aflatoxin intake seem eminently sensible.

Lung cancer is probably the most prevalent cancer in men in the world today. It is almost entirely attributable to cigarette smoking, which is very prevalent in many societies, and confers a high relative risk of disease.[5] Strategies of prevention include persuading adult smokers to quit, which would have an immediate impact on incidence and mortality, and discouraging teenagers from taking up the habit—possibly a more realistic strategy, but one unlikely to bear fruit for 30 or more years. Low-tar and filter cigarettes are known to carry lower risks, and a substantial switch to such brands could also markedly reduce disease. General air pollution may possibly confer a small additional risk in itself, but would also be synergistic with smoking, and is a factor to which relatively large segments of the population (city dwellers) are exposed. Several occupational risks are known (particularly exposure to uranium and asbestos) which carry high excess risks, also synergistic with tobacco; however, because of the small percentage of the population exposed, the proportion of lung cancers attributable to the occupations may be less than 10%.

Miller[100] ascribes 20% of breast cancer risk to dietary fat, 25% to age at first pregnancy, and 20% to familial factors. It is not at all clear that any of these could realistically be converted into preventive action—indeed, because of the more urgent priorities of many countries in the field of population control (involving delaying age at first birth), a continued rise in breast cancer incidence can be foreseen. Reduction in fat intake and in obesity may be effective decreasing incidence, and the latter may also reduce rates of endometrial cancer.

Cervical cancer presents a major challenge to prevention—epidemiological studies have strongly implicated an infectious etiology, probably sexually transmitted. In theory then, it should be feasible to reduce transmission (and subsequent disease) by advocating a return to more puritanical life-styles. Until recently, this has seemed unlikely to succeed as a preventive strategy, although the current epidemic of autoimmune deficiency syndrome (AIDS) may prove persuasive; further work on the role that certain viral infections may have (human papillomavirus[101]), with the possibility of developing effective vaccines, is clearly important.

Bladder cancer is a common tumor in men in many countries. In western societies, a substantial proportion (perhaps half) might be prevented by abandoning cigarette smoking—and, in some areas, occupationally induced tumors provide a substantial minority. The role of schistosomiasis has been described above, but prevention of this disease has proved extremely difficult in endemic areas.

Secondary Prevention

Secondary prevention is generally taken to embrace screening (the detection of unrecognized disease/precursor conditions) and early diagnosis. The objective of both is to begin treatment at an early stage in the disease process, so that a more favorable outcome is achieved. This is usually measured in terms of changes in mortality; clearly, incidence of disease is not affected, while measurement of survival or case-fatality rates is beset by problems of interpretation (see Prorok et al.[102]).

Screening tests are generally applied to large numbers of subjects, and should ideally be simple, inexpensive, safe, or free from side effects and acceptable to the population. They distinguish a group of persons who probably have the disease in question and must be further investigated from a group who probably do not. The validity of a screening test is measured in terms of its sensitivity (ability to classify diseased subjects as negative) and specificity (ability to classify disease-free individuals as negative). The yield of positive results will also depend upon the prevalence of the condition being sought in the population—this can be increased if examinations are confined to subgroups of the populations at high risk. Although such "selective screening" has an intuitive appeal, for the common screening programs for cancer (see below) it is not possible to select subgroups, on criteria other than age, that have a sufficiently high relative risk such that the majority of cases are confined to them.

The utility of screening programs has to be evaluated in terms of the benefits (e.g., the reduction in mortality or savings in person-years of life) in relation to costs. The costs of screening include not only those of providing the tests and follow-up treatment facilities, but also the lengthening of morbidity in screen-detected cases in whom the morbidity is unaltered, the probable delay in receiving treatment of cases who screen false-negative, and the anxiety and unnecessary investigation of false-positive cases.

The benefits of screening are a reduction in mortality in the population, and this is ideally tested by means of a randomized controlled trial. Unfortunately, these have rarely been carried out to test the efficacy of screening, in part because of logistic problems and partly because of ethical qualms (protagonists of screening are usually convinced of efficacy in advance and are unwilling to contemplate an unscreened group of controls). In the absence of trials, efficacy must be judged by classical epidemiological observational studies—cohort studies or case-control studies—which are subject to selection biases and confounding, or, even less satisfactory, inferences drawn from time trends or geographical comparisons.

Oral cancer would seem to be an ideal candidate for screening—lesions that appear to be precursors of squamous cell carcinoma can be detected by nonmedical workers in mass-examination campaigns.[103] However, whether such detection is effective in preventing invasive disease or mortality is unknown.

Gastric cancer screening by photofluorography has been widely used in Japan, but there has been no controlled trial. Hirayama et al.[104] reported a correlation between age-specific frequency of screening and reduction in mortality, and other studies have suggested lower mortality than expected in persons undergoing regular examinations, but selection bias cannot be excluded as an explanation.[105,106] The issue of effectiveness seems unclear and, in countries where stomach cancer is less common than in Japan, screening could hardly be considered worthwhile.

Screening for colorectal cancer by regular testing for fecal occult blood is currently being evaluated in trials in the U.S.A., the UK, Denmark, and Sweden. It is known that the test has low specificity, so that many false positives require investigation, and it seems uncertain that the (probable) small benefit from screening could offset the costs involved.

Breast cancer remains the only malignancy for which randomized trials confirm the benefits of screening. The original HIP study was started in 1963 and employed annual mammography plus palpation as the screening tests; follow-up results for 14 years are now available[107] and confirm a significant reduction in mortality, principally in women over the age of 50 at the time of entry. A second trial in Sweden employed single-view mammography alone—in women aged 50 or more (screened at intervals of 30–36 months), a mortality reduction of 40% was achieved.[108] Nonrandomized trials in the Netherlands have substantially confirmed these results. It thus seems that the maximum benefit that could be achieved in terms of a reduction in breast cancer mortality, given imperfect compliance and doubtful efficacy in younger women, is a reduction by about one-quarter. The costs involved in organizing the necessary examinations and follow-up are considerable and, even where breast cancer is of major importance, introduction of mass screening will be a contentious issue and clearly beyond the means of any but the richest nations.

For cervix cancer, there have been no controlled trials, but there is a mass of evidence now available from correlation and observational studies confirming the efficacy of regular smears in preventing invasive cancer.[109] The major concern now is to find the most satisfactory design for screening programs, in particular the ages at which screening should be offered and the frequency of testing. The protection offered by different screening intervals can be deduced from information on the relative risk of invasive cancer at different times after a negative test; results derived from the data of 10 different screening programs are shown in Table 7.[110] It appears from this table that there is a protective effect for up to 10 years, so that, even with very limited resources, a screening program concentrating upon high-risk groups (women over 35) with very infrequent tests (say, every 10 years) could prevent up to half the cases of cervix cancer (provided that compliance with screening, follow-up, and treatment of women who screen positive is satisfactory). With more abundant resources, more frequent screening and inclusion of younger women can be performed, but the ratio between benefit obtained and the costs of the program diminishes accordingly, and policies involving very frequent examinations (annual) of low-risk women (under 25) are likely to be very cost-ineffective.

TABLE 7. Relative Risk of Invasive Cancer following a Negative Cervical Smear

Months since last negative smear	Relative risk
0–11	0.07
12–23	0.08
24–35	0.12
36–47	0.19
48–59	0.36
60–71	0.28
72–119	0.63
120+	1.2
Never	1.0

Trends in Cancer Incidence and Mortality

In an earlier section, we described how the age structure of a population was the most important determinant of the number of cancer cases occurring therein. Thus, much of the current stature of cancer in the developed countries of the world is due to the progressive aging of their populations during the present century. A recent analysis of mortality data from 28 developed nations for the period 1960–1980 found that 60% of the increased number of deaths in males was explained by age changes in the countries concerned, while for females all of the observed increase was due to such demographic change—indeed the observed number of cancer cases in 1980 was slightly *less* than aging of the population alone would have accounted for.[111]

World standard population growth (1975–2000) is estimated at about 1.7% per year, but is uneven in different age groups, and an increase of 73% in the population over 65 is forecast (a 45% rise in developed countries and 103% in developing countries).[112] On this basis alone, therefore, there is likely to be a considerable increase in the number of cancers, and in the relative importance of cancer as a cause of morbidity and mortality. Based on the incidence rates in Table 2, for example, the expected number of new cancer cases in the year 2000 might be as high as 10 million. Although trends and projections of the cancer burden are an essential element in the planning of services for cancer control, the epidemiologist is more interested in changes in individual risk of cancer as an indication of changes in exposure to causative agents or susceptibility to them. This is achieved by comparisons of age-specific incidence or mortality, or by using summary statistics that have been standardized to correct for differences in the age composition of the populations being compared.

Before attributing changes in incidence or mortality to an alteration in risk of cancer, the possibility that they are due to artifacts in data collection or interpretation should be considered.

Incidence data derive from cancer registries. The incidence rates recorded will depend on the efficiency of case ascertainment, which may increase, especially during the early years of operation of a registry, giving rise to apparent increases in incidence. There have been new diagnostic techniques introduced over the years in radiology and biochemistry, so that apparent changes in frequency of certain cancers may be simply due to more accurate identification. Finally, the definition of an "incident" cancer case may change with time—there has certainly been an increasing tendency to regard all bladder papillomas as "malignant" in the last 30 years, and criteria for diagnosis of cancer for thyroid and breast have also changed.

Mortality data are similarly affected by improvements in diagnosis; there are additional problems associated with certification of underlying cause of death and its coding by the International Classification of Diseases (which itself undergoes periodic revisions in structure and nomenclature) that can introduce spurious trends in mortality rates. A more fundamental problem is the use of mortality to indicate disease risk in the face of underlying changes in survival; where there have been advances in therapy for cancer (e.g., childhood leukemia, Hodgkin's disease), mortality rates may show quite marked declines (e.g., Miller and McKay[113]) even though underlying incidence may be unchanged or even increasing.

The simplest method of assessing time trends in a population is to examine a graph of age-standardized incidence or mortality, which shows the average trend, for all ages combined. However, it is much more instructive to examine trends for individual age groups—these frequently show that the summary age-standardized rates hide marked differences at individual ages. When such differences are present, they may be due either to a change in the risk of cancer affecting successive generations (a "birth cohort" effect), or changes that affect all age groups at the same date (a "period" effect). Figure 2 shows data for mortality from carcinoma of lung in females in England and Wales between 1941 and 1978. The curve for the age-standardized rate (2a) shows a progressive rise in mortality, but, when age-specific rates are examined (2b), it is evident that this is not the case at all ages: in the young, mortality rates have been falling recently, since 1960 at ages 30–34, for example. Rearranging this figure (Figure 2) so that the x axis becomes year of birth (rather than death), it is clear that the fall in mortality affects all age groups in women born since around 1926—in other words, it is a feature of different generations or birth cohorts, rather than relating to a particular time period.

Many other cancers show trends in incidence and mortality rates that follow this pattern. A striking example is provided by stomach cancer, the incidence and mortality rates for which have been showing a decline in almost all countries and affecting successive generations, so that the overall drop in risk (all ages) is around 2–3% per year. The reverse is true for malignant melanoma of the skin, where there is a cohort-specific rise in incidence (and mortality), affecting particularly light-skinned populations. The overall rise in risk is as much as 3–7%

per year, both in males and females, making this one of the most striking "epidemics" currently observable.

The time trends in lung cancer, alluded to above, are very interesting. In many countries, at least in the developing world, there is a progressive rise in incidence and mortality in females, coincident with adoption of the smoking habit. However, in England and Wales, as noted above, there is already evidence of a drop in generations both since 1926. In males, by contrast, in those countries where the cigarette-smoking habit was adopted early (England, Finland), maximum rates occurred in generations born at the turn of the century, with evident declines since that time. This effect is seen in later generations elsewhere (e.g., U.S.A., northern Europe), and, where the tobacco habit is a relatively recent acquisition, the progressive increase between successive generations continues.[5]

Cancer of the large bowel (colon, rectum) is showing an increase in

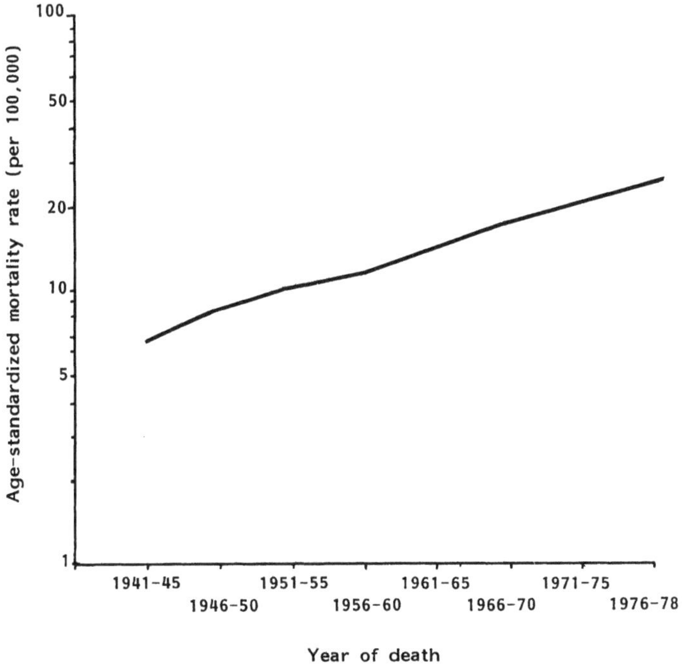

FIGURE 2. Mortality for lung cancer (ICD 162), females, England and Wales. (a) Rates standardized in population of 1951–55. (b) Age-specific rates by year of death. (c) Age-specific rates by year of birth.

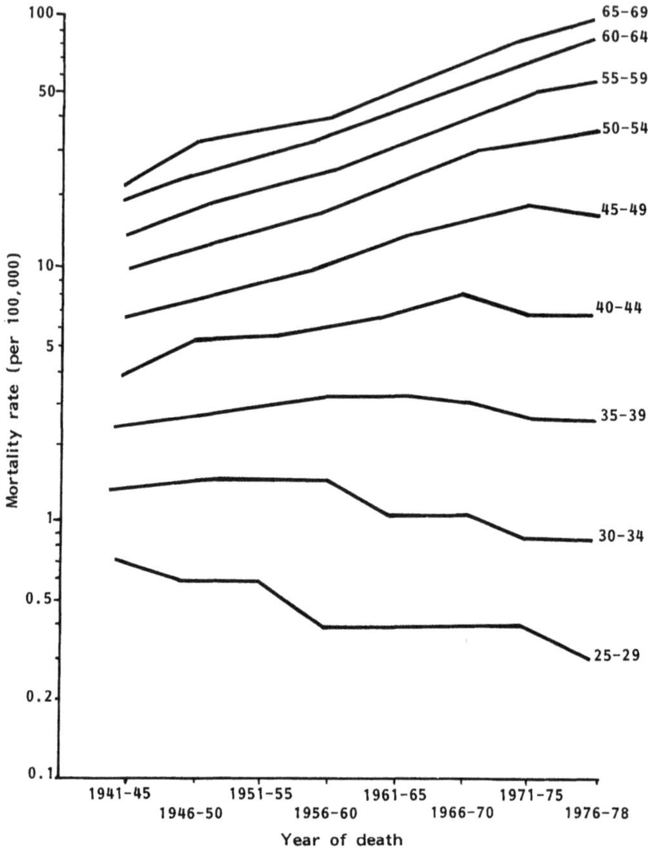

FIGURE 2. (*Continued*)

incidence and mortality in most countries—the rate of rise being in general higher where the current rates are relatively low. The same is true for pancreatic cancer and, although part of this may be due to enhanced diagnostic accuracy, this cancer is emerging as a major cause of mortality in developed countries.

The two major cancers in females show very different trends in occurrence. Breast cancer incidence is increasing almost everywhere at a rate around 2% per annum. However, in countries with high mortality (Scandinavia, U.S.A.), there is rather little change in mortality rates, though these too are rising elsewhere; the explanation for this disparity

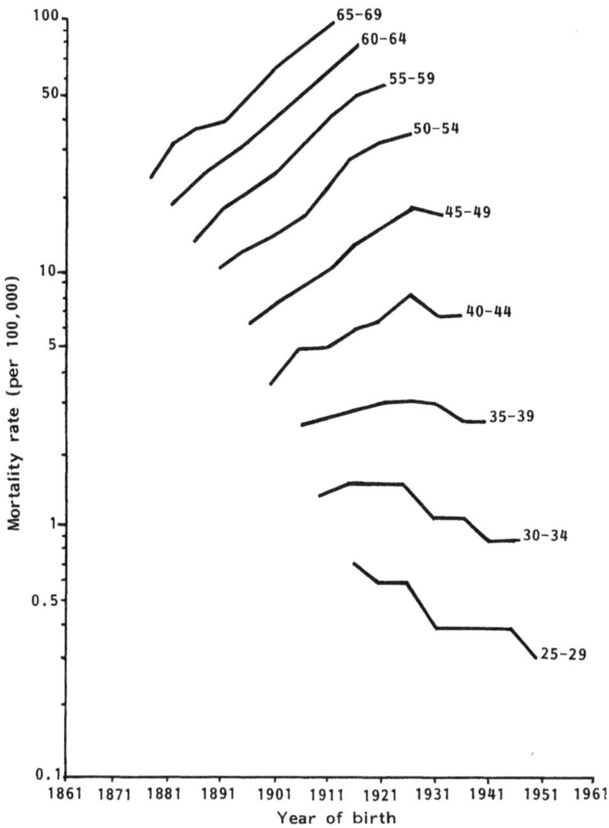

Figure 2. (*Continued*)

between incidence and mortality may lie in changing diagnostic criteria. Carcinoma of the cervix, by contrast, is showing declines in incidence and mortality rates, especially in Europe and North America. Superimposed upon the primarily cohort-specific declines is a period-related decline in rates where successful programs of cytological screening have been introduced.[114] Disquietingly, this trend has been interrupted in Britain and Australia, where young women (born since 1935) are showing a striking increase in risk.

Other than the very general outline presented here, it is difficult to summarize all of the changes in risk for different cancers in different countries of the world. However, data such as these stimulate a search for explanations or provide confirmation or cast doubt upon established hypotheses.

References

1. WHO: *World Health Statistics Annual 1984*. Geneva, WHO,1984.
2. Cook PJ, Doll RD, Fellingham SA: A mathematical model for the age distribution of cancer in man. *Int J Cancer* 1969; 4:93–112.
3. Parkin DM, Stjernswärd J, Muir CS: Estimates of the worldwide frequency of twelve major cancers. *Bull WHO* 1984; 62:163–182.
4. IARC: IARC Monographs on the Evaluation of the Carcinogenic Risk of Chemicals to Humans, Vol 37, *Tobacco Habits Other Than Smoking; Betel-quid and Areca-nut Chewing; and Some Related Nitrosamines*. Lyon, 1985.
5. IARC: IARC Monographs on the Evaluation of the Carcinogenic Risk of Chemicals to Humans, Vol 38, *Tobacco Smoking*. Lyon, 1986.
6. Walsh B, Grant M: *Public Health Implications of Alcohol Production and Trade*. WHO offset publication No 88. Geneva, WHO, 1985.
7. Tuyns AJ: Alcohol, in Schottenfeld D, Fraumeni JR Jr (eds): *Cancer Epidemiology and Prevention*. Philadelphia, PA, WB Saunders, 1982, pp 293–303.
8. Tuyns AJ, Pequignot G, Jensen, OM: Les cancer de l'oesophage en Ile et Vilaine en fonction des niveaux de consommation d'alcool et de tabac. Des risques qui se multiplient. 1977; *Bull Cancer* 64:45–60.
9. Hemminki K, Vainio H: Human exposure to potentially carcinogenic compounds, in Berlin A, Draper M, Hemminki K, Vainio H (eds): *Monitoring Human Exposure to Carcinogenic and Mutagenic Agents*. IARC Scientific Publications No 59. Lyon, International Agency for Research on Cancer, 1984, pp 37–45.
10. Doll R, Peto R: *The Causes of Cancer*. Oxford, Oxford University Press, 1981.
11. Higginson J, Muir CS: Environmental carcinogenesis: Misconceptions and limitations to cancer control. *J Natl Cancer Inst* 1979; 63:1291–1298.
12. Wynder EL, Gori GB: Contribution of the environment to cancer incidence: an epidemiologic exercise. *J Natl Cancer Inst* 1977; 58:825–832.
13. Kjuus H, Lislerud A, Lyngdal PT, et al: Cancer and polluted workplaces: A case-control study. *Int Arch Occup Environ Health* 1982; 49:281–292.
14. Kvåale G, Bjelke E, Heuch I: Occupational exposure and lung cancer risk. *Int J Cancer* 1986; 37:185–193.
15. Pastorino U, Berrino F, Gervasio A, et al: Proportion of lung cancers due to occupational exposure. *Int J Cancer* 1984; 33:231–237.
16. Pike MC, Jing JS, Rosario IP, et al: Occupation: "Explanation" of an apparent air pollution-related localized excess of lung cancer in Los Angeles County, in Breslow NE, Whittemore AS (eds): *Energy and Health*. Philadelphia, PA, SIAM Institute Mathematics Society, 1979, pp 3–16.
17. Cole P, Hoover R, Friedell GH: Occupation and cancer of the lower urinary tract. *Cancer* 1972; 29:1250–1260.
18. Davies JM, Sommerville SM, Wallace DM: Occupational bladder tumor cases identified during ten years' interviewing patients. *Br J Urol* 1976; 48:561–566.
19. Vineis P, Simonato L: Estimates of the proportion of bladder cancers attributable to occupation. *Scand J Work Environ Health* 1986; 12:55–60.

20. Armstrong B, Doll R: Environmental factors and cancer incidence and mortality in different countries with special reference to dietary practices. *Int J Cancer* 1975; 15:617–631.
21. Carroll KK: Experimental evidence of dietary factors and hormone-dependent cancers. *Cancer Res* 1975; 35:3374–3383.
22. IARC: *Cancer: Occurrence, Cause and Control*. IARC Scientific Publications. Lyon, International Agency for Research on Cancer. (in press.)
23. Jain M, Cook GM, David FG, et al: A case-control study of diet and colorectal cancer. *Int J Cancer* 1980; 26:757–768.
24. Miller AB, Kelly A, Choi NW, et al: A study of diet and breast cancer. *Am J Epidemiol* 1978; 107:499–509.
25. Potter JD, McMichael AJ: Diet and cancer of the colon and rectum. A case-control study. *J Natl Cancer Inst*. 1986; 76:557–569.
26. Braitman LE, Adlin EV, Stanton JL: Obesity and calorie intake: the National Health and Nutrition Examination of 1971–1975 (HANES). *J Chron Dis* 1985; 38:727–732.
27. Haenszel W, Berg JW, Segi M, et al: Large-bowel cancer in Hawaiian Japanese. *J Natl Cancer Inst* 1974; 51:1765–1779.
28. Lubin JH, Burns PE, Blot WJ, et al: Dietary factors and breast cancer risk. *Int J Cancer* 1981; 28:685–689.
29. IARC Intestinal Microecology Group: Dietary fibre, transit time, faecal bacteria, steroids, and colon cancer in two Scandinavian populations. *Lancet* 1977; ii:207–211.
30. Jensen OM, MacLennan R, Wahrendorf J: Diet, bowel function, fecal characteristics, and large-bowel cancer in Denmark and Finland. *Nutr Cancer* 1982; 4:5–19.
31. Evans AS: Viruses, in Scottenfeld D, Fraumeni JF Jr (eds): *Cancer Epidemiology and Prevention*. Philadelphia, PA, WB Saunders, 1982, pp 364–390.
32. Blattner WA, Gallo RC: Epidemiology of human retroviruses. *Leuk Res* 1985; 9:697–698.
33. Lenoir GM, O'Conor GT, Olweny CLM (eds): *Burkitt's Lymphoma*. IARC Scientific Publications No. 60. Lyon, International Agency for Research on Cancer, 1985.
34. Klein G: The Epstein-Barr virus and neoplasia. *New Engl J Med* 1975; 293:1353–1357.
35. Ernberg I, Kallin B: Epstein-Barr virus and its association with human malignant diseases. *Cancer Surveys* 1984; 3:51–89.
36. Thorley-Lawson DA, Edson CM, Geilinger K: Epstein-Barr virus antigens—A challenge to modern biochemistry. *Adv Cancer Res* 1982; 36:338–343.
37. Whittle HC, Brown J, Marsh K, et al: T-cell control of Epstein-Barr virus infected B cells is lost during *P. falciparum* malaria. *Nature* 1984; 312:449–450.
38. Lenoir G, Taub R: Chromosomal translocations and oncogenes in Burkitt's lymphoma, in Goldman JM, Harnden DG (eds): *Leukaemia and Lymphoma Research, 2. Genetic Rearrangements in Leukaemia and Lymphoma*. Edinburgh, Churchill Livingstone, 1986, pp 152–172.
39. de-The G, Ito Y, Davis W (eds): *Nasopharyngeal Carcinoma: Etiology and Control*. IARC Scientific Publications No 20. Lyon, International Agency for Research on Cancer, 1978.
40. Zeng Y, Zhang LG, Li HY, et al: Serological mass survey for early detection of nasopharyngeal carcinoma in Wuzhou City, China. *Int J Cancer* 1982; 29:139–141.
41. Szmuness W: Hepatocellular carcinoma and hepatitis B virus: evidence for a causal association. *Prog Med Virol* 1978; 24:40–69.
42. Munoz N, Linsell CA: Epidemiology of primary liver cancer, in Correa P, Haenszel W (eds): *Epidemiology of Cancer of the Digestive Tract*. The Hague, Martinus Nijhoff, 1982, pp 161–195.

43. Beasley RP, Lin CC, Hwang LY, et al: Hepatocellular carcinoma and hepatitis B virus: a prospective study of 22707 men in Taiwan. *Lancet* 1981; ii:1129–1132.
44. Shafritz DA, Shouval D, Sherman HI, et al: Integration of hepatitis B virus DNA into the genome of liver cells in chronic liver disease and hepatocelluar carcinoma. Studies in precancerous liver biopsies and post-mortem tissue specimens. *New Engl J Med* 1981; 305:1067–1073.
45. Summers J: Three recently described animal virus models for human hepatitis B virus. *Hepatology* 1981; 1:179–183.
46. Busby W, Wogan GN: Aflatoxins, in Searle, CE (ed): *Chemical Carcinogens*. ACS Monograph Series No 182. Washington DC, American Chemical Society, 1984, pp 945–1136.
47. Gissmann L: Papillomaviruses and their association with cancer in animals and in man. *Cancer Surveys* 1984; 3:161–181.
48. Mitchell H, Drake M, Medley G: Perspective evaluation of risk of cervical cancer after cytological evidence of human papillomavirus infection. *Lancet* 1986; i:573–575.
49. Peto R, zur Hausen H (eds): *Viral Etiology of Cervical Cancer*. Cold Spring Harbor, NY, Cold Spring Harbor Laboratory, 1986.
50. El-Aaser AA, El-Merzabani MM: Etiology of bladder cancer, in Elsebai I, Hoogstraten B (eds): *Bladder Cancer*, Vol 1, General Review, CRC Series on Experiences in Clinical Oncology. Boca Raton, FL, CRC Press, 1983, pp 39–58.
51. Schwartz DA: Helminths in the induction of cancer: *Opisthorchis viverrini, Clonorchis sinensis* and cholangiocarcinoma. *Trop Geogr Med* 32:95–100, 1980.
52. National Institutes of Health: Report of the National Institutes of Health ad hoc Working Group to Develop Radio Epidemiological Tables, NIH Publication No 85-2748. Washington DC, US Department of Health and Human Services, 1985.
53. Beebe GW, Kato H, Land CE: Studies of the mortality of A-bomb survivors. 6. Mortality and radiation dose, 1950–1974. *Radiat Res* 1978; 75:138–201.
54. Parker LN, Belsky JL, Yamamoto T, et al: Thyroid carcinoma diagnosed between 13 and 26 years after exposure to atomic radiation. A study of the ABCC-HNIH Adult Health Study Population, Hiroshima and Hagasaki 1958–71, Technical Report 5–73. *Ann Intern Med* 1974; 80:600–604.
55. Shore RE, Woodard ED, Hempelmann LH, et al: Synergism between radiation and other risk factors for breast cancer. *Rev Med* 1980; 9:815–822.
56. Webber BM: Radiation therapy for pertussis. A possible etiologic factor in thyroid carcinoma. *Ann Intern Med* 1977; 86:449–450.
57. Modan B, Ron E, Werner A: Thyroid cancer following scalp irradiation. *Radiology* 1977; 123:741–744.
58. Shore RE, Albert RE, Pasternack BS: Follow-up study of patients treated by x-ray epilation for tinea capitis. Resurvey of post-treatment illness and mortality experience. *Arch Environ Health* 1976; 31:17–28.
59. DeGroot LJ, Frohman LA, Kaplan LE, et al: *Radiation-associated Thyroid Carcinoma*. New York, Grune & Stratton, 1977.
60. National Academy of Sciences Advisory Committee on the Biological Effects of Ionizing Radiation: *The Effects on Populations of Exposure to Low Levels of Ionizing Radiation*. Washington DC, National Academy Press, 1980.
61. Beebe GW, Land CE, Kato H: The hypothesis of radiation-accelerated aging and the mortality of Japanese A-bomb victims, in: *Late Biological Effects ot Ionizing Radiation*, Vol 1. Vienna, International Atomic Energy Agency, 1978, pp 3–27.
62. Doll R, Smith PG: Mortality from cancer and other causes after radiotherapy for ankylosing spondylitis. Further observations, in: *Sources and Effects of Ionizing Radia-*

tion. United Nations Scientific Committee on the Effects of Atomic Radiation. New York, United Nations, 1977.

63. Smith PG, Doll R: Mortality among patients with ankylosing spondylitis after a single treatment course with x-rays. *Br Med J* 1982; 284:449–460.
64. Archer VE, Saccamanno G, Jones JH: Frequency of different histologic types of bronchogenic carcinoma as related to radiation exposure. *Cancer* 1974; 34:2056–2060.
65. Ham JM: Report of the Royal Commission on the Health and Safety of Workers in Mines. Toronto, Canada, Ministry of the Attorney General, Province of Ontario, 1976.
66. Sevc J, Kunz E, Placek V: Lung cancer in uranium miners and long-term exposure to radon daughter products. *Health Phys* 1976; 30:433–437.
67. McGregor DH, Land CE, Choi K, et al: Breast cancer incidence among bomb survivors, Hiroshi and Nagasaki, 1950–1969. *J Natl Cancer Inst* 1977; 59:799–811.
68. Tokunaga M, Land CE, Yamamoto T, et al: Breast cancer among atomic bomb survivors, in Boice JD Jr, Fraumeni JF Jr (eds): *Radiation Carcinogenesis. Epidemiology and Biological Significance.* New York, Raven Press, 1984, pp 45–56.
69. Baral E, Larsson LE, Mattsson B: Breast cancer following irradiation of the breast. *Cancer* 1977; 40:2905–2910.
70. Shore RE, Hempelmann LH, Kowaluk E, et al: Breast neoplasms in women treated with x-rays for acute post-partum mastitis. *J Natl Cancer Inst* 1977; 59:813–822.
71. National Research Council: *The Effects on Populations of Exposure to Low Levels of Ionizing Radiation: Report of the Committee on the Biological Effects of Ionizing Radiations.* Washington DC, National Academy Press, 1980.
72. National Research Council: *Assigned Share for Radiation as a Cause of Cancer: Review of Radio Epidemiological Tables Assigning Probability of Causation.* Washington DC, National Academy Press, 1984.
73. IARC: IARC Monographs on the Evaluation of the Carcinogenic Risk of Chemicals to Humans, Vol 40, *Some Naturally Occurring and Synthetic Food Components, Furocoumarins and Ultraviolet Radiation.* Lyon, 1986.
74. Scotto J, Fears TR, Fraumeni JF Jr: *Incidence of Nonmelanoma Skin Cancer in the United States,* NIH Publications No 83-2433. Washington DC, US Department of Health and Human Services, 1983.
75. Marino AA, Moriss DM: Chronic electromagnetic stressors in the environment: a risk factor in human cancer. *J Environ Sci Health* 1985; C3:189–219.
76. Wertheimer N, Leeper E: Electrical wiring configurations and childhood cancer. *Am J Epidemiol* 1979; 109:273–284.
77. Wertheimer N, Leeper E: Adult cancer related to electrical wires near the house. *Int J Epidemiol* 1982; 11:345–355.
78. McDowell ME: Leukaemia mortality in electrical workers in England and Wales. *Lancet* 1983; i:246.
79. Milham S Jr: Mortality from leukemia in workers exposed to electrical and magnetic fields. *New Engl J Med* 1982; 307:249.
80. Milham S Jr: Silent keys: leukemia mortality in amateur radio operators. *Lancet* 1985; i:812.
81. Wright WE, Peters J, Mack T: Leukaemia in workers exposed to electrical and magnetic fields. *Lancet* 1982; ii:1160.
82. IARC: IARC Monographs on the Evaluation of the Carcinogenic Risk of Chemicals to Humans, Vol 23, *Some Metals and Metallic Compounds.* Lyon, 1980.
83. IARC: IARC Monographs on the Evaluation of Carcinogenic Risk of Chemicals to Man, Vol 14, *Asbestos.* Lyon, 1977.

84. IARC: IARC Monographs on the Evaluation of the Carcinogenic Risk of Chemicals to Humans, Vol 35, *Some Aromatic Compounds, Part 4, Bitumens, Coal-tars and Derived Products, Shale-oils and Soots*. Lyon, 1985.
85. IARC: IARC Monographs on the Evaluation of Carcinogenic Risk of Chemicals to Man, Vol 11, *Cadmium, Nickel, Some Epoxides, Miscellaneous Industrial Chemicals and General Considerations on Volatile Anaesthetics*. Lyon, 1976.
86. IARC: IARC Monographs on the Evaluation of the Carcinogenic Risk of Chemicals to Humans, Vol 33, *Polynuclear Aromatic Compounds*, Part 2, *Carbon Blacks, Mineral Oils and Some Nitroarenes*. Lyon, 1984.
87. IARC: IARC Monographs on the Evaluation of Carcinogenic Risk of Chemicals to Man, Vol 4, *Some Aromatic Amines, Hydrazine and Related Substances, N-Nitroso Compounds and Miscellaneous Alkylating Agents*. Lyon, 1974.
88. IARC: IARC Monographs on the Evaluation of the Carcinogenic Risk of Chemicals to Humans, Vol 19, *Some Monomers, Plastics and Synthetic Elastomers, and Acrolein*. Lyon, 1979.
89. IARC: IARC Monographs on the Evaluation of the Carcinogenic Risk of Chemicals to Man, Vol 15, *Some Fumigants, The Herbicides 2,4-D and 2,4,5-T, Chlorinated Dibenzodioxins and Miscellaneous Industrial Chemicals*. Lyon, 1977.
90. IARC: IARC Monographs on the Evaluation of the Carcinogenic Risk of Chemicals to Humans, Vol 29, *Some Industrial Chemicals and Dyestuffs*. Lyon, 1982.
91. IARC: IARC Monographs on the Evaluation of Carcinogenic Risk of Chemicals to Man, Vol 1, *Some Inorganic Substances, Chlorinated Hydrocarbons, Aromatic Amines, N-Nitroso Compounds, and Natural Products*. Lyon, 1972.
92. IARC: IARC Monographs on the Evaluation of the Carcinogenic Risk of Chemicals to Humans, Vol 34, *Polynuclear Aromatic Compounds*, Part 3, *Industrial Exposures in Aluminum Production, Coal Gasification, Coke Production, and Iron and Steel Founding*. Lyon, 1984.
93. IARC: IARC Monographs on the Evaluation of the Carcinogenic Risk of Chemicals to Humans, Vol 25, *Wood, Leather and Some Associated Industries*. Lyon, 1980.
94. Waterhouse JAH, Muir CS, Correa P, et al (eds): *Cancer Incidence in Five Continents*, Vol III, IARC Scientific Publications No 15. Lyon, International Agency for Research on Cancer, 1976.
95. Waterhouse JAH, Muir CS, Shanmugaratnam K, et al (eds): *Cancer Incidence in Five Continents*, Vol IV, IARC Scientific Publications No 42. Lyon, International Agency for Research on Cancer, 1982.
96. Li JY, Liu BQ, Li GY, et al (eds): *Atlas of Cancer Mortality in the People's Republic of China*. Shanghai, China Map Press, 1979.
97. Kemp I, Boyle P, Smans M, et al (eds): Atlas of Cancer in Scotland 1975–80: Incidence and Epidemiological Perspective, IARC Scientific Publications No 72. Lyon, International Agency for Research on Cancer, 1985.
98. Haenszel W, Kurihara M: Studies of Japanese migrants. I. Mortality from cancer and other diseases among Japanese in the United States. *J Natl Cancer Inst* 1968; 40:43–68.
99. Yu MC, Ho JHC, Lai SH, et al: Cantonese-style salted fish as a cause of nasopharyngeal carcinoma: Report of a case-control study in Hong Kong. *Cancer Res* 1986; 46:956–961.
100. Miller AB: An overview of hormone related cancers. *Cancer Res* 1978; 38:3985–3990.
101. McCance DJ: Human papilloma viruses and cancer. *Biochim Biophys Acta* 1986; 823:195–205.
102. Prorok PC, Miller AB (eds): *Screening for Cancer*. UICC Technical Report Series No 78. Geneva, International Union Against Cancer, 1984.

103. Warnakulasuriya K, Ekanayake AN, Sivayoham S, et al: Utilization of primary health care workers for early detection of oral cancer and precancer cases in Sri Lanka. *Bull World Health Org* 1984; 62:243–250.
104. Hirayama T, Hisamichi S, Fujimoto I, et al: Screening for gastric cancer, in Miller AB (ed): *Screening for Cancer*. New York, Academic Press, 1985, pp 367–377.
105. Oshima A, Hanai A, Fujimoto I: Evaluation of a mass-screening programme for stomach cancer. *Natl Cancer Inst Monogr* 1979; 53:181–186.
106. Yamagata S, Sugawara N, Hisamichi S: Mass-screening for cancer in Japan—present and future, in Yamagata S, Hirayama T, Hisamichi S (eds): *Recent Advances in Cancer Control: Proceedings of the 6th Asia Pacific Cancer Conference*, Sendai, Japan. Amsterdam, Excerpta Medica, 1983, pp 33–45.
107. Shapiro S, Venet W, Strax P, et al: Ten-to-fourteen year effect of screening on breast cancer mortality. *J Natl Cancer Inst* 1982; 69:349–355.
108. Tabar L, Gad A, Holmberg LH, et al: Reduction in mortality from breast cancer after mass-screening with mammography. *Lancet* 1985; i:829–832.
109. Parkin DM, Day NE: Evaluating and planning screening programmes, in Parkin DM, Wagner G, Muir GS (eds): *The Role of the Registry in Cancer Control*, IARC Scientific Publications No 66. Lyon, International Agency for Research on Cancer, 1985.
110. IARC Working Group on Evaluation of Cervical Cancer Screening Programmes: Screening for squamous cervical cancer: The duration of low risk following negative cervical cytology and its implication for screening policies. *Br Med J* 1986; 293:659–664.
111. WHO: Cancer increases in developed countries. *Wkly Epidemiol Rec* 1985; 60:125–129.
112. United Nations: Concise Report on the World Population Situation in 1979, DIESA Population Studies No 72. New York, 1980.
113. Miller RW, McKay FW: Decline in US childhood cancer mortality, 1950 through 1980. *J Am Med Assoc* 1984; 251:1567–1570.
114. Hakama M: Trends in the incidence of cervical cancer in the Nordic countries, in Magnus K (ed): *Trends in Cancer Incidence*. Washington DC, Hemisphere, 1982, pp 279–292.

10

A Community-Oriented Approach to Surgery

LADÉ WOSORNU

INTRODUCTION

If each day of our lives is meant to be better than the day before, then the day we die must be the best of all. But, due to ill health, most human beings cannot possibly see things that way. Thus have the planners and providers of health fallen short, to say nothing of politicians and men of religion. For, although we are nowhere near the WHO goal "Health for All by 2000,"[1] in this grand scheme of things, the surgeon's role is small.

Malaria remains a threat to over half of the world's population; 450 million people suffer from malnutrition, 400–500 million from trachoma, 250 million from filariasis, and 200 million from bilharzia; 2000 million people have no access to drinking water, and 90% of women in the Third World give birth unaided.[2] By the scale of suffering that those figures show, what does it matter if the second-degree piles of a certain chauffeur-driven widow are to be anointed, snared, frozen, injected, stitched, or excised?

Paradoxically, it is in this garb as that member of the health profession who receives wages to provide primarily for the individual, and secondarily for the community, that the surgeon is so well placed to profit society if he or she practices the principles of biopsychosocial surgery. At little or great cost, the surgeon can heal or harm, by wisely or unwisely using knife, cautery, needle and thread, placebo, pill, or

LADÉ WOSORNU • Professor, Department of Surgery, Director, Residency Programmes, King Faisal University, College of Medicine, Dammam, Saudi Arabia.

even witchcraft. Perhaps at no cost at all, he or she can effectively help prevent disease or accident by personal example, advice, or a bit of opportunism. "Admission to hospital for surgery, with the general supportive atmosphere and emphasis on health and disease, provides a prime opportunity to persuade people to stop smoking."[3]

Biopsychosocial surgery is not new. It is nothing other than a surgeon's constant awareness of the timeless truth that human beings consist indivisibly of body and soul. In technical language, we may call these aspects the biologic and the psychologic. They are subject and indeed vulnerable to physical, emotional, social, and even metaphysical forces, which can be local or universal, real or imaginary, and past, present, or future.

If we are to discern more clearly some of the principles of biopsychosocial surgery at work, we must draw a bottom line for available medical resources. Otherwise, there will be no end to footnotes and parentheses as one tries to take into account the variety of constructions, health professionals, and the new breed of "physician entrepreneurs,"[4] as well as of missionaries and mercenaries, implements and so on, all purportedly geared to the care of surgical cases. The district hospital (or its equivalent) is taken here as the bottom line. And, for want of a better designation, "District Surgeon" (DS) stands for a district hospital doctor (usually a man) who has the responsibility (among many others) to manage surgical cases. (In the USSR and some other countries, most DSs are females.)

It will be assumed also that whenever patients arrive late in the district hospital, it is neither because they are impecunious, illiterate, nor stupid, nor because of muddy roads, floods, landslide, collapsed bridges, sand storms, bush fire, nor any other natural disaster barring their way. It is because they have knowingly and willfully decided to do so. Undoubtedly, money matters. "Five million people annually report that they do not seek medical care because they are unable to pay for it."[5] Although everything is relative, let it be noted that the country Dr. Mundinger[5] is referring to is neither Bangladesh or Burkina Faso; it is the United States of America.

The Outpatients Department (OPD)

It is in the OPD that the DS interviews and clinically examines most of his cases of all ages and both sexes. The DS can have problems. These include overcrowding, long and impatient waiting lines, inadequate time to examine fully each and every patient, and availability of diagnostic facilities.

In some cultures, every now and then, a female patient will refuse politely but firmly to be examined unless by a female doctor. Not only disorders of thighs, breasts, anus, and rectum evoke this degree of shyness. I have seen women in Rajasthan, India, reluctant to tell a doctor about their failing eyes and decaying teeth, let alone show their unveiled faces and, on command, intone "Ahh." The lesions of such women will become chronic, so that, by the time pain or physical disability compels them to come to the DS, their diseases can be correctly described as "neglected."

But, a particular DS I met, having much empathy, blamed not the women, their tradition, nor their total poverty. Dr. R.R. Doshi explained: "If you scold them, the word soon gets around, and no one of their age group will come to you again." This encounter was in an Eye Camp organized by the Human Service Trust (UK), in Chirawa Village, Rajasthan, India, March 1985 (Figure 1). Dr. Doshi gave figures from similar eye camps showing a 38% overall increase in the number of operations between 1979/80 and 1983/84.

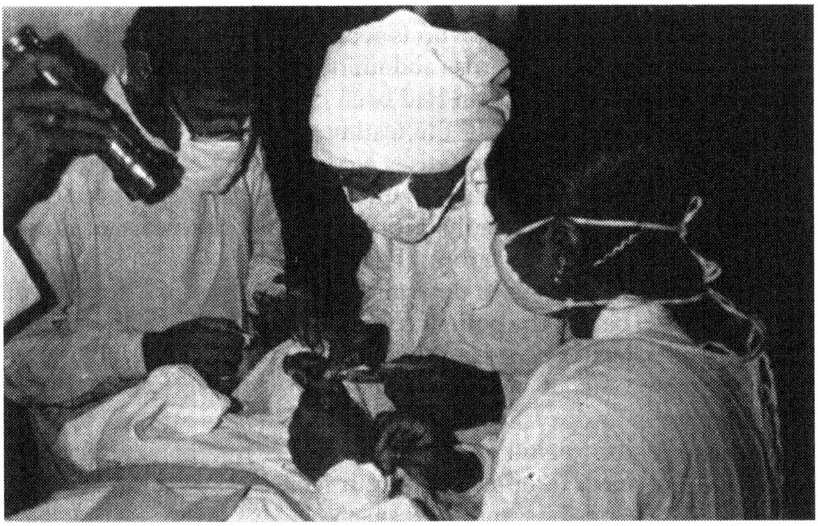

FIGURE 1. Eye operation in progress during "Eye Camp," Chirawa Village, Rajasthan, India, March 1985. Note bare hands all round—of surgeon (holding syringe) and team. A 3-dry-celled torch provides "spotlight."

Another patient may be a boy of ten accidentally kicked in the abdomen at home, with his father looking on. Boy and father make light of the central abdominal pain that would have had some men, softened by city life, whining in agony. Three weeks later, the father walks his son to the OPD because of bile vomiting and abdominal distension. The history of a kick is omitted, not out of a conspiracy of silence; it was simply forgotten, having been adjudged trivial. Eventually, pancreatic pseudocyst is diagnosed and put right.[6] Is this another example of parental neglect and ignorance, or is it perhaps that theirs is a tradition that enjoins bravery and stoicism?

A principle of biopsychosocial surgery emerges. Let us call it Number 1. The surgeon should try to understand and respect patients' traditions, beliefs, and cultural background, be it shyness, stoicism, or any behavior with which he is unfamiliar. But, this tolerance should not degenerate into negativism or indifference which precludes adequate clinical evaluation.

A surgeon accepts without much question the patient's report on symptoms, including duration. Often, the statement agrees with what is known about the prevalence of diseases in the given community, and the biology of the particular diagnosis the surgeon has in mind. For example, Burkitt's lymphoma is one of the fastest growing tumors known. (It is said that you can see the jaw double its size before your eyes.) Therefore, if a surgeon who is working in a Burkitt's lymphoma belt sees a girl of 8 or 9 with gross abdominal distension, and her mother insists that weeks earlier the girl had been climbing trees with the boys, he has little difficulty believing the testimony.

On the other hand, if there arises a conflict between patients' testimony and the surgeon's clinical judgment, he, becoming an advocate in his own court, dismisses (openly or privately) the patient as an unreliable witness. But, he can be wrong (Figure 2).

Broad groups of variables determine the duration of a surgical disease (say a lump) before the patient comes to the DS. One is the biologic. It includes the natural history of the lesion, its biological variability, and associated symptoms, if any, including pain, disability, or disfigurement. Another is the psychosocial: e.g., the patient's attitude to health in relation to his or her other commitments. A trial of other forms of treatment is the third. In other words, surgeons and patients see things differently, including time and disease.

Take other commitments first. The intention here is not to condone late attendance if early attendance is patently beneficial and cost-effective. An editorial asks: "Is Early Antenatal Attendance So Important?"[7] The answer included this: "In an audit of an antenatal care for 1975. . .

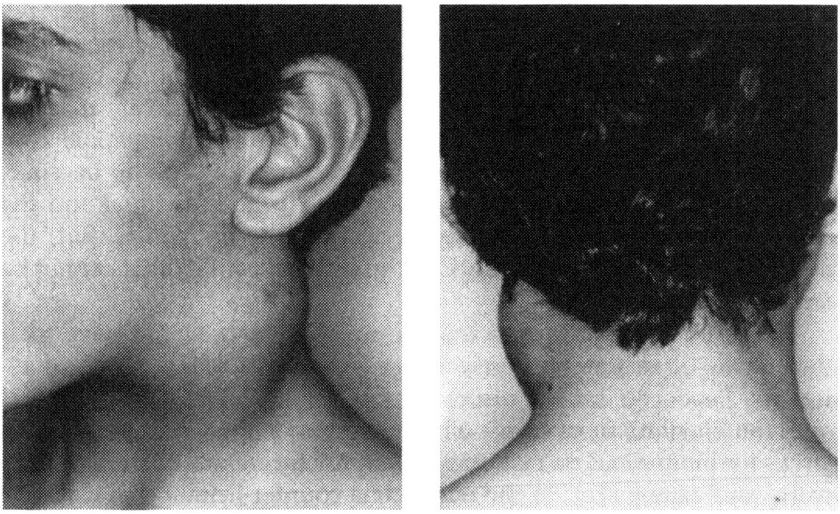

FIGURE 2. A 12-year-old pupil presented with neck swelling of, he insisted, two days' duration. He did not have the high-prevalent tuberculosis, but the rare deep-seated cavernous hemangioma. The surgeon was wrong in disbelieving the boy's testimony. The surgeon in question was LW, the author. [Courtesy Mr. Andrew Archibald, Medical Photographer.]

some salutary lessons were learnt. Late booking was common: only one third of women had attended by the 12th week, and a quarter had still not attended by the 18th week. Much of the latter group consisted of single women. But, for those who did attend the clinic the recognition of serious problems by the staff was not good." Aberdeen, Scotland, was the place audited.

Patients (single women in the Aberdeen example) do have other commitments—for example, a slippery job to hold. On the contrary, if she or he happens to be one of the millions unemployed, unemployment has health hazards of its own.[8] The *BMJ* editorial[7] continues: "In two years they screened 3479 pregnant women, of whom eight were carrying fetuses with an open neural-tube defect." Is the yield of 8 in 3479 or 0.02% cost-effective?

From a biopsychosocial approach, therefore, additional principles emerge. Number 2: Patients have other commitments and different priorities. At the same time, the surgeon should remember that the reasons for patients' dropping out might be, medically speaking, unacceptable. In other words, priorities, if set in wrong order, ought to be corrected through mass media education and guidance. [Principle Number 3].

Principle Number 4: Early presentation by all and sundry may not always be cost-effective. But with the mention of cost-effectiveness, we get into difficulties. Some surgeons have serious reservations about getting involved in the whole business. They argue persuasively that this involvement might ultimately encroach upon one's professional conduct, that ethics and cost-effectiveness do not mix. This is because, whereas ethics is concerned with the rights of the individual and the community, cost-effectiveness largely ignores the individual. But, the surgeon has obligations to both. Clearly, this is a conflict that cannot be resolved at a stroke.

Before ever presenting to the DS, most patients would have tried other forms of treatment. These range from self-administration of aspirin for headache and of multivitamins for longevity and perpetual youth (an illusion); or of castor oil, magnesium sulphate, or herbal purgatives for abdominal pain; through acupuncture, faith healing, homeopathy and osteopathy, to the ubiquitous counter-irritant therapy. The latter is called cautery in the Middle East, moxobustion in the Far East, and scarification in Africa. For better or for worse, these other forms of treatment are here to stay. The indications are that their sphere of influence will widen and their legal status become secure.

Take faith healing and Christian Science as an example. ". . . North Carolina law recognized Christian Science practitioners as professional healers and licensed them along with physicians. . . The terminology duplicates that of medical health-care system. The church trains 'nurses' and calls its healers 'practitioners,' who take 'patients,' administer 'treatments' and charge for the services on the scale of local physicians' fees."[9]

The biopsychosocially aware surgeon notes [Principle Number 5] that, before presenting to him, most patients would have tried other forms of treatment. He will do well to refrain from blaming them for presenting late because of that, and from passing judgment on the efficacy or lack thereof of the said treatment(s). There is, however, another obligation on the DS. As a highly educated and specialized member of society, he or she has to help in changing wrong medical concepts and practices, always using the most productive possible means; i.e., he or she may have to play the role of a preacher/educator: a communicator (cf. Principle Number 3).

Investigations: Pathology Tests

Show me all your bills, and I'll show you your character. . . Show me a surgeon's list of routine investigations ("diagnostic workup") and the frequency with which he repeats them, and I'll show you the extent of his medical independence. For, broadly speaking, there is a linear correlation between the two variables: the longer the list (and the more often the tests are repeated), the more dependent the man.

Editorial columns have been devoted to the issue of getting physicians to curb their appetite for long lists of routine tests, and of repeating them, including normal results. Two key examples are "Pathology tests—Too much of a good thing,"[10] and "Learning Diagnostic Restraint."[11] Reuben[11] points out: "Some physicians feel pressured to order tests that *they know are unnecessary* because the consultant has written them as suggestions in the chart. (If the patient does not do well, failure to follow the consultant's advice may be considered negligent in court.) All these might be reasonable arguments for ordering tests that do not alter therapy or outcome *if tests were inexpensive and resources plentiful*" (Author's italics).

The *Lancet* editorial[10] observes: ". . .There is no pressure on the consultant to rationalize his pattern of investigation. The facilities of the service departments are all at his or her behest. It all seems to be 'for free.'" Another *Lancet* editorial observes: "We are faced with two unpalatable facts: resources are finite and costs are rising."[12]

Before indicating the remedy, attention is drawn to another trend: the use of what has been called investigative "grab bags" (Table 1). Labels for other grab bags are the "Upper GI Series," "Lower GI Series," "Trauma I Series," and so on. "This approach may have a high diagnostic yield, but it should not be interpreted as constituting good medicine. In fact, it probably discourages analytic thinking and the development of good clinical judgment."[11]

Four reasons (among others) can be given for the popularity of this approach, inimical though it is to the development of sound clinical

TABLE 1. Components of Two Investigative Grab Bags in Terms of Label for Grab Bag and Contents, i.e., Investigations Included[a]

Clinical diagnosis	"Label"	"Contents"
Transient ischemic attacks (TIA)	"NEURO 1"	CAT scan, Doppler, occulo-plethesmography, carotid ultrasound, and EEG
Congestive cardiac failure	"CARDIAC 2"	Serial cardiac enzymes, serial EKGs, echocardiogram, and radionucleid angiography

[a]Adapted from Reuben.[12]

judgment. First, analytic thinking is difficult. One finds it easier to use ready-made checklists, especially if one is hard pressed for time, as residents and interns usually claim to be. Second, the public is enchanted by high technology and disenchanted with clinical judgment, believing "that a doctor who does many tests is simply being thorough."[13] Third (as noted by Reuben), the fear of litigation dictates that adherence to the checklist or investigative grab bag is the safer way out. Fourth, "Perhaps the main reason for over investigation is the obsessive fear of missing organic disease."[13]

The remedy is "a practice of good medicine,"[12] "a reliance on clinical wisdom."[11] No doubt, "Financial pressure may help sharpen the mind."[13] It all has to do with mental independence, which is a function of clinical stature.

On the assumption that, practicing good medicine, relying on clinical wisdom, and exercising diagnostic restraint, the surgeon has made a modest list of essential investigations (where "essential" is defined as that which is indispensable and will influence critically the choice and timing of treatment), here is what Todd[13] advises. "Every doctor before ordering an investigation should ask, 'Whatever the result of this investigation, will it influence the management of the patient?' If the answer is No, the investigation should not be done."

The next question is: Is the OPD or ward the more appropriate setting for the essential tests? Although the answer depends on several factors making generalization difficult, one practice is generally accepted and is here recommended. As many tests as possible should be completed on OPD basis.[13] Two basic reasons are given: (1) biologically (in relation to surgery), the shorter patients' preoperative stay in hospital, the lower their risk of contracting hospital infection, including postoperative wound infection; (2) financially (socioeconomically), treatment costs are cut if total inpatient days are few.

A principle [Number 6] can be stated thus: The biopsychosocially aware surgeon should exercise clinical independence, and not be swayed by trends in which tests are ordered although he believes they are unnecessary.

Preoperative Preparation of Inpatients

The broad aim of preoperative preparation is to ensure that the patients are reasonably fit for the proposed operation including anesthesia, in order that their postoperative course may be as smooth as possible. "Reasonable fitness," like health itself, includes bio- (physical), psycho- (mental), and social components.

The biologic is the easiest to describe, being more readily measurable. Attention is drawn to nutrition (including hydration and levels of hemoglobin and of serum albumin), as well as the cardiorespiratory, urinary, and endocrine-metabolic systems. A specific aim is to ensure the presence of factors that promote healing and the absence of those that impair it.

The clinical features of dehydration are well-known. They include dryness of skin (such that it feels sandy to touch), loss of skin turgor, sunken eyes with soft globes, dry and coated tongue (in the absence of mouth breathing), concentrated and scanty urine (20 ml/h or less), and, sometimes, hypotension (systolic blood pressure of 90 mm Hg or lower). The obviousness or not of these signs depends on the degree of dehydration: whether mild, moderate, or severe. When dehydration becomes severe, the patient has lost some 10% of his total body water.

In general, clinical signs are subjective and can be misleading. For example, if the patient has lost much weight recently, these skin signs can be exaggerated. On the other hand, if he is obese, or a child, they can be masked. Hence, reliance should be placed more on the objective signs, especially hourly urine output.

Pure water depletion as implied above is rare in surgical practice where the common clinical picture is due to fluid and electrolyte imbalance. Its causes include protracted vomiting, diarrhea, and enterocutaneous fistulae. The chief electrolytes lost can be predicted from the source of the loss. If electrolyte depletion becomes gross, clinical symptoms and signs ensue. These include severe muscle cramps in hyponatremia, prostration in hypokalemia, and tetany in hypocalcemia.

However, the type of imbalance should be measured using the levels of serum electrolytes and of blood urea, complemented by EKG (in hypo- or hyper-kalemia). Normal values (in mEq/L or mmol/L) are: $Na+$: 140 (135–145); $K+$: 4 (3.5–5.5); $Cl-$: 100 (95–105); HCO_3-: 25 (20–28); and blood urea : 30 mg% (20–40).

Clinical states of depletion demand replacement therapy. Crystalloids are indicated, their route of administration usually being the intravenous. Response to treatment is monitored objectively in at least two ways: estimating serum electrolytes and blood urea (until they approach normal levels) and urine output (about 0.5 ml/kg/h being considered adequate in adults).

The biopsychosocially aware surgeon [Principle Number 7] must be not only a good clinician, but also scientific in approach. He or she must be objective and numerate. This is the reason for the above details, well-known though they are.

There is little need to describe here the other biological preoperative measures. A word, though, about rectal infusion of tap water. It is a reasonable alternative to the intravenous route. Unfortunately, at present, its use is attended by an uncalled-for sense of penury and of being old-fashioned, and (which is worse, who knows?) of psychological degradation. A method of treatment deserves wide usage provided it is safe and efficacious [Principle Number 8]. It may be inexpensive and unfashionable but that should be irrelevant (cf. Principle Number 6, on clinical independence).

Of psychological preoperative preparation, the patient's needs include reassurance and a sound sleep the night before. The social component is discussed under the Consent Form.

Blood Transfusion

Nearly topping the list of overused (if not abused) commodities in surgery must come blood for transfusion (also antibiotics and oxygen by face mask). Among many other publications, editorials,[14] original articles,[15] monographs,[16] and guidelines[17] have been written on the appropriate usage of blood and its products in surgery, but apparently to little avail.

The acceptable biological "lower" limits are hemoglobin 10 g/dl, hematocrit 35%, and an estimated 25% of blood volume lost through bleeding. If a patient receives packed cells for a hemoglobin level of less than 8 g/dl, and has one of the following anemias, but without symptoms of hypovolemia or hypoxia, the surgeon should be asked to explain why. The anemias are iron lack, pernicious, nutritional, and the hereditary hemolytic anemias. Replacement therapy, including nutrition, and not the transfusion of packed cells, is their more appropriate treatment.[17] Admittedly, the urgency for a given operation is important, irrespective of the cause of the patient's anemia. In such urgent cases, if general anesthesia is required, it is acceptable to give blood transfusion to bring the hemoglobin up to 10 g% in adults. If the patient has a major hemoglobinopathy such as sickle-cell anemia, the hematocrit should be kept around 35%.

Ready availability, like familiarity, breeds contempt. For, it is chiefly because grouped and cross-matched blood is so readily available that blood is overused. The fully aware surgeon avoids unnecessary treatments, including transfusion, in order to cut treatment costs [Principle Number 9] and help reduce the incidence of lethal diseases which can be iatrogenic. Examples here are AIDS, viral hepatitis, malaria, and transfusion reactions.

As far as the recipient is concerned, the donors can be someone else or oneself. Homologous blood donated by a relative or friend (designated donor) is safe. Not so safe is the source wherein the donor is anonymous, irrespective of whether he is charitable or coerced, a conscript or a mercenary. Nor is screening donors the ready-made answer. For example, Ryder et al.[18] have shown that screening for hepatitis B virus markers is not justified in West African transfusion centers. This practice is not cost-effective due to the high prevalence of hepatitis in the subregion.

Autologous blood for transfusion, which is cheap and obviates the above complications, can be obtained by predeposit, intentionally hemodiluting the anesthetized patient, or by salvage autotransfusion. None of these methods has enjoyed the wide usage it deserves (cf. Principle Number 8).

The Consent Form

In surgical practice, fewer pieces of paper (including the pathologist's report on a paraffin section) can be more final than the consent form (CF). Although it is alleged to lack legal validity, the CF has been hallowed by tradition and protected by this standing order (whether written or spoken is irrelevant): "No valid CF, no Op." Usually, a valid CF is available and the operation (Op) gets done as planned. Sometimes it is not, and the operation is delayed, postponed, or canceled, much to the surgeon's anger, astonishment, frustration, or glee, depending on how he looks at things.

The purpose here is to examine some of the reasons for this turn of events. Straightaway, one observation is made: it is chiefly for powerful and deep-rooted psychosocial reasons that patients in the Third World delay or refuse to sign the CF. And, "No man is an island" sums up what they are trying to tell the surgeon.

It may begin with the patient asking for time to think things over and to consult the family. It can end with him or her being discharged against medical advice, and the medics dismissing the patient as ignorant, superstitious, illiterate, and ill-informed.

Mastectomy is the surgery for which permission is most often refused. Other examples are orchidectomy, amputation of limb or penis, abdominoperineal resection of rectum and anus with permanent colostomy, and total cystectomy with an ideal conduit.

Throughout the deliberations of a family in such a plight, two questions remain on their lips. (Agonizing, not deliberating, is the word, although agonizing is emotive. But to the patients, what are such operations if not emotive subjects?) Their questions are, first, is the operation really necessary? Is there no way out? They ask surgeons, junior staff, nurses, and anyone else who is prepared to listen.

The biopsychosocial way is to explain things objectively to the patient and the family without undue pressure, leave them to make up their minds, and to accept their decision without rancor. [Principle Number 10]. Sometimes, of course, reasonable pressure becomes necessary, and when applied with compassion and wisdom can be rewarding. Experienced surgeons give examples of lives saved by insisting on amputating crushed limbs infected with gas gangrene, or on thoracotomy for ruptured hydatid cyst. The thing to avoid is that the surgeon must not strut away in a huff muttering that he does not "believe" in, for example, lumpectomy (tylectomy), or in "inadequate cancer surgery."

But, before stating some currently acceptable answers to the above biological questions, let us explore the psychosocial issues involved, taking as examples mastectomy and permanent colostomy. First, consider an ostomy. The abhorrence of ostomies can be comprehensive. If it were merely repugnance at the constant smell of stool, the fear of "colostomy accidents," or of becoming a reluctant recluse, then the answers would lie with deodorants and airtight colostomy bags, adequate bowel retraining, and ostomy clubs. But, instead, the feeling is instinctive.

Socially, a mastectomized woman puts on a brave smile trying to deny her disfigurement. Psychologically, her fears are based on intangible, traditional convictions. Such a woman will never disclose to a mere surgeon her true reasons for refusal. That would be like disrobing in public. The mastectomized woman is deeply disturbed by the partial loss of femininity and the joy and pride of being a total female, which includes having two identical breasts.

Is mastectomy for cancer really necessary? Not invariably. But this is a subject on which editorials have been written[19,20] and to which whole issues have been devoted.[21] Dr. Mueller captions the *NEJM* editorial, "Surgery for Breast Cancer, Less May Be As Good As More."[20]

"Not invariably" also applies not only to amputations for diabetic gangrene,[22] but also to extensive resections for malignant melanoma.[23] LoGerfro and Coffman[22] observe: "Such patients should not be relegated to below-knee amputation, since distal arterial reconstruction may produce excellent results." They add: "Limbs should not be lost because of inappropriate diagnosis of microvascular disease."

Is that colostomy really necessary? Again, the answer is not invariably. Low anterior resections for rectal cancer are becoming lower. "A few surgeons are undertaking the sphincter-conserving operations for selected growths even lower than 6 cm."[24,25] This implies that coloanal anastomoses are being placed within 2 or 3 cm of the anal verge. For one thing, "The traditional 5 cm clearance is no longer believed necessary."[26]

Everything has its price. In this connection, the price (like life itself) is at once good and bad. On one hand, to the individual woman who refused permission for mastectomy, cancer en cuirasse can be the price she has to pay. On the other hand, to society at large, such refusals have sped the search for answers to fundamental biological questions, including other forms of effective local treatment, such as tylectomy followed by radiotherapy, or even radiotherapy alone.

Between the individual patient and society stands the surgeon. If he is biopsychosocially aware [Principle Number 11] he will develop tolerance and will refrain from insulting the patient for having been stubborn, relieve his pain as best he can, and return him to his people (society). They will certainly comfort and repossess him much as the sea repossesses a crystal of salt or the desert a grain of sand. For to them, truly, no man is an island.

Nothing material is ever static. It is the surgeon's moral duty to keep abreast with the spiral of progress in his speciality [Principle Number 12]. For example: "We can only regard these [surgeons] as the dinosaurs of their profession who are even now, like those ancient monsters, shambling on their way to extinction because their brains are too small to cope with new knowledge."[27] Furthermore, as Williams[28] points out, "these arguments [about anorectal preservation] are a precise rerun of those of the late 1930s and 1940s when anterior resection was first considered for upper-third growths."

There is another side of the CF story. Some patients are only too eager to sign up. The Munchausens apart, two eagerly accepted operations are mammoplasty and hemorrhoidectomy.[29] If it is his unshakable belief that hemorrhoidectomy enhances male libido, that man will insist on the operation and, once it is performed, his libido will be enhanced as a result. The effect may be short-lived. But this is one myth that I believe is needless to explode in a hurry.

If, on the other hand, the organ to be ablated is limb, gonad, kidney, or lung, the law in some countries and, indeed, logic itself demand the prior witnessing signatures of two consultant surgeons. One signature is not enough.

Similarly, if the treatment involves the use of cytotoxic drugs, alopecia should be discussed fully, and informed consent obtained. In some cultures, women smile with their eyes and dance with their hair. "To the psyche, hair is profoundly important, and abnormalities that arise in malignant disease cause much distress." (The source of this quotation is British.[30])

Treatment

After all is said and done, a practicing surgeon is usually paid to treat patients by operations. Technically, therefore, he must be competent. Clinically he must be wise and compassionate. He should give himself time to study patients in reasonable detail before prescribing appropriate operations to suit the particular patient. Performing all minor and as many not-so-minor ones as are safe on outpatient basis, he must maximize the use of all treatment facilities. If he is biopsychosocially aware [Principle Number 13], his approach to treatment will be holistic naturally.

In practice and in relation to patients, it is not so much what he does technically but what he refrains from doing and saying that sets him apart from his nonholistic counterparts. Thus, however subtly, he should not deny patients access to men of religion or to other forms of treatment. For example, if a patient with an ischemic foot asks to be discharged home to continue topical honey treatment, the surgeon must suppress his derision and be prepared to check it out. Unorthodox ways of treating wound infection are finding increasing acceptance in orthodox settings.[31–33]

As an old French master put it:

> What the surgeon ought to be: The conditions necessary for the surgeon are four: first, he should be learned; second, he should be expert; third, he must be ingenious and fourth, he should be able to adapt himself.
>
> It required for the first that the Surgeon should know not only the principles of surgery, but also those of medicine in theory and practice; for the second, that he should have seen others operate; for the third, that he should be ingenious, of good judgment and memory to recognize conditions; and for the fourth, that he be adaptable and able to accommodate himself to circumstances.
>
> Let the Surgeon be bold in all sure things, and fearful in dangerous things; let him avoid all faulty treatments and practices. He ought to be gracious to the sick, considerate to his associates, cautious in his prognostications. Let him be modest, dignified, gentle, pitiful, and merciful; not covetous nor an extortionist of money; but rather let his reward be according to his work, to the means of the patient, to the quality of the issue, and to his own dignity (Guy de Chauliac, 1300–1370.)

Postoperative pain can and should be anticipated and relieved effectively at all times. Is this point worth making, let alone stressing? Surprisingly, the answer is yes. Opiates, new or old, natural or synthetic, are the most potent analgesics. In some countries, rigid rules guide their use. But, once prescribed, they should be administered without the patients being made to feel contemptible for asking for pain relief.

Regarding route of administration, for simplicity combined with effectiveness, none can beat intravenous opiates. It should be remembered that postoperative pain is easier forestalled than treated. The fear of drug addiction here is unfounded. If the pain has become chronic, drug combinations should be tried.[34] [Principle Number 14—Always be merciful.]

In gastrointestinal surgery, nasogastric (NG) aspiration is another unsuspected source of argument. It is not unusual for surgeons to debate its routine use postoperatively. Some call it a nuisance; they prefer a temporary gastrotomy, or to dispense with routine postoperative gastric decompression altogether. The reason that some patients, mostly men, reject the NG tube, is that they think it could impinge on the brain, causing insanity.

Unlike a friendly myth, basic ignorance is one thing the biopsychosocially aware must dispel [Principle Number 15]. I distinguish between basic ignorance and the traditional beliefs or even misconceptions earlier alluded to. The latter involve powerful psychological overtones and intuitive mistrust of certain forms of scientific treatment. And, time is proving some of these intuitions right.

Discharge Home and Follow-up in the OPD

As soon as the patient can tolerate soft diet and make do with minimal nursing care, he can be discharged home. Nearly all patients keep the first OPD appointment. Thereafter, as they get better, attendance becomes more erratic, two patterns being discernible. Either they turn up when least expected, if at all, or complain of symptoms that, though genuine, are unrelated to the operation. In the latter event, the surgeon should be as helpful as he can.

Refusal to show up at the OPD is more significant. If a patient does this knowingly, it is by choice. He is making a statement: that he has other priorities (cf. Principle Number 2). Furthermore, it can be argued that the beneficiary of such routine OPD follow-ups is the institution, not the patient. Before refuting this argument (not convincingly, in my view), Hughes and Courtney[35] posed the rhetoric: "Is there, indeed, any advantage from regular follow up in hospital compared with leaving the patient and her General Practitioner to detect recurrence and take appropriate action?"

If the answer is no, the implication is that patients can return to the OPD with rather advanced recurrences. It is perhaps impossible to avoid such a risk altogether. We cannot predict the likelihood of this event in a particular patient, because of biological variability. One might as well try to predict the likelihood of the patient contracting a particular histologic variant of the original tumor. In any event: "The economic consequences of being ill threaten him. So there may be unreasonable delay in seeking advice, even until the illness is obvious."[36] The "him" in question is not the unlettered peasant from Tahiti. He is the doctor in "Doctors as Patients."[36]

Therefore, unless the patient is patently the beneficiary, the biopsychosocially aware surgeon should not insist on 100% follow-up in his OPD [Principle Number 16]. All the same, since a reasonably comprehensive follow-up is essential for research purposes, it should be funded as such and pursued in other ways. It can be argued that patients should show gratitude to the treating surgeon and institution by regular follow-up attendance even though they are not the primary beneficiaries.

"Doctor, how soon can I return to work?" The answer depends on several factors. The biological variables include the type of operation (appendectomy, cholecystectomy, or triple bypass); for a given operation, whether the patient (thin or fat?) has had complications such as wound infection or thromboembolism. The psychosocial variables are more complex, whether related to patient or surgeon. Therefore it helps to eliminate as many variables as possible while at the same time securing a wide range of validity for our conclusions. Inguinal herniorrhaphy seems to fit this role.

"Inguinal hernia repair remains the commonest surgical procedure undertaken in adult males in district hospitals."[37] The editorial continues: "How long off work? British attitudes are still influenced by wartime experience where hernias were commonly repaired by surgeons with little training; faced with high recurrence rates, the senior officers ordered prolonged rest in the hope of promoting sound repair. Today (cf. Principle Number 12—the spiral of progress), the evidence strongly suggests that early return to full activity in civilian and armed forces practice is followed by sound repair and low recurrence rates. We should, therefore, recommend return to work within two weeks for sedentary workers, and after four weeks for those in more strenuous occupations. Any physical activity that causes pain should be avoided, but at three months the fascia. . . . should withstand even the most vigorous activity." In short, allow patients to return to work as soon as possible [Principle Number 17].

For most surgeons, a patient's return to gainful employment ends the treatment contract, and with it all professional responsibility. It should follow that the close of this chapter is effectively at hand, and, as it began, may conclude on the note that biopsychosocial surgery (the holistic approach, Principle Number 13) is not new. Here is that note: "Such an outlook does not need to be graced with the term 'holistic medicine': it is simply the practice of treating patients as they should be treated by an adequately trained physician."[38]

But, two more topics, prevention and death, must be addressed.

Prevention

Preventive medicine we know; but, preventive surgery? By this is meant a practice of the former with particular reference to surgical diseases. It brings to mind the Chinese word for crisis which means danger and opportunity combined. The opportunities to do good that the practice of preventive surgery offers are many and beyond question, but its dangers, though fewer, are no less real.

Consider the prevention of advanced breast cancer at initial presentation. Frank and Mai[39] have questioned the cost-effectiveness of breast self-examination (BSE) in young women. They begin: "Breast self-examination (BSE) has been recommended for early detection of breast cancer for over 30 years. In a 1950 American Cancer Society monograph, Haagensen wrote: 'It is probably true that, from the point of view of the greatest possible gain in early diagnosis, teaching women how to examine their breasts is more important than teaching. . . . physicians. . . The Canadian Cancer Society has also promoted BSE for several years, listing monthly BSE as one of the 'Seven steps to Health.''" However, Frank and Mai conclude that: "BSE in younger women, by encouraging invasive and costly medical investigation of many asymptomatic benign breast lumps needing no treatment, could well do more harm than good." They are not alone; the very biological premises have been questioned.[40]

That efforts at "preventive surgery" are not always cost-effective is one side of the coin of doubt: Is our zeal misdirected? Its other side is about claims of efficacy. At best, they may fail the test of time or of numbers; they may be due to sampling errors or to type-A errors (of statistical significance). Two examples are (1) Dennis Burkitt's notion of high-fiber diet and the prevalence of acute appendicitis, and (2) psychological factors in the causation and course of cancer.

Of Burkitt's much publicized notion, need more be said than this: "But, 'Sir' Dennis, where is the evidence?" (I personally asked him this question in Lome, Togo, in 1972 during the annual conference of the Association of Surgeons of West Africa. I am still waiting for the evidence.) Psychological factors and cancer is, at present, a mushier issue. Interested readers may consult Dr. Peteet in *Cancer, Stress, and Death.*[41]

In a prepublication review, I wrote[42]: "One of the themes of *Cancer, Stress, and Death* is controversial. It can be summed up in the intuitively acceptable statement that 'Disease is a reflection of the psyche'. . . . Their (authors') god. . . . is to readvocate the holistic approach of Hippocrates and Plato which recognised the inseparability of mind, body, and soul. The trouble is that, of the evidence they (the authors) adduce so painstakingly, dismissive statements such as this shall be made for a long time to come: However, it is time to acknowledge that our belief in disease as direct reflection of mental state is largely folklore."[43]

Although articulate voices on the pages of influential journals pooh-pooh the idea that cancer is more likely in unhappy people, there is hardly a whimper against reasonable evidence. For example, there is reasonable evidence that those who habitually smoke many cigarettes have a measurably higher incidence of a number of surgical diseases. These include ischemic heart disease, chronic duodenal ulcer, peripheral vascular disease, postoperative thromboembolism, carcinoma of bronchus, urinary bladder, and of esophagus, and, incidentally, if they are women, of bearing small-for-dates babies who also may be retarded. (True, Lesko et al.[44] have concluded that: "The data suggest that women who smoke heavily may have a lower risk of endometrial cancer than non-smokers." But, the editorial on that article points out: "Even if some degree of protection from endometrial cancer is provided by cigarette smoking, a postmenopausal woman who smokes cannot take much comfort from this."[45])

In the preoperative workup, a surgeon can demand obedience, saying: "Mrs. Puffrock, if you do not stop smoking and lose a bit of weight, I shall refuse to repair your hernia." Usually but not invariably, she obeys. And, postoperative patients often ask: "Doctor, what shall I do to stop this thing from coming back?"

It is from this double vantage point that surgeons become drawn into the prevention business. First, they can suitably persuade patients. Secondly, if a patient asks (pays) for advice, he or she is likely to implement it. If this is so, then the surgeon's needs include scientific evidence for what he has to say (cf. Principle Number 7), and restraint in how he puts it. Table 2 lists a few examples of surgical diseases (excluding the sequelae of infections and infestations) for which there is reasonable evidence that suitable preventive measures reduce incidence or favorably influence course, or effect both.

Through clinically oriented research [Principle Number 18], he can point out to the community and its decision makers the epidemiology of, for example, road traffic accidents and of cancer. He can then suggest ways and means of prevention, basing his suggestions on locally gathered data. The same may apply to parasitic infestations, diseases of excesses and stresses (e.g., vascular disorders) surgical complications of diabetes mellitus, the results of parental neglect and basic ignorance, such as child battering, burns in children, and foreign bodies swallowed or inhaled by children. A surgeon should not only treat such cases; he

TABLE 2. Examples of Common General Surgical Diseases (Excluding Infections and Infestations) for Which There Is Evidence That Preventive Measures Can Make a Difference in Incidence or Course or Both

Organ	Disease	Preventive measures
Oral cavity	Squamous cell carcinoma	Avoid spices and smoking, and extract carious and jagged teeth
Esophagus	Squamous cell carcinoma	Avoid cigarette smoking, mass esophagoscopy, and brush cytology (as happened in China)
Stomach and duodenum	Peptic ulcer	Eat regular meals
	Late carcinoma	Fully investigate "maturity-onset" dyspepsia (i.e., first presentation at 40 years or older); avoid excess of smoked fish
	Severe postgastrectomy anemia	Avoid gastrectomy in patients who cannot be relied upon to attend OPD follow-up or to take prophylactic hematenics
Liver, biliary tree, and pancreas	Cirrhosis and hepatitis	Consume little or no alcohol. Eat balanced diet. Avoid herbal poisons. Improve personal hygiene and screen for Australia antigen (may not be cost-effective in Third World). Vaccinate

(*continued*)

TABLE 2. (*Continued*)

Organ	Disease	Preventive measures
Abdominal wall	Strangulated hernias	Early elective herniorrhaphy
Large gut	Recurrent volvulus	Hemicolectomy at initial presentation
	Carcinoma	Elective pancolectomy in familial polyposis coli and chronic ulcerative colitis. (CF can be hard to get)
Urogenital system	Male sterility	Early orchidopexy for cryorchidism; immediate scrotal exploration for strangulated hernias in infants, and for suspected torsion
	Penile cancer	Early circumcision
	Stones	Drink much water in areas of high prevalence. If recurrent, exlude hyperparathyroidism
Respiratory system	Bronchiectasis	Immediate removal of inhaled foreign bodies in children; vaccinate against TB and whooping cough
	Bronchogenic carcinoma	Avoid cigarette smoking
Cardiovascular system	Ischemic disease (heart and peripheral vessels)	Avoid obesity and cigarette smoking; perform vigorous physical exercise regularly, and control diabetes
	Postoperative thromboembolism	Appropriate measures (including mini-heparin) in selected high-risk cases; early ambulation in all postoperative adults
Hemopoietic system	Sickle-cell anemia	Genetic counseling
	Perioperative crises	Good anesthesia
General	Trauma from road traffic accidents	When driving, no alcohol and fasten seat belts. Evacuate victims safely and expeditiously. (But, flying squads are not cost-effective.[48]) Educate public on road safety measures
Thyroid	Late carcinoma	Assume all nodules malignant (especially in the young, or males) until proven otherwise by histology
	Hepatoma	Vaccination against type B hepatitis. Screen using alpha-feto protein (? not cost-effective in areas where cirrhosis is highly prevalent with lesions being multicentric). Avoid moldy ground nuts. (Aflatoxin may not be the sole carcinogen.)
	Gallstone-pancreatitis: recurrent attacks	Cholecystectomy and remove stones in common bile duct at initial presentation or shortly thereafter.

should also collect, analyze, and present them to the appropriate authorities, and suggest solutions.

Three more observations can be made. The biopsychosocially aware surgeon should use his opportunities at disease prevention [Principle Number 19]. Secondly, governments and corporations who pay for health should allot funds for public education aimed at the prevention not only of infections, infestations, and malnutrition, but also of surgical diseases (cf. Principle Number 3: The biopsychosocial surgeon as a communicator).

Thirdly, and on a realistic note, the practicing surgeon is perhaps justified in feeling that he is being asked to shut the stable door after the horse has bolted. To some extent this is true. However, even if he only helps to prevent a recurrence, he would have reduced or forestalled the cost of another treatment. In so doing, he would have helped the patient towards attaining that self-understanding which we believe is the other way around.[46]

Death

For the biopsychosocially aware surgeon, euthanasia is out of question [Principle Number 20]. His role is to comfort the dying and their relatives in any and every way he can for as long as necessary. He would have excluded himself from that series of omissions that have conspired to make heroin a most underused drug of our time. He will prescribe heroin and be prepared to double and redouble the dose if that is what it takes to relieve pain, always provided that the patient demands relief from pain.

If this proviso seems unexpected, it is because some patients prefer clarity of mind, with pain, to the comfort and euphoria of narcosis or even coma. Nor should the surgeon choose a course of action that might comfort patients but also bring them closer to the brink of death. The last minutes of life can be too truthful, insightful, and valuable to be marred by meddlesome narcosis. Therefore, the surgeon must know his or her patients' psychosocial makeup (cf. the holistic approach, Principle Number 13). Here, his role is to help make particular patients' last days, if not their best, then at least some of their most revealing.

Belief or unbelief in life after death neither adds to nor takes away from the truth that what we call an end is only the beginning of something else. A white and textured ceiling, for example, is the brown pebble-smooth floor of the room above. In spite of advances in therapy using laser beams, retinoic acid, monoclonal antibodies targeted with cytotoxic agents, etc., etc., there always will exist strange entities, such as an unresectable growth and the terminal phase of an illness: the end of a biological line. It is in this zone of uncertain light, this other transit lounge, at once lit but brilliantly dark, peopled with tearful activity but hearse-paced and black-silent, that a last Principle (Number 21) can be seen: Not even the hills live forever.

Postscript

The stress has been on the surgeon–patient relationship. Due to space limitations, it has not been possible to mention the following: The role of the district surgeon in relation to his or her colleagues, paramedical professionals, other administrative cadres, and to governmental bodies (social, educational, health welfare, planning, and research); nor his or her relationship with referral clinics, general practitioners, and with superspecialized centers. If the references indicate a bias towards the *Lancet* and the *New England Journal of Medicine,* it is because these two journals have recently addressed the wide issues with which an introduction, such as this has been, is concerned.

Acknowledgments

The following debts of gratitude are acknowledged: to Their Excellencies the President and Vice President of King Faisal University and the Dean of its College of Medicine, Dr. Mohamed Hisham Al-Sibai, for providing a most congenial academic atmosphere; to Professor Tawfiq Mohamed Al-Tamimi for invaluable criticism and suggestions; to Dr. Chris Grant for comments; and to Lolita Galdones-Santos for typing the manuscript.

References

1. How near is health for all? *Lancet* 1983; 2:1179.
2. *Le Monde*: Dossiers et Documents. No. 108, February 1984.
3. Jones RM: Smoking before surgery: The case for stopping. *Br Med J* 1985; 290:1703–1704.
4. Relman AS: Antitrust law and the physician entrepreneur. *N Engl J Med* 1985; 313:884–885.
5. Mundinger MO: Health service funding cuts and the declining health of the poor. *N Engl J Med* 1985; 313:44–47.
6. Grant C: Management of injuries to the pancreas and doudenum. *Tropical Doctor* 1985; 17: 23–25.

7. Is early antenatal attendance so important? *Br Med J* 1982; 284:1064.
8. Unemployment and health. *Lancet* 1984; 2:1018–1019.
9. Swan R: Faith healing, Christian Science and the medical care of children. *N Engl J Med* 1983; 309:1639–1641.
10. Pathology tests—Too much of a good thing. *Lancet* 1984; 1:1278.
11. Reuben BD: Learning diagnostic restraint. *N Engl J Med* 1985; 310:591–593.
12. High technology medicine: A luxury we can afford? *Lancet* 1984; 2:77–78.
13. Todd JW: Wasted resources. *Lancet* 1984; 2:1146–1147.
14. Horsey PJ: Blood transfusion and surgery. *Br Med J* 1985; 291:234.
15. Sykes MK: Indications for blood transfusion. *Can Anaesth Soc J* 1975; 22:3–11.
16. Petz LD, Swisher SN: *Blood Transfusion in Clinical Medicine.* New York, Churchill-Livingstone, 1981.
17. Grindon AJ, Tomasulo PS, et al: The hospital transfusion committee—Guidelines for improving practice. *JAMA* 1985; 253:540–543.
18. Ryder RW, Whittle HC, et al: Screening for hepatitis B virus markers is not justified in West African transfusion centres. *Lancet* 1984; 2:449.
19. Treatment of breast cancer—Is conservation safe? *Lancet* 1985; 1:964–965.
20. Mueller CB: Surgery for breast cancer—Less may be as good as more. *N Engl J Med* 1985; 312:712–713.
21. *Surg Clin* 1984; 64:6.
22. LoGerfro FW, Coffman JD: Vascular and microvascular disease of the foot in diabetes: Implications for foot care. *N Engl J Med* 1984; 311:1615–1618.
23. Taylor BA, Hughes LE: Width of excision of melanoma. *Lancet* 1985; 1:693.
24. Anorectal preservation. *Lancet* 1984; 2:791.
25. Goligher JC, Lee PWR, et al: Experience with the Russian model 249 suture gun for anastomosis. *Surg Gynaecol Obst* 1979; 148:517–524.
26. Williams NS, Durdey P: Recurrence of rectal cancer managed by stapled anastomoses. 1984; Lancet 2:525.
27. Faalder C: *Breast Cancer.* London, Virago Press, 1982.
28. Williams NS: The rationale for preservation of the anal sphincter in patients with low rectal cancer. *Br J Surg* 1984; 71:575–581.
29. Wosornu L, Grant C, Khwaja S, Al-Breiki H: Alternatives in the management of common anorectal conditions—1:Piles. *Tropical Doctor* 1985; 15:65–67.
30. Cancer, cancer therapy, and hair. *Lancet* 1983; 2:1177–1178.
31. Svedman P: Irrigation treatment for leg ulcers. *Lancet* 1983; 2:532–534.
32. Al-Hassan JM, Thomson Martha, Criddle RS: Accelerated wound healing by a preparation from skin of the Arabian Gulf catfish. *Lancet* 1983; 1:1043–1044.
33. Trovillet JL, Chastre Hean, et al: Use of granulated sugar in treatment of open mediastinitis after cardiac surgery. *Lancet* 1985; 2:180–184.
34. Wilkes E: Advanced malignant disease, pain, physical deterioration in patients and death, in Day (ed.) *Cancer, Stress, and Death.* New York, Plenum Publishing, 1986; pp. 149–163.
35. Hughes LE, Courtney SP: Follow-up of patients with breast cancer. *Br Med J* 1985; 290:1229–1230.
36. Doctors as patients. *Lancet* 1983; 2:201–202.
37. British hernias. *Lancet* 1985; 1:1080–1081.
38. Alternative medicine is no alternative. *Lancet* 1983; 2:773–774.
39. Frank JW, Mai V: Breast self-examination in young women: More harm than good? *Lancet* 1985; 2:654–657.
40. Skrabanek P: Screening for disease: False premises and false promises. *Lancet* 1985; 2:316–320.

41. Peteet JR: Psychological factors in the causation and course of cancer, in Day, Selye, and Tache (eds): *Cancer, Stress, and Death,* New York, Plenum Publishing, 1986.
42. Wosornu L: Prepublication review. *Cancer, Stress, and Death,* Day, Selye, Tache: (Eds.) New York, Plenum Publishing, 1986.
43. Angell M: Disease as a reflection of the psyche. *N Engl J Med* 1985; 312:1570–1572.
44. Lesko SM, Rossenberg L, et al: Cigarette smoking and the risk of endometrial cancer. *N Engl J Med* 1985; 313:593–595.
45. Weiss NS: Can not smoking be hazardous to your health? *N Engl J Med* 1985; 313:632–633.
46. Day, Selye, Tache (eds): *Cancer, Stress, and Death.* New York, Plenum Publishing, 1986.
47. Robertson C, Steedman DJ: Are accident flying squads really cleared for "take-off"? *Lancet* 1985; 2:434–436.

11

Achieving Oral Health by the Year 2000

S. Prince Akpabio

Introduction

The purpose of this chapter is to examine the contrasting trends in oral health between the technically developed and developing countries in the context of WHO/FDI's oral health goals,[1] discuss the reasons for these trends, and make suggestions on practical strategies to achieve an acceptable standard of oral health by the year 2000.

Preamble

"Our first goal is to halt the increase of dental caries in the developing countries and to bring about a decrease in the level of dental caries in developed countries—all this by the Year 2000"—WHO.[2]

That statement, made by WHO in June 1981, is still true today. But little were we then to know the magnitude of the contrasting trends in oral health continuing to take place between the technically developed and the developing countries of the world, and the global significance of such changes.

S. Prince Akpabio • Consultant, Oral Health, World Health Organization, Geneva, Switzerland; Clinical Lecturer, University College Hospital Dental School, University of London, London, England.

Indicators for Oral Health Status for the Year 2000

The Basic Global Indicator of Oral Health 2000

It was in 1979 that the World Health Assembly unanimously ratified the Alma Ata Declaration, and adopted a resolution calling for the attainment of "Health for All by the Year 2000." That Assembly urged member countries to develop coordinated plans to achieve that goal. Unlike many ideas that come and go, this one caught on. "Health for All" also means "Oral Health for All"—by the year 2000.[3,4,5]

In 1981, the 34th World Health Assembly adopted the first global indicator of oral health status: that there should be no more than an average of three decayed, missing, and filled permanent teeth at the age of 12 years by the year 2000.[4] Holding this initial indicator as a beacon, a workshop was organized in 1981 with the active collaboration of the FDI (International Dental Federation), which represents the dental profession internationally. This workshop defined four other indicators for oral health for the year 2000:

- *At 5–6 years of age* 50% of children should be caries free.
- *At 18 years of age* 85% of the population should retain *ALL* their permanent teeth.
- *At 35–44 years of age* there should be a 50% reduction in the present levels of edentulousness. What this really means is that at least 90% of the adult population in this age group should be dentate, and that at least 75% should have a minimum of 20 functional teeth.[6,7]
- *At 65 years of age,* at least 50% of the population should have 20 functional teeth.

The workshop further recommended that a data bank should be established to monitor changes in oral health throughout the world.

Table 1 shows these oral health goals.

Global Goals—Objectives

It is important to emphasize that in establishing these global goals, it was expected of each country to formulate its own subgoals and its oral health target. It is equally important to emphasize that these goals were established with the idea that they should:

1. Be simple in terms of data needs and interpretation;
2. Serve as reference points against which countries and populations could be compared at different times; and

TABLE 1. WHO Global Indicators of Oral Health for All by the Year 2000

Goal 1	At 5–6 years	50% to be caries free
Goal 2	At 12 years	Only three DMF teeth
Goal 3	At 18 years	85% should retain all their permanent teeth
Goal 4	At 35–44 years	50% reduction in present level of edentulousness (i.e., 75% should have at least 20 functional teeth).
Goal 5	At 65 years	25% reduction in present level of edentulousness (i.e., 50% should have at least 20 functional teeth).
Goal 6	Data bank to be established	

3. Stimulate each country to take stock, set its own goals, and develop plans to reach them.

Finally, these goals recognized that some countries might have difficulty in achieving them. Other countries, already having a high level of oral health, might have to reverse current trends (if this is deteriorating) in order to stay at, or ahead of the goal levels, while others might be stimulated to set goals representing even better levels of oral health.

Trends in Oral Health between Technically Developed and Developing Countries

Since WHO's global goals for oral health were set in 1981, there has been a basic difference in trends in oral health between the technically developed and the developing countries.

Briefly, the important differences in trends in oral health that have taken place and continue to take place between the technically developed and the developing countries of the world are as follows.

Dental Caries

There is a dramatic reduction in dental caries in many of the technically developed countries, because of effective preventive measures.[8] In fact, a 10% reduction in the annual intake of university dental undergraduates has been imposed by the governments of some of these countries, with some dental schools closing. Figure 1 shows this decreasing trend in dental caries in the technically developed countries.

In the developing countries, on the contrary, there continues to be an increase in dental caries,[9–19] with some exceptions. In a few coun-

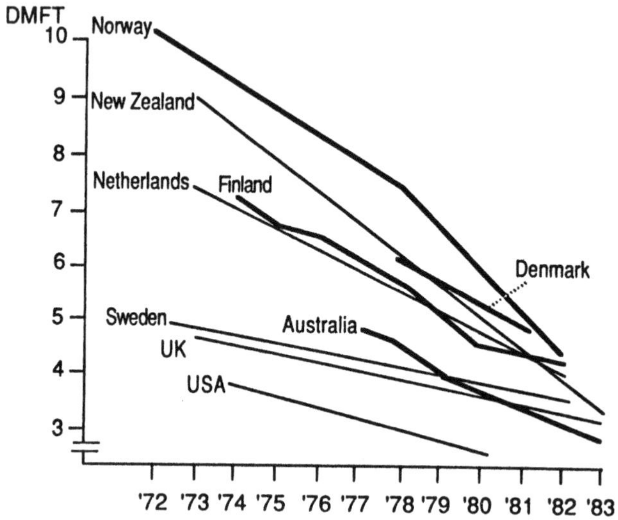

FIGURE 1. Trends in dental caries in technically developed countries.

tries, such as Singapore and Hong Kong, effective preventive measures, such as community water fluoridation, has led to a gradual reduction. Increase in caries varies from one country to the other: rapid in some, such as Mexico, the Central African Republic, Indonesia, and Nigeria; but slow in others such as Kenya, Tanzania, India, and Korea. A few developing countries, such as Singapore, Cuba, Barbados, and Syria, show the welcome trend of a gradual decrease in caries prevalence.[20]

Figure 2 (a–c) shows the trend of increasing caries in countries in Africa, Asia, South America, and parts of the Middle East.

Periodontal Disease

Periodontal disease occurs in both the technically developed and developing countries. It is totally preventable, but extremely costly to treat. Periodontal disease has always been prevalent and more severe in the developing countries, because of the poor standard of oral hygiene.[21–25] Other factors, of course, can modify the severity of periodontal disease. In the technically developed countries, because of the improved standards of oral hygiene, we are now receiving reports that indicate a continued reduction in the level of the disease and improved periodontal health. In the developing countries, on the contrary, there is

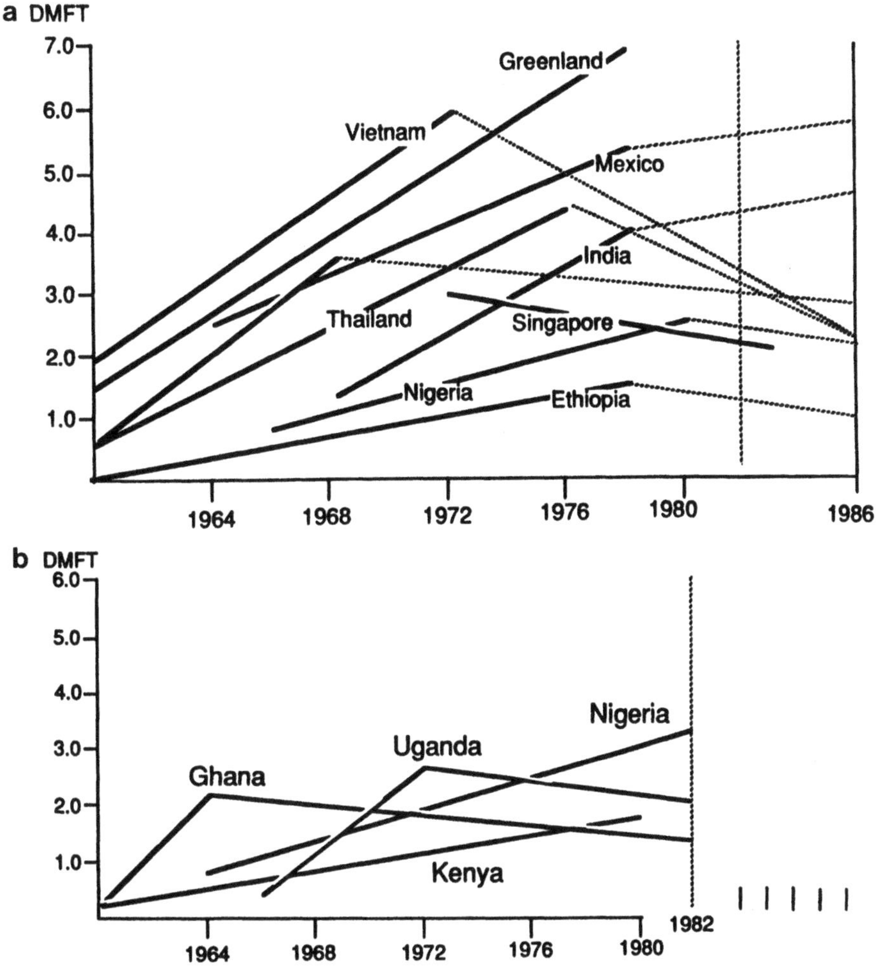

FIGURE 2. (a) Increasing dental caries in various developing countries (1958–1986). DMFT at 12 years. (b) Increasing dental caries in developing African countries (1960–1986). DMFT at 12 years. (c) Increasing dental caries in developing countries in the Middle East and South America (1962–1986). DMFT at 12 years.

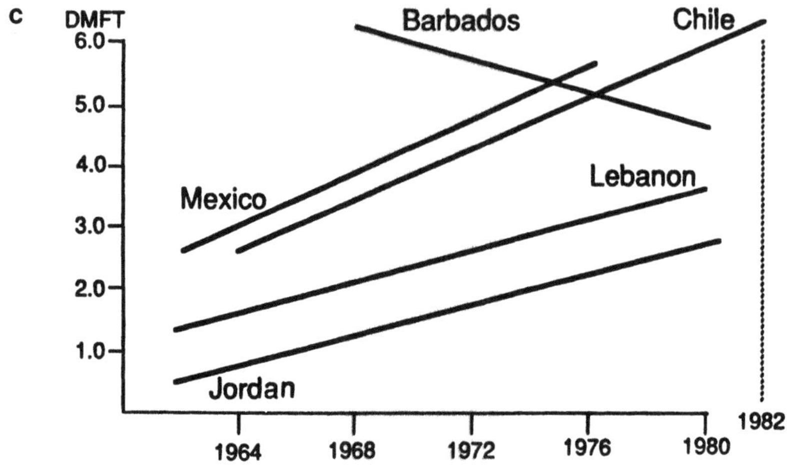

FIGURE 2. (*Continued*)

still severe periodontal disease. This affects children, often at a very early age. Poor oral hygiene is again the principal causative factor.[21–26]

Figure 3 (a, b) was taken in Africa and shows severe periodontal disease affecting a youth aged only 18 years. There is already marked mobility and migration of teeth, even at such a young age.

Figure 4 is a histogram prepared from the WHO 1986 data. It shows the mean number of sextants, i.e., sections of the mouth, affected by shallow periodontal pockets as a result of different levels of periodontal disease. Calculus has always been found to be more severe in the Third World countries. This histogram illustrates the greater prevalence of periodontal disease in the developing countries.[27]

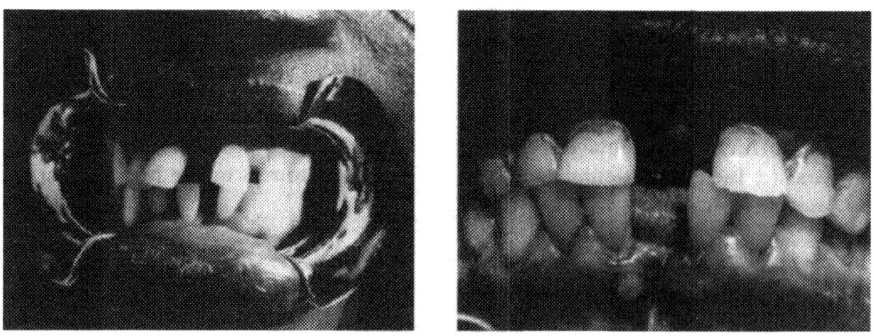

FIGURE 3. Periodontal disease in African youths, aged only 18 years (gross mobility, spacing, and migration of upper and lower incisor teeth).

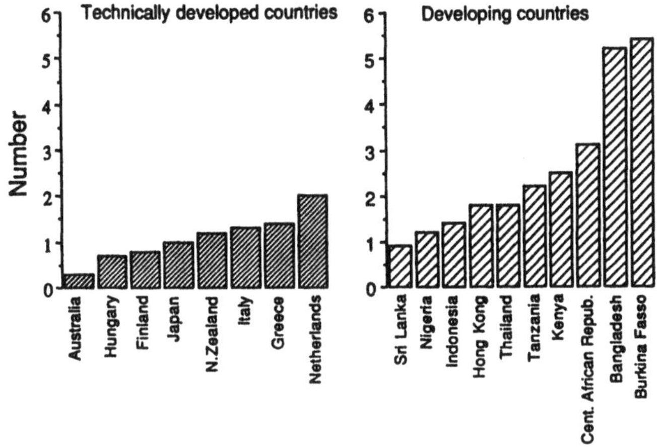

FIGURE 4. Histogram showing shallow periodontal pockets at 35–44 years age group between technically developed and developing countries (WHO data 1986).

Oral Health Trends in Context of Global Goals

The first WHO oral health goal is that at least 50% of the 5–6 year old children should be caries-free. In the technically developed countries, recent data indicate that between 10–50% of the 5–6 year-olds are caries-free, and this improving trend is continuing. In the developing countries, between 30–91% of the 5–6 year-olds are caries-free.[8]

The danger here, however, is that if the present trend of increasing caries in the developing countries continues, we will shortly have less than 50% of the 5–6 year-olds being caries-free, instead of the present 30–91%. There is, therefore, need for the governments in these countries to take appropriate, effective, preventive community measures to halt, and indeed reverse, the present trend of increasing dental caries among the young.

The second WHO oral health goal is that at 12 years of age, the global average will be no more than three decayed, missing, or filled teeth. Data available at WHO's Data Bank[28] in 1986 indicated that:

1. In 58 developing and 7 technically developed countries, caries prevalence was equal to or less than 3 DMF at 12 years of age.
2. In 32 developing countries and 21 technically developed countries, caries prevalence was more than 3 DMF teeth at 12 years of age.

3. A further 11 technically developed countries were on the verge of reaching 3 DMF teeth as the present decreasing caries trend continues. On the other hand, and rather disturbingly, 16 developing countries were in danger of reaching that level of 3 DMF teeth at 12 years of age, because of their caries prevalence levels continuing to increase.

Again, the obvious strategy of governments in these countries is that appropriate, effective, preventive community measures against caries should be instituted.

The third WHO oral health goal is that at 18 years of age, 85% of the population should retain all their permanent teeth. No baseline data for this age group has been published yet. Nevertheless, there are indirect pointers.

In some developing countries, such as Nigeria, Kenya, and Tanzania, recent survey data have shown that more teeth are now being lost among this age group through untreated, increasing dental caries of the first permanent molars, and sometimes the second molars. To quote the report of a recent epidemiological study in Kenya and Tanzania: "*Dental caries was the principal reason for loss of teeth in all age groups (and not periodontal disease).*"[29]

In the technically developed countries, the early diagnosis of dental caries, the fact that treatment facilities are readily available, and current effective, preventive community programs mean that, in these countries, there will be a progressive reduction in tooth loss through dental caries among this age group. The technically developed countries, therefore, seem to be in a position to achieve WHO's oral health goal.

In the developing countries, on the other hand, if the increasing loss of first and permanent molars through untreated caries continues, it seems that these countries will gradually fall behind, and not be able to achieve WHO's goal for this age group. Governments in these countries should, therefore, undertake effective, preventive measures to halt and eventually reverse the increasing loss of the first or second permanent molars through untreated caries.

The fourth WHO oral health goal is that at 35–44 years of age, 75% of the population should retain a minimum of 20 functional teeth.

WHO's 1986 publication of observed periodontal conditions, measured by CPITN index, and estimated national percentages of edentulousness at 35–55 years of age described the situation in 24 countries.[27] Ten of the countries listed were technically developed; 14 were developing countries. The 10 technically developed countries had a range of 1–19% levels of national edentulousness at that age group, whereas 14 of the developing countries had a range of 1–4% levels of national edentulousness. A significant observation in that publication was:

"The conclusion must therefore be that, for a large majority in most of the populations observed, the *progress of periodontal disease has been slow, and seems compatible with the retention of a natural dentition until at least the age of 50,* i.e., a few years older than the upper age limit for the data presented."[27]

It would seem that for this adult age group, the prevention of periodontal breakdown should constitute the main dental challenge in the technically developed countries. In the developing countries, the strategy to prevent progressive periodontal breakdown should be combined with measures to reduce the loss of teeth through untreated dental caries.

The fifth WHO oral health goal is that at 65 years of age, more than 50% of the population should retain at least 20 functional teeth.

Until the latter 1980s, for this age group, published data were available for only 8 technically developed countries. The levels of edentulousness in these countries ranged from 28 to 80%. Then some interesting studies were carried out in Kenya and Tanzania. In one such study, which investigated the pattern of tooth loss in adult rural populations in Kenya, the author concluded:

"The study found that the majority of the population retained most of their dentition in a functional state even up to the age of 65 years: in all age groups, more than 50% had at least 26 teeth present, and more than 90% had at least 16 teeth present. The prevalence of edentulousness was less than 0.3%." This worker found that "the principal cause of tooth loss in all age groups was dental caries, and this was true for all tooth-types except incisors for which periodontal diseases accounted for the main pathological cause of tooth loss."

Similarly, in another recent study in Tanzania, the authors concluded that:

"The number of teeth present in both the Tanzanian and Kenyan population was remarkably high, even among the older age groups. Dental caries was the principal reason for loss of teeth in all age groups (and not periodontal disease)." These authors remarked "these findings indicate that periodontal diseases in African populations do not lead to tooth loss to the extent hitherto thought."[29]

For the 65-year-old age group, the strategy must therefore be for the prevention of progressive periodontal breakdown in the technically developed countries. Whereas in the developing countries, at least in some of the African countries (for which some data are available), the strategy must be the prevention of loss of teeth through untreated caries as well as prevention of progressive periodontal breakdown.

Achieving Oral Health by the Year 2000—Preamble

What are the factors that have brought about this remarkable improvement in the standard of oral health in the technically developed countries, and how can the developing countries attempt to achieve comparable improvements, in order to attain a reasonable standard of oral health, for their people, by the year 2000. If increasing dental caries and severe periodontal disease are the two most common oral disease that we have to deal with in order to attain WHO's goals of oral health by the year 2000, then we must discuss the important factors that are responsible for these two diseases. We should then examine practical ways to control, and indeed prevent them.

National Oral Health Goal—The Need for Definite Objectives

To deal effectively with any national health problem, there must be planning. This should be done by the government or its ministry of health, and preferably in consultation with the professional body directly involved. Such national government planning should have clearly stated, measurable objectives, which can be critically evaluated at definite intervals. In the absence of any stated goals or objectives, evaluation is difficult. Without a definite, well-defined oral health policy and stated objectives, the oral health policy becomes fluid. It may change quite easily with a change of either the minister of health or the outgoing principal government dental surgeon. Thailand has already formulated its "Strategies to Achieve Thailand's National Oral Health Goal for HFA 2000," which is realistic, not too ambitious, and capable of being achieved within the economic resources of the country.

Table 2 shows Thailand's national oral health goals.

Dental Caries

Dental caries cause pain and misery. Figure 5 shows a patient with dental caries which, if untreated, will progress to form a dental abscess (Figure 6). Dental caries are expensive to treat, and cause a great financial drain on the health budget and resources of any country.

Table 3 and Figure 7 show the cost of running the general dental

TABLE 2. Thailand's National Oral Health Goals for Health for All by the Year 2000

Goal 1	At 5–6 years	30% to be caries free.
Goal 2	At 12 years	DMFT 1.5
Goal 3	At 18 years	75% should retain their permanent teeth.
Gingival health		
Goal 4	At 18 years	CPI = 0 (i.e., normal) in at least 2 sextants.
Goal 5	At 33–44 years	95% of population should have at least 20 functional teeth.
Goal 6	At 60 years	50% of population should have at least 20 functional teeth.

services within the National Health Service in the United Kingdom. It can be seen that the cost of such services has increased each year. The current improvement in the dental health in the United Kingdom was brought about not solely by the expenditure of millions of pounds sterling each year to train dentists and to provide curative treatment, but almost certainly through cumulative preventive measures, such as the use of fluoride in toothpastes.

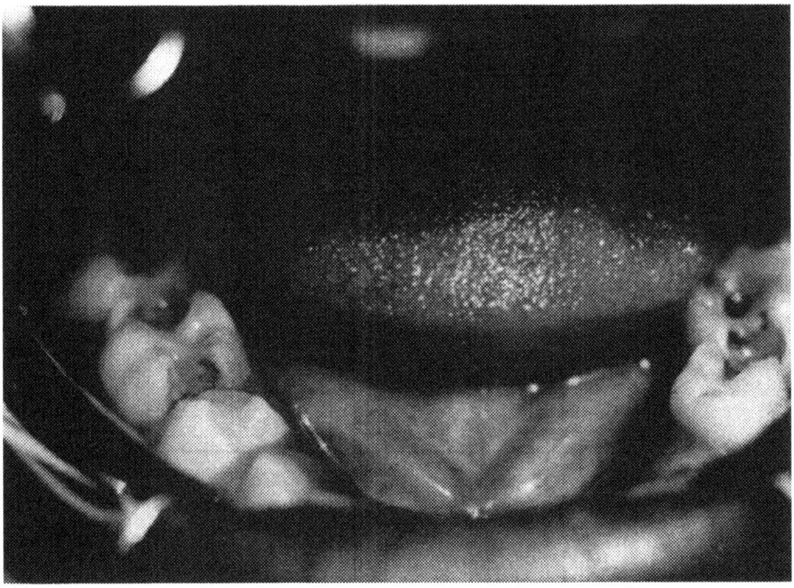

FIGURE 5. Dental caries in an African mouth (Nigeria) affecting 76|67, i.e., the lower right and left, first and second permanent molar teeth.

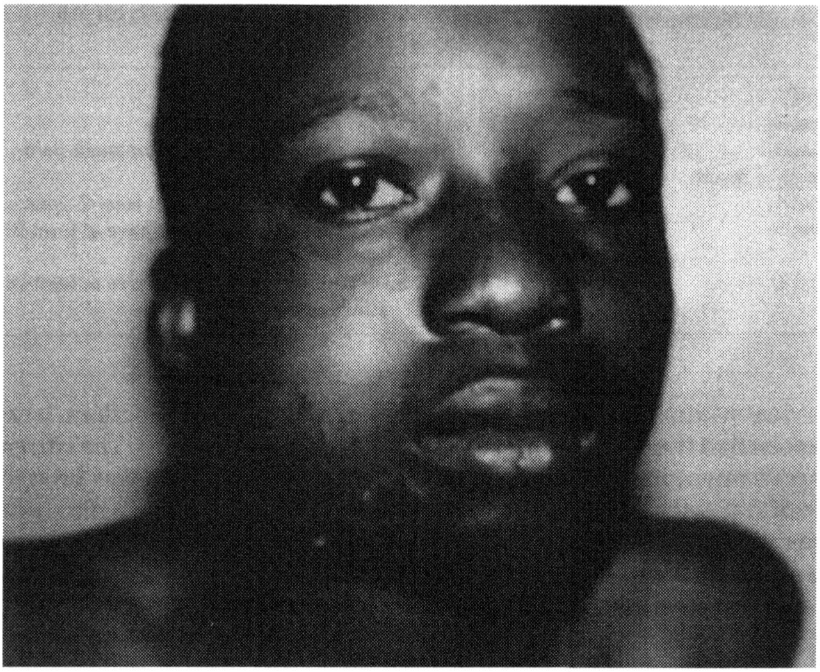

FIGURE 6. Dental abscess from untreated dental caries (Nigeria) from 6|, i.e., from untreated maxillary first molar teeth.

ETIOLOGY

Dental caries is a sugar-dependent disease, and any discussion of the changing pattern of dental caries in the developing countries must consider the changes in sugar consumption in these countries. Sugar consumption in all developing countries is rising, and continues to rise.

TABLE 3. National Health Service (United Kingdom) General Dental Service Cost

Year	Courses of treatment	Cost (millions sterling)
1968	20,065,772	71.5
1970	20,747,678	88.0
1972	23,418,337	106.5
1975	27,068,684	191.5
1977	28,276,234	230.0

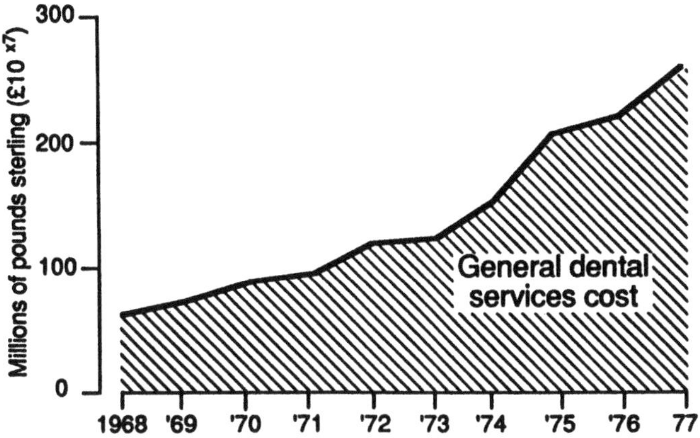

FIGURE 7. Cost of general dental services (NHS) in the United Kingdom 1968–1977.

Figure 10 shows the total sugar consumption in Nigeria between 1969 (95 million kg) and 1975 (137 million kg). This represents an increase of 70% in the amount of sugar consumed in Nigeria within those years.

It is not sugar, which is consumed as such, that is the only problem. The "hidden sugar," consumed in soft drinks, sweet biscuits, cakes, sweetened condensed milk, sweets, and other confectionery constitute a greater problem. Sugar is one of the first foods to respond to a rise in income in low-income countries. The percentage of hidden sugars consumed rises progressively with rising income, and thereby increases the total sugar consumption.

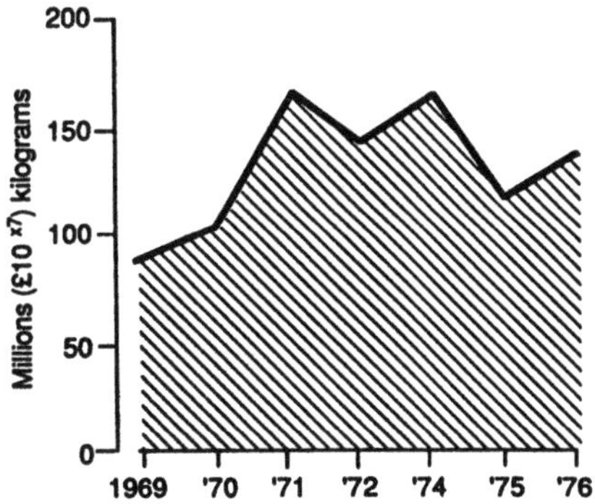

FIGURE 8. Sugar consumption in Nigeria between 1969 and 1976.

SUGAR AND DENTAL CARIES The consensus opinion on the cause of the increase in dental caries in many developing countries is that refined sugars and, in particular, sucrose, is the principal dietary cause. Dental surveys in many African countries have already shown that children from the higher socioeconomic groups have more dental caries than children from poorer homes, simply because the former have greater access to sugars in one form or another. At school, a permanent secretary's child can easily be identified from that of an artisan farmer during dental examination.[11–13]

COMMUNITY MEASURES TO COUNTER CARIES INCREASE

REDUCE SUGAR CONSUMPTION If the increase in dental caries in many developing countries is directly related to the increased consumption of refined sugar, and particularly sucrose, the obvious countermeasure is to reduce sugar consumption. The traditional African or Asian food contains little refined sugar. Such traditional food is in such total contrast to the now popular sweet biscuits, cakes, sweets, and soft drinks, which are all laden with "hidden sugars," and which one sees our African or Asian children consume during school breaks, or along the streets of Lagos, Nairobi, Delhi, Bangkok, or Manila. Figure 9 shows

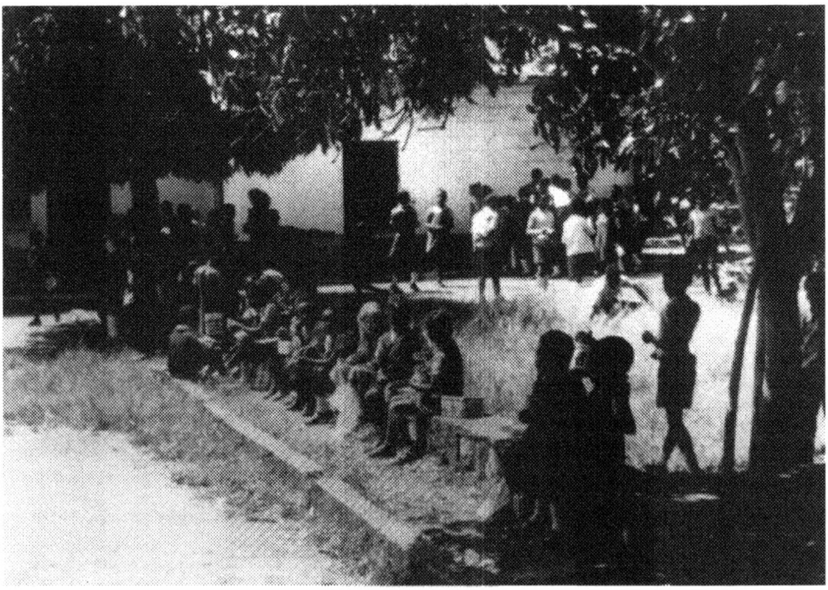

FIGURE 9. School break at Jos, Northern Nigeria.

a school break at Jos in Northern Nigeria. Each of those sandwich boxes has either sweet biscuits or some form of confectionery. Since it is not easy to change children's or adults' habits overnight, it is suggested that in addition to initiating appropriate health education programs at schools, at health clinics, and through village health workers, the government, through their ministry of health, should seriously consider implementing the following food policy, for a start, in many developing countries:

1. No sugars should be added to infant and baby foods, pediatric medicines, fruit juices, and vitamin preparations.
2. The levels of added sugars in commonly used foods should be reduced, and more alternative brands of foods with no added sugars should be made available.
3. The sugar content of confections and drinks should be reduced, and sugar-free snacks and drinks made available.
4. Sugar consumption should be discouraged; the level should not go above 10 kg per person per annum.
5. A community health education program focused on community involvement and school health education should be introduced as a matter of urgency.

Fluoridation

Community Water Fluoridation Community water fluoridation has been shown, over and over again, to be the most effective, and the cheapest, tested method of preventing the onset and the progression of dental caries. Where the fluoride content of community drinking water supply is minimal, that is, less than 0.7 ppm in the tropics or 1 ppm in the temperate countries, the government should investigate first and then seriously consider water fluoridation. Between 40–60% caries reduction has been reported in many parts of the world through community water fluoridation. In England, the current 32–57% reduction in the level of caries seen among the 12-year-old children (1970–1983) has been attributed, *not* to the increased number of dentists, but simply to the greater exposure to the use of fluoride toothpastes. Community water fluoridation is *not* advocated in areas such as parts of East Africa, Kenya, Tanzania, and other parts of the world where there is severe endemic dental fluorosis, and a high fluoride content in the natural drinking water supply.

Alternative Methods to Water Fluoridation Where there is minimal fluoride, but water fluoridation is not feasible, it is suggested

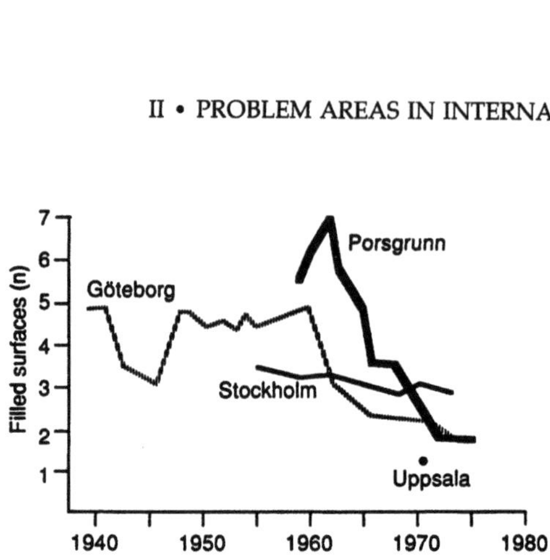

FIGURE 10. Sweden—Reduction in caries from water fluoridation.

that the government could consider other simple alternative methods of using fluorides, such as:

1. Salt fluoridation—as is done in parts of Switzerland and France,
2. Supervised fluoride rinsing at school—as is carried out in Norway and Sweden,
3. Supervised use of fluoride tablets, and
4. The use of fluoride toothpastes—as in the United Kingdom.

Figures 10, 11, and 12 show the beneficial effect of using fluoride to reduce dental caries in several countries.

Since every ministry of health is cost-conscious, and rightly so, it

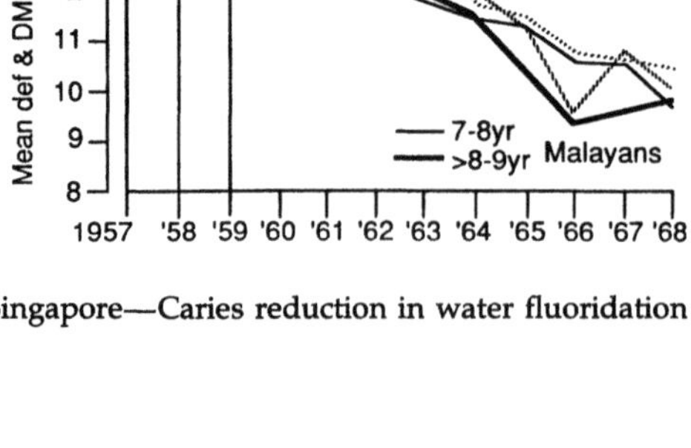

FIGURE 11. Singapore—Caries reduction in water fluoridation (1959–1968).

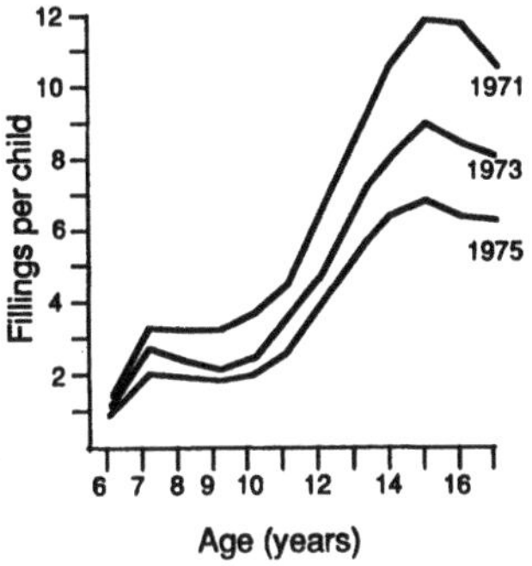

FIGURE 12. Norway—Caries reduction from regular fluoride rinsing at school.

should be pointed out that the initial cost of installing a fluoride plant in any community will be paid back, several times over, in the saving that will be made in the cost of treating dental caries and training appropriate dental personnel to provide such treatment. The cost of treating the ravages of dental caries in the United Kingdom, which is illustrated in Figure 7, is an eloquent testimony to the very expensive commitment involved in treating dental caries at a national level.

PERIODONTAL DISEASE

DENTAL PLAQUE AND PERIODONTAL DISEASE

The severity of periodontal disease (Fig. 13) in developing countries because of poor oral hygiene (Fig. 14) has already been referred to. There is indisputable evidence of a positive correlation between the level of dental plaque and the severity of periodontal disease. Reporting from a 1986 study in East Africa on the "Patterns of Periodontal Diseases in East African Populations,"[31] the research workers involved recorded that: "The oral hygiene was generally poor, with abundant deposits of gingival plaque and calculus."[30] Similarly, a section of the Report of the Dental Survey in Nigeria in 1982[12] recorded that: "One of the most striking findings in this Survey was the prevalence and severity of periodontal disease in Nigeria. Between the ages of 6–21 years, there was the urgent and *almost universal* need to improve the standard of oral

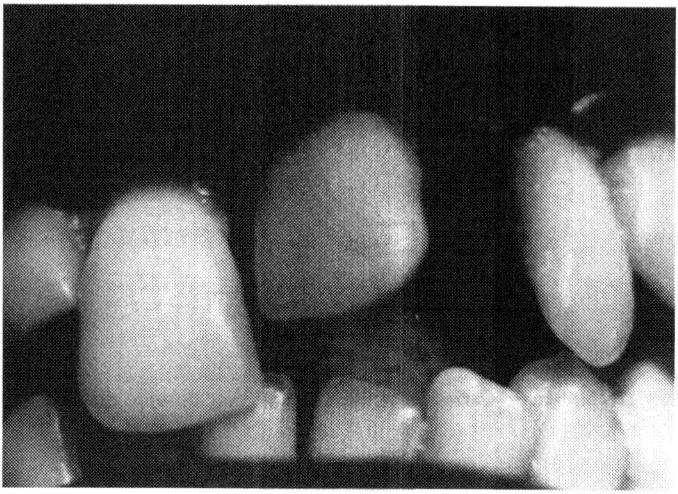

FIGURE 13. Severe periodontal disease (Nigerian—aged 18 years).

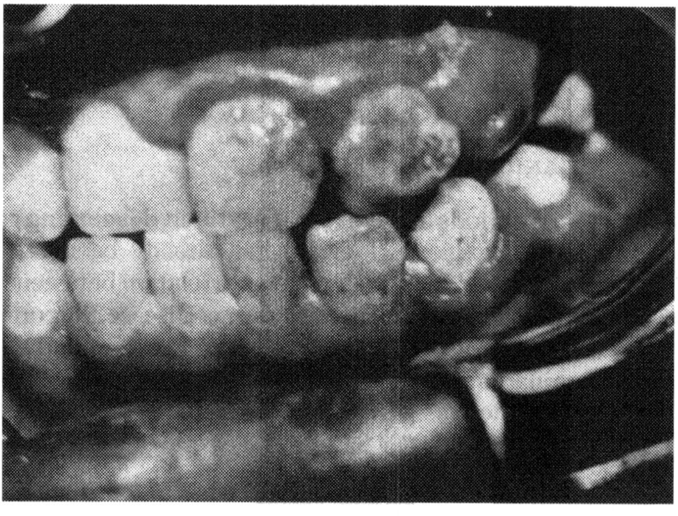

FIGURE 14. Poor oral hygiene (African).

hygiene amongst the children, and to prevent the heavy deposition of supra and subgingival calculus" (Akpabio 1983) (Fig. 15).

Those observations from Kenya and Nigeria are applicable to many other developing countries in Africa, Asia, parts of the Middle East, and the Western Pacific. How can children in developing countries be taught and encouraged to improve their standard of oral hygiene, and thereby bring about improvements in their periodontal health?

Dental Health as Part of Primary School Education

If improved oral hygiene is one of the keys to improved periodontal health, then it is reasonable to suggest that dental health education should be taught:

1. At the antenatal clinics to expectant mothers;
2. At primary schools to the school children, preferably at the commencement of their primary school education, when they are most impressionable;

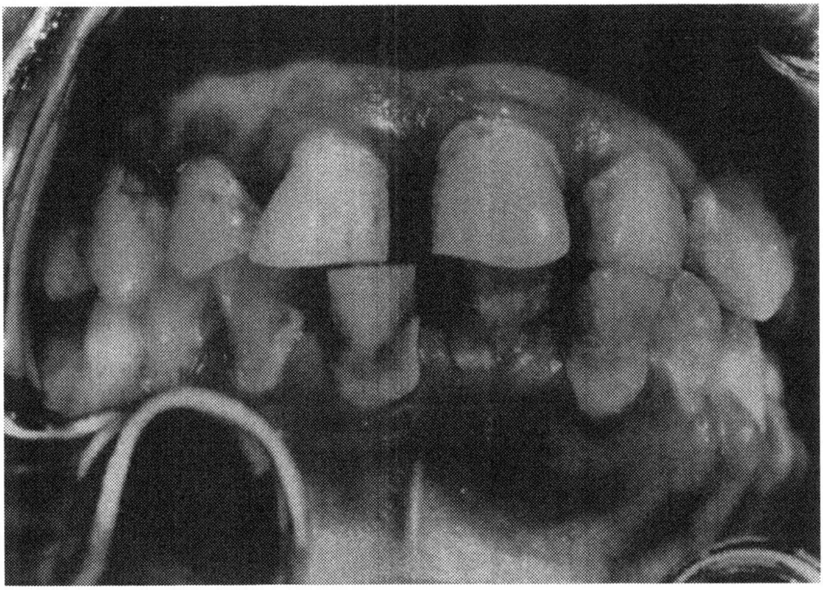

Figure 15. Heavy calculus deposition (Nigeria).

3. As an integral part of the school curriculum. This is already being done in some countries, such as Hong Kong and Tanzania. A regular period should be set aside in the timetable for dental nurses to visit the schools, teach, and then demonstrate to the children how to clean their teeth *effectively*—whether with toothbrush or with a chewing stick—whichever method the child uses at home.

Figure 16 shows dental nurses demonstrating tooth cleaning at a government primary school in Hong King.

Use of Locally Produced Materials

During travels to South East Asia and Africa, I had the opportunity to study some oral health strategies totally different from the traditional treatment-oriented approach. They seemed effective for what they were intended to do.

Chiang Mai Alternative Model—Thailand The WHO Collaborative Inter-Country Centre for Oral Health offers a unique alternative

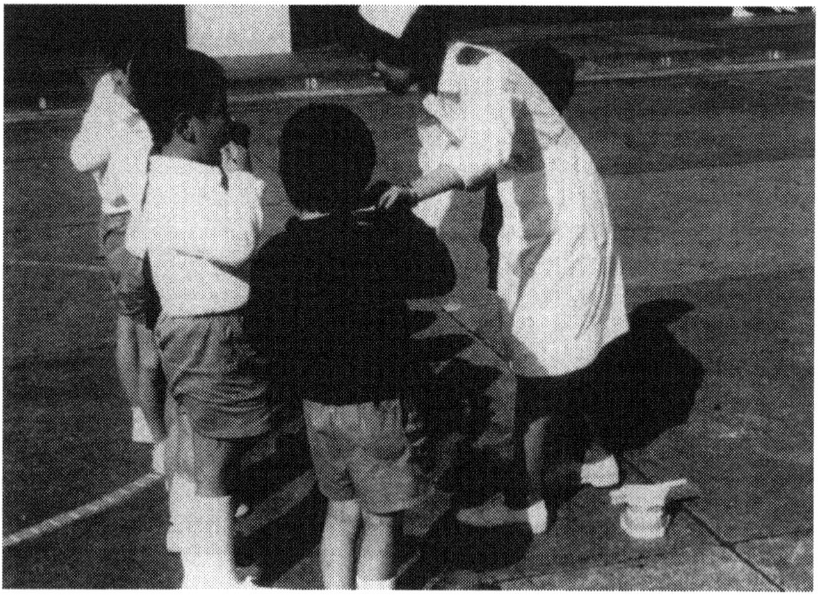

Figure 16. Hong Kong—School dental nurse teaching tooth cleaning at a primary school.

method for providing dental care and dental health education to the rural villages around Chiang Mai. In the Chiang Mai Alternative Oral Care Model, the significant innovation is that specially, locally trained dental auxiliaries are used to provide treatment and dental health education, after special training at the WHO Center, using simulators for training, and using locally made materials to carry out treatment in the villages. The local community is involved in the whole health care process, and there is emphasis on prevention and self-help. Figure 17 shows a Chiang Mai TA scaler, using locally made bamboo beds and stools to carry out scaling and oral health education.

DENTAL HEALTH EDUCATION—TANZANIA In Tanzania, under a Tanzania DANIDA Dental Health Program, dental health education is now actively taught at primary schools, maternity and antenatal clinics, and through village nurses and village midwives. Figure 18 shows a maternal child health aide giving dental health education to mothers at a

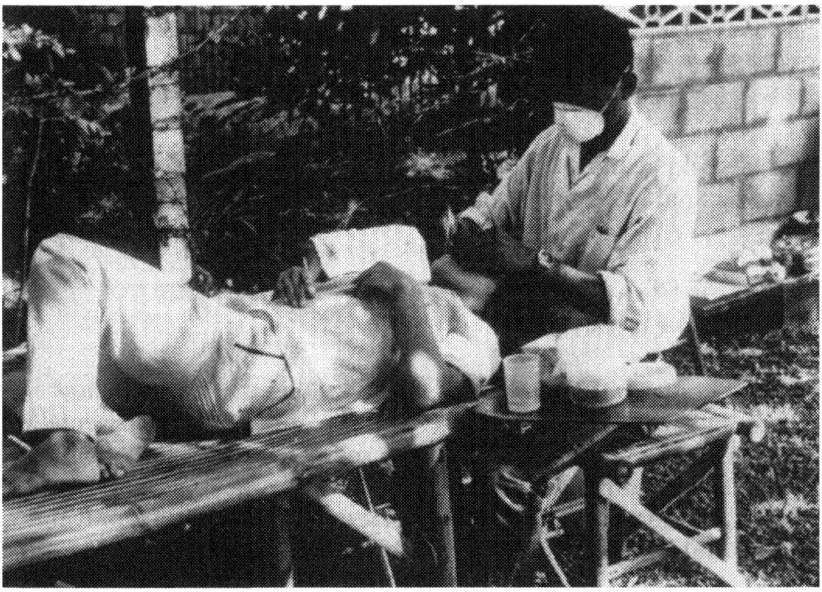

FIGURE 17. Thailand—TA Scaler at Chiang Mai, northern Thailand, using locally made dental equipment for scaling of teeth. (Emphasis on locally made equipment, not on expensive imported dental equipment, which often breaks down due to lack of recommended care.)

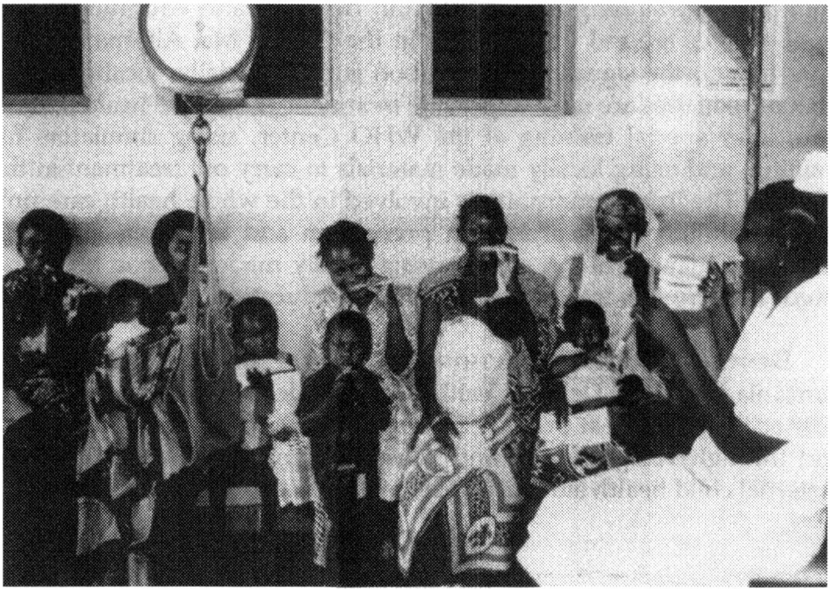

FIGURE 18. Tanzania—Maternal child health aides giving dental health education. (Emphasis on use of local chewing sticks for oral hygiene.)

maternal child health clinic. Figure 19 shows dental health education at a primary school in Hong Kong. Figure 20 shows an excellent dentition.

Change of Strategy—From Treatment-Oriented to Prevention-Oriented

From the content of this chapter, it is obvious that there is now very serious doubt about the effectiveness of a treatment-oriented dental policy. Such a policy has been shown in many countries to be expensive and totally ineffective because it does not tackle the real cause of dental diseases. A strong plea is therefore made for a change to a prevention-oriented oral health policy in developing countries.

Conclusion

I have attempted to discuss strategies to achieve oral health for all by the year 2000, in the course of which, indicating the causes of dental

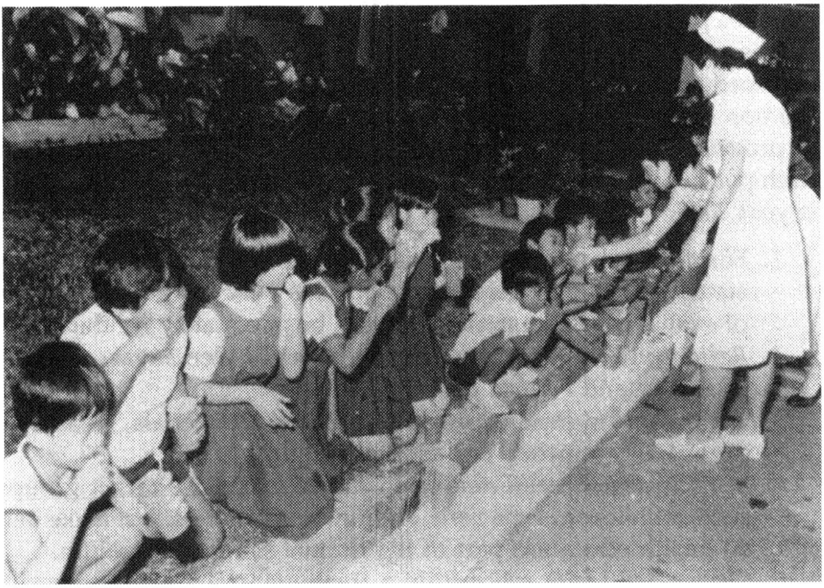

FIGURE 19. Singapore—Practical dental health education taught to primary school children.

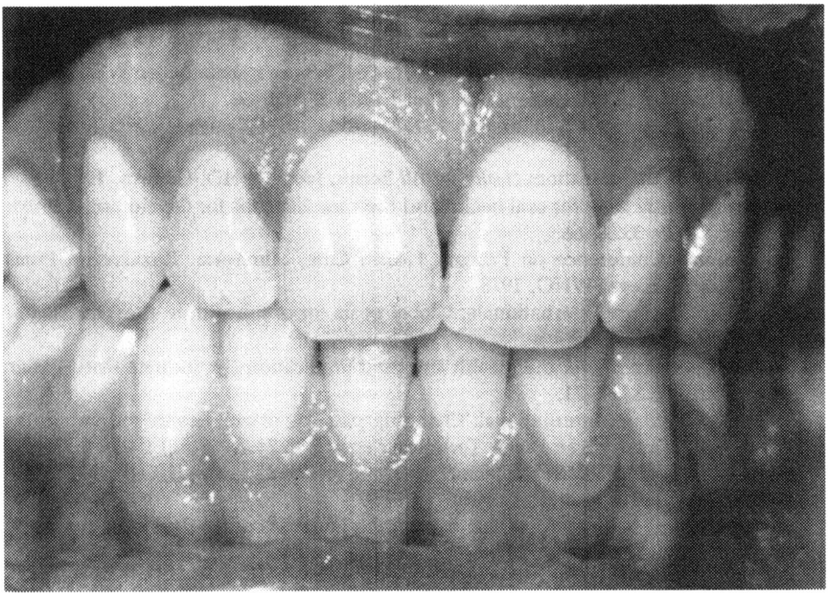

FIGURE 20. Excellent dentition.

decay and periodontal disease. Also discussed have been the reasons for the present contrasting trend of improving oral health in the technically developed countries, with increasing dental caries and poor periodontal condition in the developing countries. It is hoped that the presentation has provided food for thought for those who control medical and oral health policies in their various countries. To achieve oral health for all by the year 2000, the basic strategy is that each country should:

1. Formulate a *national oral health policy*—with a definite, clearly stated, realistic, measurable goal. This policy should be capable of evaluation. The strategy should be adequately funded.
2. *Reduce sugar consumption*, especially the hidden sugars, in order to reduce and control dental caries.
3. *Improve oral hygiene*—using available local materials, in order to control and improve periodontal health.
4. *Institute dental health education*—aimed at special target groups, such as children, expectant, and nursing mothers, but make dental health education part of the normal school curriculum.
5. *Change oral health policy* from a treatment-oriented to a prevention-oriented strategy.

References

1. Aggeryd: Goals for oral health in the Year 2000: Co-operation between WHO, FDI and the national dental associations. *Int Dent J* 1983; 33:1:55–58.
2. Barmes DE: "Oral Health in the Year 2000" World Health, Geneva, WHO (June 1983), p 3.
3. World Health Organization: *Health for All* Series, No 3, WHO, Geneva, 1981.
4. Barmes DE: Indicators for oral health and their implications for developing countries. *Int Dent J* 1983; 33:60–66.
5. International Conference on Primary Health Care, Alma-Ata, Kazakhstan *Primary Health Care*, Geneva, WHO, 1978.
6. Federation Dentaire Internationale: Global goals for oral health in the Year 2000. *Int Dent J* 1982:32:74.
7. Greene JC: Indicators for oral health and their implications for industrialised nations. *Int Dent J* 1983; 33:67–71.
8. Federation Dentaire International: Changing patterns of oral health and implications for oral health manpower: Part 1, Technical Report No. 24. *Int Dent J* 1985; 35:235–251.
9. Barmes DE: Oral Health in the Year 2000. *World Health*; Geneva WHO (June 1981), pp 3–5.
10. Barmes DE: Indicators for oral health and their implications for developing countries. *Int Dent J* 1983; 33:60–66.
11. Henshaw NE, Adenubi JO: The increase in dental disease in the northern states of Nigeria and its implications *Int J Dent*. 1975; 3:243–250.

12. Akpabio SP: Dental epidemiological and orthodontic survey—Nigeria. Report of study sponsored by WHO and the Federal Government of Nigeria.
13. Henshaw NE: A survey of dental caries and oral hygiene in the southern zone of Nigeria. *Nig Med J* 1974; 3:243–250.
14. Enwonwu CO: Oral diseases in Africa. *Int Dent J*, 1981; 32 (1): 29–32.
15. Sheiham A: Dental caries in underdeveloped countries, in Guggenheim B (ed): *Cariology Today*. Zurich, Kargar, 1983, pp 33–9.
16. Akpata ES: The pattern of dental caries in urban Nigerians. *Caries Res* 1979; 13:241–249.
17. Hobdell MH, Cabral JR: Dental caries and gingivitis experience in 6 and 12 year old school children in 4 provinces of the People's Republic of Mozambique (1978). *Odontol Stom Trop* 1980; III (3):111–126.
18. Baelum V, Fejerskov O: Tooth loss as related to dental caries and periodontal disease breakdown in adult Tanzanians. *Commun Dent Oral Epidem* 1986; 14:353–357.
19. Moller IJ: Pindborg JJ, Roed-Peterson B: The prevalence of dental caries, enamel opacities, and enamel hypoplasia in Ugandans *Arch Oral Biol*, 1972; 17:9–22.
20. *Dental Health Survey—Singapore, 1984*. A Report, Ministry of Health, Singapore, 1984, pp 23–24.
21. Sheiham A: The prevalence and severity of periodontal disease in rural Nigerians. *Dent Practit* 1966; 17 (2):51–55.
22. Akpabio SP: Dentistry—A public health service in East and West Africa. *Dent Pract Dent Rec* 1966; 16:412–421.
23. Akpabio SP: Thesis. University of London, 1970.
24. Enwonwu CO: Thesis. University of Bristol, 1966.
25. MacGregor IDM: Patterns of alveolar bone loss in Nigerian Yorubas. *Trop Dent J* 1980; 1(3):49–55.
26. Enwonwu CO: Socio-economic factors in dental caries prevalence and frequency in Nigerians. An epidemiological study. *Caries Res* 1974; 8:155–171.
27. Pilot T, Barmes DE, Leclercq MH, McCombie BJ, Sardo Infirri J: Periodontal conditions in adults, 35–44 years of age: An overview of CPITN data in the WHO Global Oral Data Bank. *Comm Dent Oral Epid* 1986; 14:310–312.
28. World Health Organization: *Oral Health Global Indicator for Year 2000*. Annual Publication, WHO, Geneva, May 1986.
29. Baelum V, Fejerskov O: Tooth loss as related to dental caries and periodontal breakdown in adult Tanzanians. *Comm Dent J* 1986; 14:353–357.
30. Manji F, Bealum V, Fejerskov O: The pattern of tooth loss in an adult rural population in Kenya—The primary oral health project. Presentation by Dr Manji at KEMRI Symposium on Oral Health in Africa, Nairobi, Kenya, 8 November 1986.
31. Baelum V, Fejerskov O, Karring T: Oral hygiene, gingivitis and periodontal breakdown in adult Tanzanians. *J Periodont Res* 1986; 21:221–232.

12

Trends in Managing Hereditary Diseases

N. P. Bochkov and V. E. Bulyzhenkov

Introduction

The recent development of theoretical and clinical medicine is characterized by increasing attention to the hereditary disorders. Modern trends in the changing of the morbidity structure show an increasing role of genetic conditions in human pathology. Hereditary diseases cover a wide spectrum of conditions, ranging from severe congenital disorders to complex and variable genetic predisposition (Fig. 1). The general birth incidence of infants with congenital disorders is estimated to be about 40/1000 and approximately half of them have severe conditions which can cause early death of lifelong chronic diseases, though the total number varies widely in different countries (Table 1).[1]

The following data indicate the importance of genetic services in health care systems. In developed countries, congenital disorders now account for the majority of physical and mental handicaps in childhood. It was shown that 5% of all children at age seven suffer from some kind of impairment and that 88% of these handicaps are congenital in origin.[2] In developing countries where undernutrition and infectious diseases can be prevented, congenital disorders have emerged as a major residual cause of infant mortality and morbidity. Health statistics in such countries indicate that 20.8% of the infant mortality is due to congenital malformations and hereditary diseases.[3,4] In addition, many infants

N. P. Bochkov • Director, Institute of Medical Genetics; USSR Academy of Medical Sciences, Moscow, USSR. V. E. Bulyzhenkov • Hereditary Diseases Programme, Division of Noncommunicable Diseases, World Health Organization, Geneva, Switzerland.

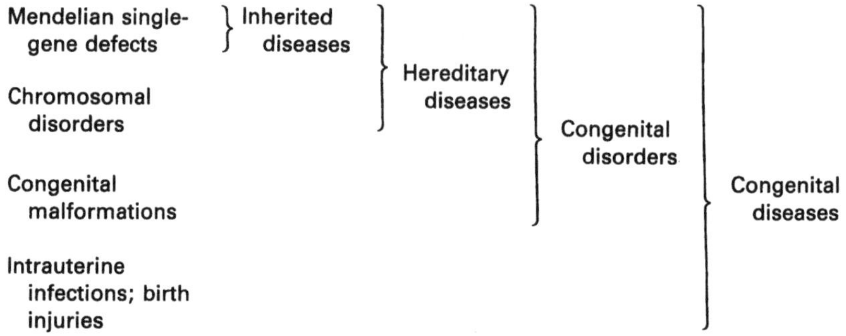

FIGURE 1. Categories of congenital diseases. "Common diseases" are not included. From Ref. 1.

with a severe congenital disorder are usually susceptible to infections, and, thus, most affected children simply disappear in infant mortality without attracting special attention. For example, in West Africa 2% of newborns have sickle-cell disease and most die from infections in the very early years, so this inherited disease contributes about 14% of the general infant mortality.[1]

Apart from this, progress in understanding the etiology and pathogenesis of a number of common diseases (such as coronary heart disease, hypertension, diabetes, some oncological and mental disorders) pointed out that genetic factors and genetic predisposition are also important in their appearance and manifestation.

Therefore, clinicians should pay attention to the genetic aspects of these diseases and genetic services, which should be an integral part of international health care.

The further development of clinical medicine and human genetics makes it possible to improve the genetic services available to the families with hereditary disorders. Previously existing points of view of dooming patients with hereditary diseases and members of their families should be disregarded. Genetic services are to help those with a hereditary disadvantage to live as normally and as responsibly as possible. It involves a comprehensive approach combining diagnosis, counseling, and appropriate technical interventions, as well as possible treatment of affected individuals and preventive approaches that range from selective abortion of a fetus to protective alteration in life-style. Modern diagnostic treatment and prevention approaches allow us now to mitigate the burden of inherited diseases.

TABLE 1. Estimated Incidence and Recurrence Risk of Different Types of Congenital Disorders[a]

Type of disorder	Incidence/1,000
Congenital malformations	
Congenital heart defects	6–8
Cleft lip/palate	0.5–2
Spina bifida aperta	0.5–4
Anencephaly	0.5–4
Other	10–12
Subtotal (approx.)	17–30
Chromosomal aberrations	
Sporadic	
Sex chromosomes in males	2.3–5.0
Sex chromosomes in females	1.2–2.9
Other	1–2
Inherited	
Unbalanced translocations	0.63
Subtotal (approx.)	6–13
Mendelian disorders	
Autosomal dominant	1.9–2.6
Huntington's chorea	0.4
Deafness or blindness	0.2
Osteogenesis imperfecta	0.04
X-linked recessive	0.8–2.0
Duchenne muscular dystrophy	0.14
Hemophilia	0.1
Autosomal recessive	0.9–2.0
Cystic fibrosis	0–0.4
Phenylketonuria	0.08
Mucopolysaccharidoses	0.04
Hemoglobinopathies	0–20
Global mean	1.8
Subtotal (approx.)	5.4–26
Total (approx.)	28–69

[a]From Ref 3.

APPROACHES TO THE DIAGNOSIS OF HEREDITARY DISEASES

Possibilities in diagnosis of genetic diseases have greatly increased in recent years. Diagnosis of hereditary diseases cannot be based only on clinical approaches, as it was in the past. Modern diagnostic methods, including genetic engineering, allow us to identify diseases rapidly and accurately. Achievements in general and in human genetics allow us to extend every year the list of hereditary diseases that can be punctually diagnosed.

It is now possible to point out two main peculiarities of modern methods in the diagnosis of hereditary diseases: first, the precision in diagnosis of a genetic defect, not only at the level of its clinical manifestation but also at the level of a gene or gene products; second, the essential feature of diagnosis is concerned with its timeliness. The number of hereditary diseases that can be diagnosed not by using (later) clinical disorders, but by gene action or an expression of gene products, is constantly increasing. This makes it possible to formulate the concept of preclinical diagnosis of hereditary diseases. For example, mutation of the thalassemia gene can be detected in a fetus before development of the specific hemoglobinopathies traits. Therefore, prenatal diagnosis, widely penetrating into modern practical medicine based on cytogenetic and biochemical researches, is one of the best examples of preclinical diagnosis.

It was shown, using the analysis of a special contingent of patients, that even different forms of hereditary diseases had not always been diagnosed in specialized clinics. The difficulties of diagnosis arise first from the variety of the nosological forms of hereditary diseases (more than 2000) each of which is characterized by the features of their phenotypic variation, on clinical polymorphism. At present, approximately 4700 different variants of Mendelian (monogenic) inheritance (nonobligatory diseases) have been recognized[5] and the early diagnosis of monogenic diseases is facilitated by the fact that in 10% of cases, the protein defect has been elucidated.[5,6]

As a whole, diagnosis of hereditary diseases is based on clinical, paraclinical, and special genetic research approaches. Main genetic methods are as follows:

1. *Pedigree studies.* These studies are especially important in a genetic evaluation and should be applied to any suspicious case of hereditary disease. They are concerned with thorough clinical examination of family members and genetic analysis of their data.

2. *Cytogenetic studies.* This type of analysis is performed on any fetus, proband, parents, or relatives having the increased risk of chromosomal disorders, which is the most frequent indication for prenatal diagnosis. As a rule, karyotyping is carried out when traits of chromosomal diseases (multiple congenital malformations) appear, as well as in the case of advanced maternal age, mental retardation, and spontaneous abortions in anamnesis. The detection of chromosome abnormalities using the banding techniques makes chromosome analysis more sensitive.

3. *Biochemical methods.* This approach is widely used for diagnosis of inborn errors of metabolism where the defects of primary gene products are revealed. The primary biochemical products more correctly reflect the pathogenesis of diseases than could be achieved on a clinical level and provide the basis for specific diagnosis and therapy. This is why biochemical methods are now playing the leading role in diagnosis of Mendelian (single-gene) hereditary diseases. In contrast to cytogenetic methods, the biochemical methods are not only diverse but complex, due to the expressed genetic heterogeneity as the wide clinical polymorphism. In connection with that point, a biochemical examination to diagnose precisely a hereditary disease should be made for probands as well as their relatives, i.e., combining biochemical and pedigree studies.

4. *RNA Technique.* With the development of new methods of molecular biology and genetic engineering for diagnosis of hereditary diseases, there is now the possibility of analyzing the gene structure instead of its products or its reactions. This approach, based on either close linkage of mutant genes with restricted fragment length polymorphisms, or by direct identification of the mutant site, permit the diagnosis of genetic disorders when gene products are not available in cells and chromosomal and biochemical levels are not feasible either. Thalassemia and sickle-cell disease are classic examples. Since, among the genes that have been cloned, there are many (several hundred) that cause hereditary diseases, the diagnostic procedures can be rapidly developed.

5. *Immunogenetic methods.* These methods are used for studying patients with suspicious immunodeficiency status, immunological incompatibility between fetus and mother, and genetic predisposition to diseases according to their HLA-antigen association.

6. *Genetic linkage method.* This method makes it possible to demonstrate the presence of one gene using the manifestation of the other one. It can be useful when each of the two genes has more than one allele and members of the family should be polymorphic concerning the marked gene.

Thus, combining the different approaches, it is possible now accurately to diagnose hereditary diseases and, therefore, to solve a primary task for the clinical geneticist.

For practical health care and its preventive orientation, mass *screening programs* have been elaborated. The programs are constantly being perfected and developed according to the medical peculiarity of the national health care. Screening for genetic diseases may have two objectives that are, although more or less distinct, related to the improvement of health. One of them may be aimed at the collection of genetic information on frequency, heterogeneity, and natural history of the mutant genes; others, at the diagnosis, counseling, and treatment when preventive and therapeutic measures are available. Mass screening on a public health basis was not recommended if there were no facilities for patient retrieval, diagnosis, counseling, and treatment.[7,8] In fact, in the frame of screening, the precise diagnosis, treatment, counseling, and prenatal diagnosis should be organized.

Since the screening methods are preliminary, they should be simple, inexpensive, and provide relatively little of the false-positive data. It is necessary that express methods to detect the patient with hereditary diseases be provided because large contingents should be examined. As a rule, elaboration of the express methods has been worked out to diagnose the common diseases appearing (no less than 1/20,000 in general, or in specific populations).

At the basis of world health care systems, two approaches are known to be used for mass screening programs:

1. Neonatal newborn screening for conditions such as phenylketonuria, galactosemia, hypothyroidism, adrenogenital syndrome, cystic fibrosis.
2. Detection of the heterozygote carrier in screening programs for hemoglobinopathies and Tay–Sachs disease among certain populations.

Apart from this, there are screening programs on familial hyperlipoproteinemia, adenosine desaminase deficiency, and some other forms.

The following examples are the most common neonatal screening programs carried out:

Phenylketonuria (PKU, one of the forms of hyperphenylalaninemia) is a classic example of the control of a relatively rare, severe, and easily treated inherited disease. It occurs in European populations with a frequency óf 1 in 13,000–20,000 live births,[1] and is detected in the neonatal period by a test using obtained blood spots. These blood spots are now used for the neonatal diagnosis of not only PKU but also congenital hypothyroidism, sickle-cell disease, galactosemia, and some amino acid disorders in different populations.

Cystic fibrosis (CF) is a common, recessively inherited genetic disorder that presents a widespread health problem throughout the world. Among Caucasian populations, about 5% of those who are heterozygous, the reported incidence of CF patients ranges from 1 : 1500 to 1 : 15,000 live births. CF is a generalized exocrinopathy resulting in obstruction or abnormal secretions in ducts of the respiratory tracts, salivary glands, pancreas, and digestive and genitourinary tracts. Screening techniques include the testing for increased albumin content in meconium, radioimmunoassay for testing elevated levels of serum trypsin/trypsinogen, and enzyme immunoassay, which has several advantages over the radioimmunoassay. Although further research is required to develop simpler and less expensive tests, at present the measurement of trypsinogen in dried blood spots has recently been applied in many parts of the world.[9]

For detecting heterozygotes among populations with a relatively high incidence of particular mutations, the examples of screening programs are Tay–Sachs diseases among Ashkenazi Jews[10] and hemoglobinopathies among certain populations.[11,12]

Tay–Sachs disease is a severe recessively inherited condition, classified as sphingolipidosis, and connected with the progressive neurodegenerative disorder, which was the first monogenic disease to be prevented by heterozygotes screening. Among the Ashkenazi Jewish populations, the carriers of the gene are consistently 3–5%. Heterozygotes for Tay–Sachs disease can be easily identified by quantitative analysis for activity of hexosaminidase A (Hex-A) using the synthetic fluorogenic substrate. Carriers have a significant reduction in Hex-A activity in their serum and leukocytes; by developing automated techniques the high-volume screening can readily be achieved.

There are two main groups of inherited disorders of hemoglobin production (*hemoglobinopathies*). First, there are conditions that result from a rate of production of one or more of the globin chains called, in general terms, *thalassemia*. Secondly, there are the structural hemoglobin variants, most importantly represented by the sickle-cell disease. Nearly 200 million people (about 4% of the world population) carry a potentially pathological hemoglobinopathy gene.[13] Over half of these are thalassemia genes. Both thalassemia and sickle-cell disease can be managed with reasonable success and prevented by heterozygote diagnosis and genetic counseling. The strategy to be adopted in heterozygote testing depends on the hemoglobinopathies that are most prevalent in the community. Three possible approaches to screening can be used: Automated measurement of the red cell parameters, the mean cell hemoglobin (MCH) is recommended as the most sensitive index; MCH determination and cellulose acetate electrophoresis at alkaline pH; and MCH and electrophoresis and Hb A_2 quantification. There are two main tests for sickle-cell disease: hemoglobin electrophoresis (cellulose acetate membrane electrophoresis) and the sickle test detecting the characteristic sickle shape of red cells. Therefore, a test for sickle-cell heterozygotes is simple, cheap, and should be incorporated into the routine so that each center acquires a picture of the distribution of heterozygotes in its district.

Thus, diagnosis and basic care for homozygous children should be included in the developing medical health care system. Ideally, this should be based on prospective identification of couples at risk of producing homozygotic children, so that a neonatal diagnosis can be made and optimal care offered from the outset.

The recommended laboratory strategy for population screening should be adopted to local conditions on the basis of an initial study of carrier frequency of diseases. Further research is strongly indicated for the development of techniques for fetal diagnosis and for understanding the social aspects of population screening. In initiating a strategy to control hereditary diseases, fetal diagnosis should be offered first to retrospectively detected couples. A community program of prospective heterozygote diagnosis and counseling should follow a successful retrospective approach as a distinct second phase.

Due to the implementation of various and improving approaches in health care systems, the early fetal diagnosis is at present available. Prenatal diagnosis is an important part of the counseling, allowing the congenital disorders during the early fetal development to be revealed. During the last 15 years, several hundreds of thousands of pregnancies have been monitored by the methods of prenatal diagnosis followed by cytogenetic or biochemical analysis obtained from fetal cells. The scope of prenatal diagnosis includes approximately 60 inborn errors of metabolism, over 30 other monogenic disorders, and an increasing number of chromosomal aberrations (see Table 2).[14] The overall rate of fetal abnormalities detected among pregnancies screened has been 3–5% and in most instances, termination of the pregnancy was requested, thus avoiding the birth of a handicapped child. The world counseling experience shows that many counseled couples need prenatal diagnosis because they are at risk (10% or more) of bearing abnormal children.[15]

The current approaches to prenatal diagnosis include:

1. *Amniocentesis* at 16–17 weeks of pregnancy involves a minimal risk to the fetus and woman. Several centers report a fetal loss rate of 0.5%.[3,16] Fifteen or 20 ml of amniotic fluid is needed to obtain sufficient viable fetal cells and it usually takes approximately 2–3 weeks of cultivation for reliable karyotyping on biochemical studies. Chromosomal observations, fetal sex, and some genetic metabolic diseases can be detected in this way.[17]

2. Recent technical developments are opening new perspectives in fetal diagnosis. The introduction of *chorionic villus sampling* (CVS) for fetal diagnosis in the first trimester of pregnancy is particularly impor-

TABLE 2. Inherited Disorders Diagnosed Prenatally

Disorder	Method of diagnosis	Mode of inheritance[a]
Conditions with known biochemical defects		
Disorders of amino acid metabolism		
Arginosuccinic aciduria	Deficient arginosuccinase	AR
Citrullinemia	Deficient arginosuccinic acid synthetase	AR
Cystinosis	Cystine accumulation in amniotic fluid	AR
Glutaric aciduria	Deficient glutaryl-CoA carboxylase	AR
3-Hydroxy-3-methylglutaryl coenzyme A lyase deficiency	Elevated 3-hydroxy-3-methylglutaric acid in maternal urine	AR
Hyperammonemia	Deficient omithine transcarbamylase in liver	X
Isovaleric acidemia	Deficient isovaleryl-CoA carboxylase	AR
Maple syrup urine disease	Deficient branched-chain ketoacid decarboxylase	AR
Methylmalonic aciduria	Deficient methylmalonic CoA mutase	AR
Multiple carboxylase deficiency (neonatal)	Deficient carboxylases (biotin responsive)	AR
Propionic acidemia (ketotic hyperglycinemia)	Deficient propionyl CoA carboxylase	AR
Tyrosinemia, type I (tyrosinosis)	Elevated succinyl acetone in amniotic fluid	AR
Disorders of carbohydrate metabolism		
Aspartylglucosaminuria	Deficient β-aspartylglucosaminidase	AR
Fucosidosis	Deficient α-fucosidase	AR
Galactokinase deficiency	Deficient galactokinase	AR
Galactosemia	Deficient galactose-1-P uridyl transferase	AR
Glycogen storage, Type I (von Gierke disease)	Deficient glucose-6-phosphatase	AR
Glycogen storage, Type II (Pompe)	Deficient 1, 4 glucosidase	AR
Glycogen storage, Type IV	Deficient branching enzyme	AR
Pyruvate dehydrogenase deficiency	Deficient pyruvate dehydrogenase	AR
Disorders of lipid metabolism		
Adrenoleukodystrophy	Accumulation of C26 fatty acids	X
Fabry disease	Deficient ceramidetrihexoside galactosidase	X

(continued)

TABLE 2. (*Continued*)

Disorder	Method of diagnosis	Mode of inheritance[a]
Familial hypercholesterolemia	Deficient LDL cholesterol receptors	AR/AD
Farber disease	Deficient ceramidase	AR
Generalized gangliosidosis G_{MI} gangliosidosis, Type I	Deficient β-galactosidase	AR
Gangliosidosis, G_{MI}, Type II (juvenile)	Deficient β-galactosidase	AR
Gaucher disease	Deficient glucocerebrosidase	AR
Hypercholesterolemia	Deficient HMG CoA reductase	AD
Krabbe disease	Deficient galactocerebroside β-galactosidase	AR
Metachromatic leukodystrophy	Deficient arylsulfatase A	AR
Mucolipidosis, Type I	Deficient α-neuraminidase	AR
Mucolipidosis, Type II (I-cell disease)	Deficiency of multiple lysosomal enzymes	AR
Mucolipidosis, Type IV (Bermann disease)	Electron microscopy	AR
Neimann–Pick disease A	Deficient sphingomyelinase	AR
Neimann–Pick disease B	Deficient sphingomyelinase	AR
Sandhoff disease	Deficient hexoxaminidase A and B	AR
Tay–Sachs disease	Deficient hexosaminidase A	AR
Wolman disease	Deficient acid lipase	AR
Disorders of mucopolysaccharide metabolism		
Hunter syndrome (MPS II)	Deficient α-L-iduronic acid-2 sulfatase	X
Hurler syndrome (MPS I H)	Deficient α-L-iduronidase	AR
Maroteaux–Lamy syndrome (MPS IV)	Deficient arylsulfatase B	AR
Morquio syndrome	Deficient N-acetylgalactosamine 6-sulfate sulfatase	AR
Sanfilippo syndrome A (MPS III A)	Deficient heparin sulfatase	AR
Sanfilippo syndrome B (MPS III B)	Deficient N-acetyl-α-D-glucosamindase	AR
Other metabolic disorders		
Adenosine deminase deficiency	Deficient adenosine deaminase	AR
Adrenogenital syndrome (21-hydroxylase deficiency)	Elevation of amniotic fluid steroids	AR
Alpha-1-antitrypsin deficiency	Deficient α-1-antitrypsin, or restriction endonuclease DNA analysis	AR
Hyperoxaluria	Increased amniotic fluid oxalate	AR

TABLE 2. (*Continued*)

Disorder	Method of diagnosis	Mode of inheritance[a]
Hypophosphatasia	Deficient alkaline phosphatase; ultrasound	AR
Lesch–Nyhan syndrome	Deficient hypoxanthine guanine phosphoribosyltransferase	AR
Lysosomal acid phosphatase	Deficient lysosomal acid phosphatase	AR
Menkes disease	Copper incorporation increased	AR
Nucleoside phosphorylase deficiency	Deficient nucleoside phosphorylase	AR
Osteopetrosis with renal tubular acidosis	Deficient carbonic anhydrase II	AR
Placental (steroid) sulfatase deficiency	Deficient placental steroid sulfatase	X
Porphyria, acute intermittent	Deficient uroporphyrinogen I synthetase	AD
Porphyria, congenital erythropoietic	Deficient uroporphyrinogen III cosynthetase	AR
Hematologic and immunodeficiency disorders		
Glucose phosphate isomerase deficiency	Deficient glucose phosphate isomerase	AD
Hemophilia A	Deficient factor VIII	X
Hemophilia B	Deficient factor IX	X
Sickle cell disease	Restriction endonuclease DNA analysis	AR
α Thalassemia	Molecular hybridization DNA analysis	AR
β Thalassemia	Fetal blood by fetoscopy: decreased synthesis of β-chain	AR
Von Willebrand disease	Deficient factor VIII	AD
Conditions with unknown biochemical defects		
Central nervous system disorders		
Cockayne syndrome	Increases sensitivity to UV light	AR
Fragile X syndrome	X-chromosomal fragility	X
Meckel–Gruber syndrome	Ultrasound, AFT	AR
Myotonic dystrophy	Linkage analysis in some families	AD
Seckel syndrome	Ultrasound	AR
Aqueductal stenosis	Ultrasound	X/AR
Hematologic and immunologic disorders		
Chronic granulomatous disease	Nitroblue tetrazolium slide test; hemiluminescence test	X

(*continued*)

TABLE 2. (*Continued*)

Disorder	Method of diagnosis	Mode of inheritance[a]
Fanconi anemia	Detection of chromosome breakage	AR
Severe combined immunodeficiency disease	Fetal blood: T-cell incompetence	X/AR
Renal disorders		
Finnish nephrosis	Elevated amniotic fluid AFP	AR
Polycystic kidneys	Ultrasound (some)	AD
Polycystic kidneys, infantile type	Ultrasound	AR
Skeletal disorders		
Achondrogenesis	Ultrasound amniography	AR
Achondroplasia	Ultrasound	AD
Asphyxiating thoracic dystrophy	Ultrasound	AR
Camptomelic dysplasia	Ultrasound	AR
Diastrophic dwarfism	Ultrasound	AR
Ectrodactyly	Ultrasound	AR
Ellis–van Creveld syndrome	Ultrasound	AR
Osteogenesis imperfecta congenita (Type II)	Ultrasound: femur growth	AR
Roberts syndrome	Ultrasound: chromosome analysis	AR
Thrombocytopenia-absent radii (TAR) syndrome	Ultrasound	AR
Skin disorders		
Albinism, oculocutaneous (tyrosinase negative)	Fetal skin biopsy	AR
Congenital bullous ichthyosiform (epidermolytic hyperkeratosis)	Fetal skin biopsy	AD
Epidermolysis bullosa letalis	Fetal skin biopsy	AR
Hypohidrotic ectodermal dysplasia	Fetal skin biopsy	X/AR
Ichthyosis, lamellar (harlequin)	Fetal skin biopsy	AR
Sjögren–Larsson syndrome	Fetal skin biopsy	AR
Xeroderma pigmentosum	Defective DNA repair in fibroblasts	AR

[a]AR, autosomal recessive; AD, autosomal dominant; X, X-linked.

tant. Because amniocentesis has to be performed in the second trimesters, the CVS method offers a greater benefit in terms of a reduced waiting period for results and a safer method of abortion if it becomes necessary. The biopsied material of fetal chorionic villi can be cultured or used directly for cytogenetic, biochemical, or DNA analysis. The latter technique has become a powerful tool for the prediction of hereditary diseases in cases where diagnosis of the chromosome or gene product level is not feasible or even when the mutant gene products are not expressed in examined cells.[22]

3. *Ultrasound examination* is important not only for guiding sampling techniques for fetal diagnosis, but its impressive and continuing improvement also means that more and more fetal malformations can be diagnosed in the second trimester of pregnancy.[20,21] The main risk in an ultrasound examination is misdiagnosis, which can lead to either therapeutic abortion of a normal fetus or the continuation of a pregnancy with a seriously abnormal fetus. Therefore, unless special expertise and equipment is available, screening for fetal malformation in all pregnant women is not recommended because of the high risk of false-positive or -negative results.

4. *Fetoscopy* was initially concerned with direct visualization of the fetus. It is now mainly used to obtain fetal blood for diagnosis of disorders that are only expressed in blood cells or plasma, as in hemoglobinopathies, hemophilia, and some immune deficiencies. Fetal skin, liver biopsies, and intrauterine transfusions may also be performed through a fetoscopy.[18] The obstetric risk involved is in general about 7% but can be as low as 1–3% in expert centers. The need for fetal blood sampling will decrease as DNA probes become available for the diagnosis of disorders that at present can only be detected by protein analysis of fetal blood.[19]

The main indications for prenatal diagnosis are as follows (see Table 3): Increased maternal age (>35 years); a previous child with a chromosomal abnormality; one parent carrying a chromosomal abnormality or dominant disorder; both parents are heterozygous or mutant gene or mother only is a carrier of mutant gene in x-chromosome; effect of teratogenes or X ray on pregnant women.

Diagnosis of chromosomal abnormality leading to termination of the pregnancy occurs in about 1.5 to 3% of older mothers and the risk of a recurrence in subsequent pregnancies is relatively small. Amniocentesis for the maternal age indication is therefore viewed by many women as a reassuring procedure.

The main means of diagnosing single-gene defects in the fetus is by biochemical analysis of the amniotic fluid, fetal blood cell, or chorionic villus sampling. Some Mendelian conditions associated with physical abnormalities can be diagnosed directly by ultrasound. The range of conditions that can be diagnosed at present is shown in Table 3. Individuals carrying dominant conditions, such as achondroplasia, may now be diagnosed in the fetus. The new DNA technology also offers

TABLE 3. Examples of the Pattern of Fetal Diagnosis for Congenital Disorders[a]

Indication	Proportion total number pregnancies monitored: Rotterdam, 1973–83	Proportion total number pregnancies monitored: Denmark, 1980–82	% Affected fetuses detected
Maternal age ≥35–38 years	40%	61%	1–3%
Previous child with chromosomal abnormality	14%	33% (both rows)	1.2%
Chromosomal translocation in parents	3%		8–15%
Risk X-linked disease	3%	1.6% (both rows)	20–25%[b]
Risk metabolic disease	5%		20–25%
Risk open neural tube defect	35%	4.2%	1–6%

[a]From Ref 3.
[b]The percentage of affected fetuses is usually lower than theoretically expected because of the monitoring of pregnancies where heterozygosity has not been demonstrated with certainty.

possibilities for others, such as Huntington's chorea. For female heterozygotes with sex-linked conditions (hemophilia A and B, Lesch–Nyhan disease), the prospective fetal diagnosis can be offered. The genetic conditions diagnosable by these methods are indicated in Tables 4–6.[23] DNA probes have already been used in the fetal diagnosis of thalassemia and sickle-cell diseases. A limiting factor in the widespread use of DNA technology is the complication of P32 radioactivity. Simplification of DNA analysis and the development of nonradioactive probes are essential for large-scale prevention programs involving carrier screening, genetic counseling, and fetal diagnosis.

The present limitation in the application of fetal diagnosis is its unavailability in many parts of the world. Ideally, there should be one center to provide genetic services, including fetal diagnosis, for every 2–3 million people;[24] but this level is reached in only a few countries.

Thus, everything mentioned above makes clear that the possibilities for diagnostic and prophylactic measures are wide and available. They allow diagnosis of the heterozygous and pathological conditions before their clinical manifestation. Some widespread diseases can be prevented at present due to existing and developing screening programs. Prenatal diagnosis approaches, combined with the attention of physicians to the hereditary diseases and provision of skilled counseling, could lift the burden of hereditary pathology and thereby prevent the birth of affected children.

TABLE 4. Direct Analysis of a Genetic Disease Using Gene Probes to Detect Intragenic Defects[a]

Disease	Gene probe
Achondroplasia	Collagen (type II)
Adenosine deaminase deficiency	Adenosine deaminase
Adrenal hyperplasia	Steroid 21-hydroxylase
Amyloidotic polyneuropathy	Albumin
Antithrombin III deficiency	Antithrombin III
α_1-Antitrypsin deficiency	Synthetic oligonucleotide
Atherosclerosis	Apolipoprotein A-1
Chorionic somatomammotropin deficiency	Chorionic somatomammotropin
Diabetes mellitus (maturity-onset diabetes of the young)	Insulin
Ehlers–Danlos syndrome	α1(1) collagen
Factor X deficiency	Factor X
Growth hormone deficiency (type A)	Growth hormone
Hemophilia A	Factor VIII
	Factor VIII and synthetic oligonucleotide
Hemophilia B	Factor IX
Hereditary persistence of fetal hemoglobin	β-Globin
Hypercholesterolemia	Low-density-lipoprotein receptor
Hypoxanthine-guanine phosphoribosyltransferase (HPRT) deficiency	HPRT
Immunoglobulin K-chain deficiency	Immunoglobulin C_k
Lesch–Nyhan syndrome	HPRT
Leukemias and lymphomas	T-cell antigen receptor
Marfan syndrome	α2(I) Collagen
Ornithine transcarbamylase deficiency	Ornithine transcarbamylase
Osteogenesis imperfecta (type II)	Pro 1(1) collagen
Phenylketonuria	Phenylalanine hydroxylase
Sickle-cell anemia	β-Globin
	Synthetic oligonucleotide
Thalassemias	α- and β-globin
	Synthetic oligonucleotide

[a]From Ref 3.

ARE HEREDITARY DISEASES CURABLE?

The more the community and health care system has been developed, the more attention has been provided to patients with congenital disorders. The concern is not only with providing medical services but also the social adaptation of the affected patients. Rehabilitation of those

TABLE 5. Indirect Analysis of Genetic Disease Using Gene Probes to Detect Closely Linked Polymorphisms[a]

Disease	Gene probes
Amyloidosis	Albumin
α1-Antitrypsin deficiency	α1-Antitrypsin
Apolipoprotein CII deficiency	Apolipoprotein CII
Atherosclerosis	Apolipoprotein A-1
Carbamyl phosphate synthetase I deficiency	Carbamyl phosphate synthetase
Diabetes mellitus (type II)	Insulin
Growth hormone deficiency type I	Growth hormone
Hemophilia A	Factor VIII
Hemophilia B	Factor IX
Hypothyroidism	Thyroglobulin
Hypercholesterolemia	Low-density-lipoprotein receptor gene
Hyperlipidemia	Apolipoprotein A-1
Hypertriglyceridemia	Apolipoprotein A-1
Sickle-cell anemia	β-Globin
Lesch–Nyhan syndrome	HPRT
Ornithine transcarbamylase deficiency	Ornithine transcarbamylase
Osteogenesis imperfecta types I, IV (mild autosomal dominant)	proα2(1) collagen
Phenylketonuria	Phenylalanine hydroxylase
Thalassemia-beta	β-Globin, γ-globin
Thrombosis	Antithrombin III

[a]From Ref 23.

TABLE 6. Indirect Analysis of Genetic Disease Using Linked DNA Segments to Examine the Co-inheritance of DNA Polymorphisms[a]

Disease	Probe	Distance between marker locus and disease locus (cM)
Adrenoleukodystrophy	St14	<10
Adult polycystic kidney disease	α-globin	~5
Alport syndrome-like hereditary nephritis	DXS3	~22
	DSX1	~25
Charcot–Marie–Tooth disease	DXYS1	a
	DXYS1	~7
Choroidemia	DXYS1	<9
Cystic fibrosis	LAM4-917	15
	c-met	Very close
	pJ.3.11	Very close
	T-cell receptor beta	10
	α-2(1) collagen	10

(*continued*)

TABLE 6. (*Continued*)

Disease	Probe	Distance between marker locus and disease locus (cM)
Fragile X mental retardation syndrome	Factor IX	10–30
	St14	<18
	Factor IX	<23
	DXS15	~12
Hemophilia A	DX13	<12
	St14	<6.5
Hunter disease	DXS15.DXS52,F9	~25
	F8	~15
Huntington's chorea	G8	<10
Hypercholesterolemia	Low-density-lipoprotein receptor	Very close
Menkes kinky hair	LI.28	16
Muscular dystrophy Becker	782	20
	λRC8	19
	99.6	15
	D2	24
	754	18
	OTC	15
	L1.28	18
	C7	Very close
Duchenne	782	25
	λRC8	17
	99.6	17
	D2	16
	754	21
	OTC	12
	L1.28	22
	99.6	~3
	C7	12
Myotonic dystrophy	Complement C3 gene	7
	Apolipoprotein CII gene	4
	D19S7	Very close
Neuropathy, X-linked	DXYS1	10
Norrie's disease	L1.28	Very close
	L1.28	Very close
Ocular albinism (X-linked)	DXS85	Very close
Osteogenesis imperfecta (type IV)	proα2(I) collagen	Very close
Retinitis pigmentosa	LI.28	<15
	DXS7	12.5
	L1.28	15
Retinoschisis	λRC8	15
	DXS85	20
	DXS16	10
Steroid-sulphatase-X-linked ichthyosis	λRC8	25

[a]From Ref 23.

already afflicted with a handicap due to a genetic disorder must also be considered in any comprehensive health program. While clinic-based facilities are needed for many purposes, in order to reach and help the vast number of handicapped, including those genetically determined, community approaches are necessary. The recent concepts developed by the WHO that aim at involving the community in helping a person with a handicap are some of the most promising concepts to emerge in recent times.

The presence of a severe chronic handicap, and the prospect of an early death due to a congenital disorder, not only affects the quality of life of the patient but often means a heavy burden for the whole family. During the last decade, there has been much progress in understanding the etiology of various categories of congenital disorders and their manifestation on clinical, cytogenetic, biochemical, and molecular levels. In some cases, the prevention of physical and mental handicaps can be achieved by early dietary management or drug administration after newborn screening. Well-known examples are phenylketonuria and congenital hypothyroidism[25]; in others, surgical methods permit the connection of various congenital malformations.

At present, due to progress of genetics and general medicine, it is possible to state that many hereditary diseases have already been treated. Like other well-known diseases, the treatment of hereditary diseases and diseases with hereditary predisposition can be divided into the three approaches—symptomatic, pathogenetic, and etiological therapy. At the modern level of medical genetics development, the main approach for treatment is a pathogenetic one, including the various types of therapy: drugs, diet, surgical methods, radiology, physiotherapy, and so on.

Symptomatic Therapy

This kind of therapy can be used in treating practically all hereditary diseases to prevent their clinical manifestations and, for many disorders, there is no alternative to this treatment as yet. Drug symptomatic therapy is used more frequently: for example, specific tranquilization for mental disorders, unguents for skin diseases, and so on. Understanding the causes of symptoms provides more delicate correction of diseases. When it was realized that cystic fibrosis led to obstruction of the respiratory system due to abnormal secretions in ducts and bronchus, affected children were prescribed dilutants with broad-spectrum antibiotics to prevent pneumonia.

Apart from drug therapy, a great many genetically determined conditions, especially congenital malformations, can now be effectively treated by surgical methods. For example, blood transfusion in hemoglobinopathies; plastic surgery for cleft palate and pyloric stenosis, heart diseases and meningomyelocele, hip dislocation, and osteoporosis; and bone marrow transplantation in the immune deficiency diseases. In general, surgical treatment for affected children can be of three types—correction, removal, and transplantation; and its possibilities are far from being exhausted. Thus, improving the method of renal transplantation could provide patients with polycystic kidneys, which would enable them to live a normal life due to the replacement of the affected organ. The same could apply to patients with hemophilia or agammaglobulinemia by transplanting spleens.

It should be stressed that symptomatic therapy will be available and helpful in conjunction with the most perfect pathogenetic or even etiological treatment of hereditary diseases.

Pathogenetic Therapy

During the last few years in the treatment of hereditary diseases, a new approach based on the recent progress of molecular and biochemical genetics has appeared, allowing the realization of all biochemical links that are responsible for the development of the pathological process from the abnormal gene product to the clinical manifestation of diseases. Thus, it is possible at present purposefully to implicate these approaches in the pathogenesis of disease.

Pathogenetic approaches to the treatment of hereditary diseases are based on the assumption that the affected patients have had abnormal product (protein), or the concentrate of the normal product is less or absent altogether. This point of view can be traced to the treatment of hereditary metabolic diseases. Briefly, these approaches are summarized as: correction of metabolism, treatment of the gene product, and enzyme replacement.

Correction of metabolism is one of the commonest forms of treatment combining different methods. Patients with phenylketonuria are put on a low phenylalanine diet at an early age. Special diets with limitations of the appropriate components are also provided in the cases of aminoacidopathies, galactosemia, and other disorders with known biochemical abnormalities. It should be emphasized that the specific limitation of the diets that restrict the manifestation of diseases is a widely used method of treatment for genetically determined metabolic disorders.

Apart from this, if the substrate is toxic, or participates in another pathological metabolic pathway, therapy can involve removing the toxic products. For example, thalassemias lead to iron overload and pathological iron deposition in the tissues. Care should be taken in prescribing disferrioxamine-B which, during the reaction with the iron ion, results in a water-soluble complex that can easily be excreted via the kidneys. The same approach is involved in the treatment of Wilson's disease with copper accumulation or cholesterol accumulation in familial hypercholesterolemia and these products can be removed by D-penicillamine or cholesterolamine.

Metabolic correction concerned with deficiency of a metabolic or biosynthetic product can be carried out by artificial replacement of metabolite. The usefulness of hormonotherapy is well known to patients suffering from adrenogenital syndrome, hypothyroidism, replacement treatment in some aminoacidopathies, mucopolysaccharidoses, and immunodeficiency disorders.

Following the progress of molecular biology, genetic engineering, and biotechnology, the necessary prerequisites for the production of specific proteins and hormones have now been created, such as insulin, somatotropichormones, and interferon.

Treatment of the gene product is useful for the correction of hereditary disorders where the abnormal enzyme of a gene product is known. With that purpose in mind, cofactor supplementation could be done[26,27] as, for example, pyridoxine for the enzyme cystathionine synthetase for patients with homocystinuria, vitamin B_{12} for methylmalonil isomerasa in the cases of methylmalonic aciduria, vitamin B_1 for ataxia or megaloblastia anemia, and vitamin D for familial hypophosphatemia.

In the cases where disorders are limited to one organ or tissue, the prospective approach could be the cell, tissue, or organ transplantation containing the normal DNA and allowing the supply of enzymes, hormones, or immunological factors. Within the different hereditary diseases are the examples of the modern trends for the treatment: blood transfusion and bone marrow transplantation in the immune deficiency conditions; hypodermic transplantation of fibroblastic cells in mucopolysaccharidosis; and transplantation of liver, kidney, pancreas, thymus. However, the major limitation of transplant experiences is the transient effect of the supplied proteins and the development of antibodies against them.

Enzyme replacement is supposed to be done at the level of the primary gene product (protein). Some examples of replacement have already been mentioned above: insulin to diabetic patients, factors VIII to hemophilia-A patients, etc. The main problems of the modern enzymotherapy are concerned with the enzyme sources and the delivery of the normal enzyme to the appropriate substrate in specific cells or tissues. In the latter, there is a hazard of immune intolerance to the introduced enzymes, if they are not encapsulated, that complicates this approach to therapy. At present, one of the prospective methods for delivering the enzyme to the target cells is the elaborating of artificial microcapsules—lyposomes, loaded with specific enzymes. Lyposomes could be captured by cells, their lipid covers destroyed, and the enzymes could interact with the substrate. Reassuring results have been obtained with respect to treatment of a number of diseases such as Fabry disease, Gaucher disease, and some glycogenoses.

Etiological Therapy

This is the optimum means, because it removes the cause of a disease. One way to correct the hereditary disease conditioned by a single-gene defect is to ferry into cells a copy of the functioning gene compensating for malfunctioning or nonfunctioning genes. This approach, called gene therapy, will initially be attempted in quite rare hereditary disorders: adenosine deaminase (ADH) deficiency and Lesch–Nyhan syndrome.[28] Gene therapy for thalassemia and sickle-cell disease can consist of two approaches: replacement of the defective gene with a normal one or extension of fetal hemoglobin synthesis into adult life.[11] The recent advances in molecular biology and genetic engineering do offer some promise to replace abnormal genes in the near future. The major difficulties are to insert normal genes into the correct cell population and getting them to express themselves in the appropriate progeny and in appropriate amounts. However, reasonable hope can be offered in using bone marrow cells as carriers of vectors with the new genes and developing vectors specific to particular target cells, and therapeutic gene replacement may become a reality within the foreseeable future.

Some mention should be made in respect to fetal therapy. Prenatal treatment for some of the hereditary diseases, due to improvement in the technique of early fetal diagnosis, is now leading to a new in utero approach to therapy. Vitamin B12-responsive methylmalonic acidemia and biotin-responsive multiple carboxylase deficiency have already been treated prenatally.[14] Although this approach is not widespread, there is no doubt about its usefulness.

Thus, many genetic disorders benefit from treatment and a steady advance may be expected in the range of conditions for which treatment is possible. Certainly, treatment of many inherited diseases (as more and more treatable genetic diseases are being recognized) is palliative and is likely to remain so until the molecular basis of each individual disease is known. However, it does not mean that a molecular understanding will necessarily lead to effective therapy, or that present approaches are ineffective. Treatment of genetic diseases is not always the direct responsibility of the geneticists. Many children with common inherited diseases, such as Down's syndrome, the hemoglobinopathies, or cystic fibrosis are managed by general pediatricians. Not all congenital diseases are of genetic origin, but the geneticist is nearly always involved in its differential diagnosis and works together with pediatric and obstetric colleagues. Most geneticists develop a particular interest in managing one or another group of diseases and should retain responsibility for centralizing information on the frequency, natural history, and treatment of genetic conditions in their area of responsibility.

Hereditary Diseases Must and Can Be Prevented

Prevention of hereditary diseases as a goal of all practical applications of medical genetic research could be achieved by measures including: prevention of new mutations appearing; limitation of the number of affected children delivered; and nonmanifestation of the hereditary sickly status. During the last 20 years, the condition of the prevention of hereditary diseases has been changed. If previously the limitation of the newborn was the main approach in preventive measures to couples at risk for bearing offspring with an inherited disease, in recent years preclinical and prenatal diagnosis are the main links to prevention of hereditary diseases.

In general, the preventive measures aimed at the three types of hereditary pathology are: (1) newly created diseases resulting from spontaneous mutations in the gonads of a parent; (2) diseases inherited from previous generations; and (3) diseases developing as a result of genetic predisposition combined with revealing environmental factors.

In other words, the preventive measures to deal with genetic diseases may be primary or secondary. Primary measures refer to actions taken to prevent the conception of a fetus with a genetic disorder, including either preventing mutation, or, if the latter has occurred, preventing its spread. This is provided through advice of the risks to offspring of known carriers, through properly integrated counseling services. Secondary measures refer to actions taken after conception, including early diagnosis of an affected fetus, genetic counseling, and the possibilities of suitable treatment to prevent disability.

The possibility of primary prevention, i.e., avoiding the occurrence of chromosomal aberrations and gene mutations, is very limited.[24,29] All environmental factors known as mutagenic agents should be avoided and a reduction in the rate of artificially induced mutations requires knowledge of the types, consequences, and frequencies of mutational events. Natural mutagens, including radiation, are widespread and there are few clear data on the frequency of spontaneous mutations in humans.[24] There is no possibility of freeing the environment completely from mutagens and the preventive measures to minimize the risk should be based on realistic goals.

Following these objectives, genetic services are most effectively delivered on a regional basis for a population of 2–3 million. It should be responsible for diagnosis of genetic diseases, treatment of genetic conditions that are not provided for by the general medical service, prenatal and neonatal screening programs concerning diseases or heterozygote conditions of the general population, counsel on the natural history, recurrence, risks, and social burden of a given genetic disease, and centralization of information about common conditions that are treated by general pediatricians and physicians.

Prophylaxis of hereditary diseases as an integral part of genetic services is best expressed in genetic counseling, which is the most effective and popular approach for measures of prevention. The essence of genetic counseling, observed as a kind of specialized medical care, consists of determining the risk of the affected child, giving an explanation of the risks to counseled couples at risk, and helping the family to make a decision. For couples at high risk (10% or more), two possibilities should be recommended as preventive measures: deterring them from childbearing (or pregnancy) or prenatal diagnosis, if it is possible for a given pathological condition.

The approach to avoiding the births of affected children can be focused on families at high genetic risk through the early diagnosis of the index patient in a family. Progress that has been made with the technology of cytogenetic, biochemical, and molecular diagnosis of genetic diseases, permitting genetic counseling for family members. Formerly, most requests for genetic counseling came from parents who already had an affected child and who were afraid of a recurrence (i.e., *retrospective counseling*). Now, about 50% of the requests for genetic counseling in some developed countries come from couples who have not yet reproduced and want to be informed about the risk because of relatives with congenital disorders.[16] Only genetic counseling delivered prospectively (i.e., before the birth of an affected child) can decrease the birth rate of affected children. *Prospective counseling* depends on prospective carrier detection, population screening, and counseling prior to reproduction, as well as early fetal diagnosis. The latter is concerned with the problem of the decision to limit reproduction and is a difficult one, especially for couples who have not yet had a child. Fetal diagnosis in early pregnancy with the possibility of selective abortion offers, for couples at risk, not only the possibility of preventing the birth of an affected child, but the possibility of having a normal child. It has led to the result that an increasing number of centers for fetal diagnosis have been established and many tens of thousands of amniocenteses are performed annually, preventing the birth of affected fetus through selective abortion.[3,30,31]

Prospective genetic counseling also requires community education, which should be directed towards informing the population about the conditions necessary to ensure the birth of healthy children. Ideally, pregnancies should be planned in an age range of between 18 to 30. The health and nutrition of the mother should be controlled during pregnancy. Avoidance of drugs, smoking, and alcohol that are harmful to the fetus should be recommended. Apart from this, about 19% of the world's births are located in areas where consanguineous marriage occurs by choice rather than by accident. The available data indicate that the incidence of recessively inherited diseases has fallen with the decline in numbers of consanguineous marriages and vice versa. The effect of the consanguineous marriage is also revealed in the appearance of rare conditions. Similar results could be traced in small populations where high frequencies of different genetic disorders are found due to a founder effect combined with isolation.

The other way to reduce the incidence of birth defects is to advise against pregnancy, those at an advanced maternal age (35 and over), since the various chromosomal aberrations, including trisomy 21 (Down's syndrome) increase with maternal age. These incidences in the newborn population can also be significantly reduced by termination of the pregnancy where such abnormalities have been identified.[3]

At present, the best way to avoid birth defects is detection and counseling of mothers at risk either prior to or during pregnancy. Since every pregnancy is at low risk for the sporadic congenital disorders, the approach must involve large-scale screening, using relatively simple methods, either of all pregnant women or of those who are at higher risk. Examples of such large-scale programs are as follows.

The neural tube defects (anencephaly, spina bifida) were the first group of serious congenital malformations to be diagnosed in the fetus due to increasing the level of *alpha-fetoprotein* (AFP) in both amniotic fluid and maternal serum. Most affected pregnancies can be identified by a raised maternal serum AFP level at the 16th week of pregnancy, and screening programs can detect more than 90% of anencephalies and about 80% of spina bifida.[30,32,33,34] The maternal serum AFP may be raised by many factors (multiple gestation, gastrointestinal atresia, fetal death) that can be detected by routine ultrasound, and about 5% of pregnant women with a positive result are carriers of a fetus with a neural tube defect. Therefore, a testing procedure should be developed to detect the cause of increased maternal AFP level, including genetic counseling, amniocentesis (if the reason cannot be clearly seen, a raised amniotic fluid AFP level in its turn can be confirmed by amniotic fluid acetylcholinesterase assay,[35] and ultrasonography. It should be stressed that the newborn incidence of neural tube defects vary from 1–2 per thousand to as much as 4–8 per thousand in some parts of the world, pointing out that maternal serum AFP screening should be implemented at least in high-incidence areas.

Increased maternal age (35 and over) is one of the main indications for prenatal screening because of the increased number of chromosomal abnormalities, including Down's syndrome, in fetus. In many developed countries, amniocentesis, CVS, and selective abortion are offered to older mothers. The incidence of Down's syndrome in many countries has been decreased from 1.7 to 1.2 per thousand live births due to the decrease in number of pregnancies among older women. However, only about 37% of Down's syndrome infants are born to mothers of 35 years or more because the total number of births at advanced age is less than at younger ages[36] and, therefore, it is necessary to develop new approaches of identifying mothers at risk. Now there is evidence of the correlation between a low maternal serum AFP level and the presence of Down's syndrome in the fetus. Thus, introduction of maternal serum AFP screening means the establishment of a system through which women may be offered genetic information about their reproductive life. In many developing countries the birth rate of Down's syndrome remains above 2 per thousand because so many "older" women go on reproducing. Education of older women about their risk, combined with family planning programs, would be a useful and inexpensive strategy.

Fetal malformations may be diagnosed by *ultrasound*, either by demonstrating abnormal growth of a fetal part or by visualization of a structural defect.[37] Routine scanning in early pregnancy is now widely accepted, allowing every patient to have a detailed scan to exclude anomalies. Apart from craniospinal defects, trained operators can diagnose fetal tumors, gastrointestinal anomalies, and congenital heart disorders that can be corrected by intrauterine surgery or early neonatal surgery.

The early diagnosis of monogenic diseases is complex. Biochemical abnormalities have been identified in an increasing number of Mendelian disorders, allowing improved fetal diagnosis, newborn screening, and treatment and carrier detection.[14] There is no doubt that every hereditary disease control program should, starting with public education, include heterozygote testing before marriage or during pregnancy, counseling at-risk couples on their reproductive behavior, fetal diagnosis, and termination of affected pregnancies. More satisfactory data are available for the common condition where prospective heterozygote diagnosis is possible, including hemoglobinopathies and Tay–Sachs disease.

Thalassemia control programs that combine optimal treatment with a community-based approach to prevention are now established in many Mediterranean countries. The thalassemia major birth rate has fallen to zero in the Ferrara district of northern Italy, to about 6% of expectation in southern Cyprus, and to 30% of expectation in Greece.[1,3] The introduction of first-trimester fetal diagnosis by chorionic villus sampling (CVS), combined with gene mapping, has largely extended the prevention possibilities of the program, because it allows the termination of affected pregnancy before 12 weeks of gestation, which is acceptable in some ethnic minorities and in several Middle Eastern and Asian countries that could not accept second-trimester diagnosis.[3,38]

It should be stressed that the vast majority of diagnoses for hemoglobinopathies are now done by DNA technique after CVS at several European centers.[1] DNA methods [cloned gene or oligonucleotide probes, restriction fragment length polymorphisms (RFLPs)] are widely used at present to diagnose and prevent inherited diseases (Tables 5–7).[23]

The prevention of *sickle-cell disease* (SCD) should be based on prospective identification of couples at risk, so that a neonatal diagnosis can be made and optimal care offered from the outset, since much evidence points to high mortality in the first two years of life.[11,12] Though the neonatal diagnosis, together with appropriate treatment, can reduce the early mortality and morbidity, SCD control programs based on neonatal screening have been established only in North America, some of the Caribbean islands, and a few districts in Europe. Diagnosis of SCD can be done by gene mapping in the first trimester of pregnancy and this approach, combined with heterozygote screening and neonatal diagnosis, is established at present in some Caribbean countries.

Other programs for prevention of *Tay–Sachs* disease, where heterozygotese carriers can be detected, have been established in the Jewish communities in North America. The implementation of the program with heterozygote screening, counseling, and fetal diagnosis has brought about a reduction of up to 90% the number of affected births between 1970 and 1980.[10,39]

At present, apart from above-mentioned diseases, carrier detection at the individual level is limited to X-linked disorders, such as hemophilia, Duchenne muscular dystrophy, Fabry disease, Lesch–Nyhan syndrome, and mucopolysaccharidosis.[3] For example, hemophilia could be prevented by fetal diagnosis detecting the sex of the fetus by amniocentesis and if the fetus is a male, a definitive diagnosis can be done by fetal blood sampling.

At the population level, neonatal screening for phenylketonuria, galactosemia, hypothyroidism, or cystic fibrosis, combined with effective treatment, results in the development of a normal child. *Phenylketonuria* is a classic example of a severe but easily treated hereditary disease, with a frequency of 1 in 13,000–20,000 in European populations. Neonatal screening is possible and widely used in the Guthrie test. At present, for many families with phenylketonuric children, prenatal diagnosis and identification of carriers by DNA analysis can be applied.[40,41] It should be said that establishment of the Guthrie test in screening programs can be used as a starting point for the control of other conditions, because Guthrie blood spots are also available for neonatal diagnosis of congenital hypothyroidism, SCD, galactosemia, and some amino acid disorders.

Cystic fibrosis (CF) is the commonest inherited disease. Among Caucasian populations the incidence of CF ranges from 1 per 1,500 to 1 per 15,000 live births.[9] Neonatal screening technique, based on testing for increased albumin in meconium or trypsinogen in dried blood spots, is being used in many parts of the world.[9] Due to the absence of reliable tests for detecting heterozygotes and affected fetus, diagnosis of cystic fibrosis as a rule could be made only after birth. However, the recent identification of genetic markers associated with the CF gene, as well as of the CF gene itself, has improved the situation[42,43,44] and there is a hope to use it in the prenatal diagnosis of CF.

The possibilities of DNA analysis permit the diagnosis of a significant number of genetically determined diseases as well as carriers of abnormal genes (Tables 5–7); but in the case where no cure is available, but diagnosis is possible, screening for the disease can be recommended only on a research basis.

In spite of the progress in the prenatal diagnosis, most disorders can be diagnosed only retrospectively. In the absence of genetic advice a family usually realizes that disease is inherited only by having more than one affected child. In countries where most families consist of 2–3 children, this effect is very minimal, but in countries where the average size of a family includes 6–7 children, the consequences are more serious. There is evidence that genetic counseling, taking into account the problem of family planning, could reduce birth defects by up to 50%.[24] Thus, a family planning service could be the first step toward controlling genetic diseases in many developing countries.

The prospect of prevention of inherited diseases is limited to preventing their increase rather than eradication, which is a necessary attribute to the communicable preventive programs. It depends on the natural mutation rate which is the essential characteristic of every human being. At present, sporadic congenital malformations are diagnosed only rarely prior to birth and most of them are based on ultrasound equipment, maternal serum AFP programs, and advanced maternal age. Improved diagnosis in the future will depend on the development of new approaches to identify populations at risk and to evaluate the consequences of the various types of mutational events.[29]

Conclusion

The diagnosis, treatment, and prevention of genetic diseases at present should be an integral part of every health care system. Health education, early recognition of risk, and utilization of a structured system of genetic services play an important role. The health burden varies between ethnic groups within the same country or among countries, due to genotypic differences at the population level; therefore a single strategy is not realistic. Genetic services should recognize this variability and be developed within the national health care systems.

There is a need, accordingly, for the physician to be aware of basic concepts of genetics so that he can recognize individuals at risk of genetic disease and refer them to institutions with more specialized services, or give appropriate advice. In developing countries, it would be helpful if the elements of diagnosis in genetic disorders common in an area could be reduced to a few simple components so that the primary health worker could be more easily trained to identify the individual who requires further evaluation.[23]

Thus, the geneticist contributes to improving the delivery of medical care through providing genetic services, incorporating it into the existing health care system to ensure effective delivery to the population, advising on the genetic aspects of general health care programs, contributing to community health education, and thereby carries out the prevention and control of genetic diseases.

References

1. World Health Organization: *Community Approaches to the Control of Hereditary Disease.* Report of a WHO Advisory Group. Unpublished WHO document HMG/HG/85.10, 1985.

2. Wells N: *British Impairments*. Office of Health Economics, No. 63 London, White Crescent Press Ltd, 1978.
3. World Health Organization. Report of a WHO/SERONO meeting. Perspectives in fetal diagnosis of congenital disorders. Unpublished WHO document HMG/SERONO/84.4.
4. Oakley GP: Antenatal diagnosis potential for major reduction in pediatric morbidity. *Ped Ann* 1981; 10: 13–21.
5. McKusick VG: *Mendelian Inheritance in Man*, ed 8. Baltimore and London, Johns Hopkins University Press, 1988.
6. Stanbury JB, Wyngaarden JB, Fredrickson DS, Goldstein JL, Brown MS (eds). *The Metabolic Basis of Inherited Disease*, 5. New York, McGraw-Hill, 1983.
7. World Health Organization. *Screening for Inborn Errors of Metabolism*. Report of a WHO Scientific Group. WHO Technical Report Series, No. 401, Geneva, WHO, 1968.
8. Vogel F, Motulsky HG (eds): *Human Genetics*. Berlin: Springer-Verlag, 1986.
9. World Health Organization. Report on a Consultation. Proposal for joint WHO/m(A) Programme for neonatal screening for cystic fibrosis. Unpublished WHO document WHO/HDP/COUS/88.2, 1988.
10. Kaback M (ed): *Tay-Sachs Disease: Screening and Prevention*. New York, Alan R. Liss, 1977.
11. World Health Organization. Report of a WHO Working Group on Hereditary anaemias: Genetic basis, clinical diagnosis and treatment. *Bulletin of the World Health Organization* 1982; 60: 643–660.
12. World Health Organization. Memorandum from a WHO meeting. Community control of hereditary anaemias. *Bull WHO* 1983; 61: 63–80.
13. World Health Organization. *Report of the Third and Fourth Annual Meeting of the WHO Working Group on the Community Control of Hereditary Anaemias*. Unpublished WHO document HMG/WG/85.8, 1985.
14. Epstein CJ, Cox DR, Schonberg SA, Hogge WA: Recent development in the prenatal diagnosis of genetic diseases and birth defects. *Ann Rev Genet* 1983; 17: 49–83.
15. Bochkov NP, Zakharov HF, Ivanov VI: *Medical Genetics. Moscow*, Medicina, 1984.
16. World Health Organization. Report of a WHO Working Group on Fetal diagnosis of hereditary diseases. *Bulletin of the World Health Organization* 1984; 62: 345–355.
17. Turnbull AC, Mackenzie IZ: Second-trimester amniocentesis and termination of pregnancy. *Br Med Bull* 1983; 39, No. 4: 315–321.
18. Rodeck CH, Holman CA, Karnicki J, Kemp JR, Whitmore DN, Austin MA: Direct intravascular fetal blood transfusion by fetascopy in severe rhesus isoimmunisation. *Lancet* 1981; i: 625–627.
19. Rodeck CH, Nicolaides KH (eds): *Fetal Diagnosis*. Royal College of Obstetricians and Gynaecologists of the U.K. London, John Wiley & Sons, 1984.
20. Hausmann M: Prenatal diagnosis of fetal malformation by sonar, in H Galjaard (ed): *The Future of Prenatal Diagnosis*. Edinburgh Churchill-Livingstone, 1982.
21. Campbell S, Smith P: Routine screening for congenital abnormalities by ultrasound, in C. H. Rodeck and R. H. Nicolaides (eds): *Prenatal Diagnosis*. Royal College of Obstetricians and Gynaecologists of the U.K. London, John Wiley & Sons, 1984.
22. Rodeck CH, Morsman JM: First-trimester chorion biopsy. *Br Med Bull* 1983; 39(4) 338–342.
23. Cooper DN, Schmidtke J: Diagnosis of genetic diseases using recombinant DNA. *Hum Gen* 1986; 73: 1–11.
24. World Health Organization. *Report of a WHO Advisory Group on Hereditary Diseases*. Unpublished WHO document, HMG/AG/82.4, 1982.
25. Bickel H, Guthrie R, Hummersen G (eds): *Neonatal Screening for Inborn Errors of Metabolism*. Berlin & New York, Springer-Verlag, 1980.

26. World Health Organization. *Report of a WHO Scientific Group on Genetic Disorders: Prevention, Treatment and Rehabilitation.* Technical report series, 1972; No 497: 1–48.
27. Desnick RJ, Krivit W, Fiddler MR (eds): Enzyme therapy in genetic diseases: Progress, principles and prospects, in *The Prevention of Genetic Disease and Mental Retardation.* Philadelphia, WB Saunders 1975, pp. 317–342.
28. Walters L: The ethics of human gene therapy. *Nature* 1986; 320: 225–227.
29. World Health Organization. Memorandum from a WHO meeting on prevention of avoidable mutational diseases. *Bull WHO* 1986; 64, (2) 205–216.
30. Ferguson-Smith MA: Prenatal chromosome analysis and its impact on birth incidence of chromosome disorders. *Br Med Bull* 1983; 39 (4) 355–364.
31. Galjaard H (ed): *The Future of Prenatal Diagnosis.* Edinburgh, Churchill-Livingstone, 1982.
32. Wald NJ, Cucle HS, Boreham J, Turnbull AC: Maternal serum alphafetoprotein and birth weight. *Br J Obstet Gynaecol* 1980; 87: 860–863.
33. Fuhrmann W, Weitzel H: Maternal serum alphafetoprotein screening for neural tube defects. *Hum Gen* 1985; 69: 47–61.
34. Korner H, Rodriguer L, Fernandezyero JI, Schulze M, Horn A, Heredero L, Witkowski R, Tinschert S, Oliva J, Sommer D, Solis R, Zwarhr Ch, Prenzlau P, Gobet G, Günter H: Maternal serum alphafetoprotein screening for neural tube defects and other disorders using an ultramicro-ELISA. *Hum Genet* 1986; 73: 60–63.
35. Smith AD, Wald NJ, Cukle HS, Starrak GM, Bobrow M, Laugerkrantz H: Amniotic fluid acetylcholinesterase as a possible diagnostic test for neural tube defects in early pregnancy. *Lancet* 1979; i: 665–668.
36. d'A Crawfurd M: Ethical and legal aspects of early prenatal diagnosis. *Br Med Bull* 1983; 39 (4): 310–314.
37. Campbell S, Pearce JM: Ultrasound visualization of congenital malformations. *Br Med Bull* 1983; 39 (4): 310–314.
38. Modell B, Berdoukas V: *The Clinical Approach to Thalassaemia.* London, Grune and Stratton, 1984, p 453.
39. Kaback M (ed): The utility of prenatal diagnosis, in Rodeck CH, Nicolaides KH (eds) *Prenatal Diagnosis.* Royal College of Obstetricians and Gynaecologists of the U.K., London, John Wiley & Sons, 1984.
40. Woo SCL, Lidskey AS, Guttler F, Chandrda T, Robson KJH: Cloned human phenylalanine hydroxylase gene allows prenatal diagnosis and carrier detection of classical phenylketonuria. *Nature* 1983; 306: 151–155.
41. Lidskey AS, Guttler F, Woo SCL: Prenatal diagnosis of classic phenylketonuria by DNA analysis. *Lancet* 1985; i: 549–551.
42. Tsui LC, Buchwald M, Banker D, Braman JC, Knowlton R, Schumm JW, Eiberg H, Mohr J, Kennedy D, Plavsic N, Zsiga M, Markiewicz D, Akots G, Brown V, Helms C, Gravius T, Parker C, Rediker K, Donis-keller H: Cystic fibrosis locus defined by a genetically linked polymorphic DNA marker. *Science* 1985; 120: 376–383.
43. White R, Woodword S, Leppert M, O'Connell P, Holf M, Herbst J, Labonel JM, Dean M, Van de Woude G: A closely linked genetic marker for cystic fibrosis. *Nature* 1985; 318: 382–384.
44. Kerem B, Rommens JM, Buchanan JA, Markiewicz D, Cox TK, Chakravarti A, Buchwald M, Tsue LC: Identification of the cystic fibrosis gene: Genetic analysis. *Science* 1989; 245: 1073–1080.

III

Approach to Problem Solving in Developing Countries

13

Education for Health

Stacey B. Day

Paradigm and Paradox

As this century turns, and after almost two decades of increasingly obsessive preoccupation with the costs of medical care, health educators remain faced with the problems of how to develop some suitable consensus that will realistically guarantee equitable access to health not only for the poor in this nation, but that will pave the way to appropriate basic health for the global population at large.

Certainly the need to improve the quality of life for fellow inhabitants of the planet earth is unassailable, yet in looking to the next century there is inevitably anticipation, even fear, of the various vicissitudes in the global, social, cultural, and political environments that will shape the lives of peoples and nations to come. Some of these changes are predictable, others are unforeseen.

Although disconcerting, the 21st century, like every century before it, while signifying a new era, offers mixed images largely of its own unique stability—instability equations borne on the waves of post-World War II technology and the contemporary communications–information explosion. At first glance these dynamics appear not so much to pose a challenge as to provide paradigms of opposites for the problem-solving skills of international health proponents.

We are obliged to consider, side by side, the health needs of several worlds. This charge and the broadening of international commitment is certainly not due alone to the recent numerous and diverse groups of national and international conferences and committees to define new approaches to the overwhelming problems of disease and poverty with which we are faced in the developing world.

Stacey B. Day • Professor of International Health, Founding Director, World Health Organization Collaborating Center for Community-Based Education for Health, Nashville, Tennessee 37208.

These conference committees, while often providing fascinating background reading, haven fallen far short of the real thrust of the problem of global health education, which by and large has been led by the World Health Organization. It is sobering to realize that John Stuart Mill long ago placed contemporary issues in perspective when he said, "No great improvements in the lot of mankind are possible until a great change takes place in the fundamental constitution of their modes of thought."

The Apostle Paul put it no less directly: "Do not be conformed to this world but be transformed by the renewal of your mind"; and though an ethic is not a policy, much less a system of organization, the Stockholm Declaration of 1972, reserved to the human environment, admonished *all* men to be responsible in the care of their community. As this prudence for care for man and his environment was expressed: ". . . A point has been reached in history when. . . we will demand the acceptance of responsibility by citizens and communities and by enterprises and institutions at every level, all sharing equitably in common efforts."

Understanding basic human needs does not require deep spiritual motivation; but it does require understanding of change. National development agency strategists, international negotiators, and global organizations now realize that they must be affected by the simple notion that the purpose of economic development and international cooperation is to meet the human requirements of people, and especially the minimum needs of the neediest.

If the developing world stands out as exceptionally in need, it may be observed that the poor and disenfranchised are not unknown in the industrialized technocracies, where in the midst of the rich and the affluent a new poor, including blue-collar and middle-class citizens who have lost their employment and, consequently, their health insurance, represent a compelling challenge to those faced with concern to find ways of assuming the costs of paying for the health care of citizens who now are unable to do so themselves.

Broadly, however, so vast and geographically, sociologically, politically, and culturally separate are the two worlds, that for all essential practical purposes, it is difficult to contrast them. Comparisons at best are imperfect exercises, yet notwithstanding diversity, all people have one shared need—an equitable guaranteed access to basic health.

Around this need are focused the many formulations deemed appropriate to alter the macroeconomic, political, and structural elements in the society in question in order to resolve the questions *Who will pay for decent human health?* and *How will this be done?*

By and large in the western industrialized technocracies it has become accepted that illness is the expression of a relationship or transaction of the individual, and that health is an entity or commodity that could be purchased, or distributed, rather than an essential primum mobile upon which the whole biopsychosocial construct of the society is founded.

In these industrialized countries, the dramatic improvements in health that are now so much taken for granted, in fact, date to the first half of this century, widely followed in train of social medical advances—pasteurization of milk, chlorination of water, fluoridation, childhood immunization programs, improvements in maternal and child care, and control of infectious diseases. Practically all these advances were made by public health measures. It was not until post-World War II, as a spin-off from military–industrial research and development technology that the notion of curative medicine, based on biomedical research, gained force. New World technology provided the vehicle for advancement to molecular biology, molecular pathology, and molecular pharmacology, and the impact of "health" became increasingly focused at the frontline of the entire human genome.

This magnificent thrust for a short time spawned new medical schools, new hospital plants, new technological equipment, new "health industries," and new health curricula. Pari passu, almost imperceptibly and at first almost unnoticed, the information–communications revolution gained momentum until biosciences communications and informatics have virtually exploded upon societies, so much so that there is an acute problem in terms of sifting through material to retrieve needed information. This rate of change of information per se will continue to be a major problem in industrialized societies for some time to come. Information produced in the Third World regarding socioeconomic, scientific, and technical fields is usually poorly organized, incomplete, and rarely connected to any centralized data system. The developing nations need access to the data bases of the industrialized world and must simultaneously begin to develop bases and banks of their own.

It is in precisely the communications area that one fears most for the developing world. As communications become a more complex and technical enterprise, the power to disseminate information is becoming controlled by fewer and fewer organizations. The power to inform has become a key to both politics and economics, and imbalances are daily growing. "The gargantuan disparities between developing and industrialized countries are growing, and are further aggravated by even greater disparities between urban and rural areas," notes the UNESCO plan of action "for building a better world." The responsibility for keeping open channels of communication between all nations—east and west, north and south, is crucial. Training and costs of installation are enormous; linkups demand training too, and search fees and transmission costs are considerable. Yet the development of integrated national systems for information and access to knowledge is one evolution indispensable for the uplifting of the developing world and collaboration towards the objectives of international peace and the common welfare of all mankind.

Nor have the western industrialized societies escaped the cost factor. Paradoxically, as their innovative technology opened up new vistas for enhanced human health and life, so did it fuel rising health care costs. In 1970, health care cost $369 per American. By 1986 this cost has climbed to $1896, and increasingly contemporaneous issues of cost containment generate controversy and debate among diverse concerned groups—physicians and academicians, researchers, business and industry, hospitals, patients, third-party payors, and so forth. How much money is *too* much for health? How much money is too little to save life?

Some policy leaders argue that the only long-term means to control the rising cost of health care is to slow the development and diffusion of medical technologies, change the practice of medicine, and revise the role that hospitals and health care providers have assumed. All these indications are "shifts in the way of doing business," and bespeak rumblings that some of the gains of the post-World War II era may be in peril.

Nor do current behavioral patterns in industrialized societies give assurance that all is right with national health—at least in America. Indeed, many social indicators sound alarms that the health of the society might be going in the wrong direction—stress, mental health deterioration, violence, suicide, chemical and narcotics addiction, teenage pregnancy, and uprooting, to name only a few.

Uprooting is the social metaphor of modernization and increasingly is becoming a dominant trend underlying all societies. The World Health Organization has identified uprooting as "the common factor in a number of psychological high-risk situations, such as migration, urbanization, resettlement, and rapid social change."

Few international health problems require the compassion of educators and administrators as uprooting. Humankind is becoming a single global ecological system—yet grudgingly so, assailed on all sides by national tendencies, parochial interests, and fixed and rigid cultural habits. In the industrialized societies, particularly, man's biological nature is confronted by unrelenting social and environmental pressures.

Uprooting, in both the developed world and the developing world, has to do with one of the fundamental properties of human life, the need to change, and with the personal and societal mechanisms for dealing with that need. Whether such growth into new capacities leads to new social health, whether the outcomes will be destructive or constructive, is a further option for man.

With respect to defining new approaches to the overwhelming problems of the developing countries, few agencies in the industrialized nations are prepared to acknowledge that "development" is to be viewed as a process that embraces all life and is therefore a global process. So-called "assistance" to the developing world, particularly when offered in the name of "education," or "technical and vocational education," or when "transferred as technology," has in the past had an appalling history of serving not so much the socioeconomic environment of the beneficiary countries, but rather the international economy and alien world markets fostered by foreign population, environment, technology, and development needs. Funding with strings attached is as often as not destructive to the developing world as it has been useful.

The keystone to advances in Asia, Africa, Latin America, and other parts of the developing world is biosocial development directed towards satisfying the needs and aspirations of their peoples, taking into account their actual circumstances—geoclimatic, sociological, cultural, and *their* development choices, utilizing as frequently as possible *their* experts and *their* people.

While there is no intent in this chapter to suggest technical models or to discuss theories of practical application in the light of different cultural and geographical settings—the integration of policies for the training of personnel or the involvement of women, for example—note should be made of the conditions that are determining so many third world national orders.

The degree of civil and social development considerably affects the major causes of morbidity and mortality, and biosocial conditions directly or indirectly are associated with constraints in health and in progress.

Of those biosocial conditions that exert a priority demand in determining community development the following are critical:

- Control of infectious and parasitic diseases
- Amelioration of defective nutrition states
- Improvement in maternal morbidity and closely spaced and too frequent pregnancies

- Reduction in infant mortality due to poor nutrition and unavailability of social services
- Banishment of apathy and reduced vitality to poor social, environmental, and economic conditions

Social dimensions and environment relate specially to many diseases:

- Malnutrition
- Malaria
- Measles
- Tuberculosis
- Tetanus
- Meningitis
- Dysentery
- Cholera
- Avitaminoses
- Helminthoses
- Filariasis
- Leprosy
- Guinea worm
- Poliomyelitis, and so forth

Further, these dimensions and diseases relate to the quality of life. We may well ask *What controls the quality of life?* and respond:

- Quality of the environment
- Quality of the water supply
- Quality of waste disposal
- Quality of housing facilities
- Quality of sewage and drainage
- Quality of power supplies available
- Quality of communications facilities
- Educational threshold of the society, including roles for women and youths

It is obvious at a glance that few educators in the developed world have reasonable *experiential* skills or familiarity with these problems in their environment, nor the expertise to set up priority agendas or prescriptives to single-handedly solve the situations at hand. Development has to be clarified as an economic, social, and cultural process in both a national and international aspect. Participation of the people is a most important factor in the success of health development, and training and potential improvement in life-styles must begin in the home, in the schools, and in the communities.

The technical implications in transferring health technology to the developing worlds are staggering and, even if appropriate, must be guarded. At best, communications are poor, infrastructure and planning capacity weak, and public awareness, especially in rural regions, uninformed. Political will to understand and use appropriate limited technologies, to resolve uneven distribution of resources, and fully to comprehend that the imperative must be for change induced *by* the nation and people itself and not simply be *in* it, is still a hope rather than a reality.

It is now some years ago (March 23, 1983), that in an address by invitation to the 12th Nigerian Medical Students Annual Conference at Calabar, I pointed out that many of the traditional western objectives of medicine and education, when transferred to institutions in developing countries, have failed to improve education and training of students, and critically have been of little or no use in rural communities where the great majority of people live. This point has been reemphasized by Professor Walter J. Kamba, Vice-Chancellor of the University of Zimbabwe, at Harare, when he remarked: "Much of the curriculum was similarly oriented to Britain, with little historical and cultural reference to Zimbabwe. Customary law, for example, was taught as an option—and a half course at that. In Zimbabwe there are two legal systems in effect, the indigenous (customary) and the Roman-Dutch on which the statutory law is based. Yet the rights of the overwhelming majority of the people are determined by customary law." "How," Kamba asked, "can one claim to understand the legal system in Zimbabwe without knowing the law that regulates the right of the majority?"

This perception is underlined by the words of another senior African educator, Professor Makany, Secretary General of the Association of African Universities, who in 1983 proclaimed that "the African University in the year 2000 is first of all a philosophy, an idea to assert ourselves as Africans." Given the enormous spectrum of problems, whatever approach to education for health is sanctioned, it should rest upon biopsychosocial integration of the biobehavioral sciences. This approach best offers improvement in the quality of life, protects the environment, and preserves the cultural integrity of the society, promoting education of women and children, and enhancing communication, including interactions at the international level.

Prudent and wise basic assumptions must guide this international interaction with the developing world. While we recognize that most of the people live in rural villages; that 80 percent have little or no access to health care; and that widespread poverty and illiteracy add to their vulnerability, nevertheless:

- Even though poor or illiterate or unemployed, people are intelligent.
- People are capable of defining their own needs. They are capable of defining their own problems, and given opportunities, they are capable of solving these problems.
- The satisfaction of basic human needs, both material and nonmaterial, implies the development of each and every human being.
- Such development as we have expressed is the right of *every* person, in all societies, in the developed countries as well as in the developing world.

As a matter of record I have seen conditions in the United States that are as lamentable as any I have seen in tropical west Africa, both in urban ghettos and in the fragile and difficult living conditions of the Navajo Reservation in Arizona.

In an effort to face "first-floor" standards in moving to change these situations, the U.N. has urged the following goals for the year 2000:

- *Food:* At least 2200 calories for every adult, with appropriate variations for hard physical workers and for children. Dietary standards for protein and fat have also been specified.
- *Life:* Not more than 30 infant deaths per 1000 live births, and a range of 55–65 years of age for life expectancy at birth for those born in 1985, 1992, and 2000.
- *Education:* A literacy rate of 98 percent for those born after 1970, 1975, and 1985.

Through national action and international cooperation these approaches to international health may at least attempt to satisfy fundamental human values in life.

The Rural Imperative

In the developing world, the underserved live in rural areas. They may, or they may not, reflect the understanding of the term "rural" in developed countries, where probably the single most important characteristic distinguishing rural from urban areas is low population density. This factor is particularly important in terms of its impact on communication and transport patterns, the individual persons' "sense of community," and the availability of specialized services and complex organizations and institutions. Further, in the *developed* countries a serious misconception is that of equating agriculture with rurality. While most farmers live and work in rural areas, only a fraction of rural Americans, for example, are engaged in agriculture. In the developing world, on the other hand, nearly everyone is a "farmer," and a "farm" in general may be little more than a garden plot of land.

In terms of health needs, the priorities in the developing world are as discussed—essential public services, primary health care provisions, clean water, and basic education combined with improved shelter and nutrition.

Developing for this broad range of features to enhance quality of life can hardly be focused on single-issue resolutions. In the developing world, and especially in the rural areas, any comprehensive strategy must aim at chain reactions. Such advances can only be made in a climate of economic growth; but growth alone and its advantages, essential as it is, cannot assist the people unless it in fact reaches them. All too often in the developing world the rural areas are passed by, and the mechanistic technocratic approach to development promising trickle-down effects has been without benefit. Rural problems must therefore be considered in an integrated way. Poverty and ill health will remain unless problems of population increase, health, employment, nutrition, housing, sanitation, and communications are all tackled simultaneously.

Regarded from this perspective, rural development may be defined as "a process of change in societies whereby poverty will be reduced and the creativity and existing knowledge of the poor fully utilized. The poor should be enabled access to the resources of society and the environment and encouraged to achieve control of resources that are introduced at reasonable cost from outside their rural environment in order to make available resources and goods required and wanted by the poor and their governments."[4]

Another useful definition considers rural development as the optimum utilization of the natural and human resources of a given rural area for the enrichment of the quality of life and the population.[11] This optimum utilization should take into account not only production but also distribution, employment, uplift above the poverty line, and environmental harmony.

The deepest underlying fundamental is low productivity, and it is this that characterizes largely the developing world.

In these relationships health is both an objective of and an instrument for development. In rural or in urban areas it is difficult to have a productive population if people are seriously ill or incapacitated; and this is especially true for labor-intensive farm areas.

To the extent that health is affected by poor nutrition and illness, rural people become less productive, the circumstances setting in train a critical cycle of low production, poverty, and malnutrition, which ultimately limits their ability to grow in the future. As often as not, characteristics attributed to apathy in the villages of the developing world, among rural people, could in many cases be better ascribed to poor health. A rural community is the best exemplar that in order to have a productive society we must recognize and deal first with its health problems.

Once a community learns to deal with health problems and their interrelationships, it almost invariably improves its ability to deal with other problems. Thus lowered morbidity in adults is usually evident in increased productivity and concomitant with lower mortality in infants. In programs against tuberculosis, trachoma, filariasis, and nutritional deprivation, the net economic impact of lowered morbidity is a positive increase in productivity.

Good health and freedom from disease contribute to economic development. Poor health imposes economic costs in rural populations by:

- Reducing the availability of labor
- Impairing the productivity of workers and capital goods
- Wasting resources
- Impeding development by new growth.

It might also be remarked that it is difficult to increase per capita income in a high-birthrate society. Consequently health and living standards remain low. One of the compelling reasons for high birthrates is the high mortality rate among infants in unprovided rural communities. Clearly, the entire spectrum of health services must be an integral part of any rural development program.

Health for All—All for Education for Health

Notwithstanding the magnitude of the task of improving global health, often in the face of conflicting social, economic, and political orientation, numerous health educators, academicians, technicians, and administrators, including some in government and parliamentary committees, as well as others in international agencies and organizations, have devoted time and effort to problem solving over the last 20 years. Prospects for health have appeared in many guises—curative, preventive, rehabilitative, holistic, traditional (native) and sociomedical, yet gradually a biopsychosocial–biobehavioral thrust has appeared from this input. Further, the need for a consolidated leadership, authoritative and responsible in a global sense, capable of harnessing political will, and with the organizational management background to integrate diverse socioeconomic groups everywhere, all bent on improving health, and all consciously involved with "community," has emerged. It was inevitable and fortuitous that the World Health Organization developed the leadership role for this movement and assigned a priority urgency to resolving international problems of health. Over the last ten years this leadership was manifest through three strategies and a number of support programs:

1. Adoption by the Thirtieth World Health Assembly in 1977 of the concept of "Health for All by the Year 2000," as a common goal of WHO and all its member states.
2. Formulation by the 1978 International Conference at Alma-Ata of the concept of *primary health care* as a leading strategy in achieving "health for all."
3. Adoption by the Thirty-fourth World Health Assembly in 1981 of the "Global Strategy of Health for All by the Year 2000."
4. Program to evaluate the implementation of the health-for-all strategy at national, regional, and global levels, 1985.
5. WHO's Health Manpower Development program to assist countries in formulating *health manpower policies*—goals, priorities, main directions aimed at the achievement of health for all through primary health care.

The first two of these concepts implied that there should be an equitable distribution among populations of whatever health resources were available, both nationally and internationally. Further, it urged that essential health care should be accessible to all individuals and families in an acceptable and affordable form, and with their full involvement, so that all people of the world would have the opportunity to attain, by the year 2000, a level of health permitting them to lead a socially and economically productive life.

This global strategy explicitly indicated that achievement of the health-for-all goal would require relevant reorientation of national health systems so that each might develop an appropriate organizational infrastructure based on primary health care. Such reorientation would have to be motivated by a basic regard for equity, social justice, and human rights, as well as comprehension of the political and economic conditions influencing the reorientation process towards the desired changes.

These imperatives led, among most workers, during the past few years to philosophies of interdisciplinary integration and various intersectoral coordination mechanisms advancing health manpower development objectives. Underlying these advances was the realization that optimum health care, even self-health, must involve the community in its own development—planning, training, and managing health workers, and evaluating their performance at all levels.

There cannot be health care without health workers to provide support and care. Planning for these workers, training them, deploying them in the health system, managing them, and evaluating their performance and their relevance to the actual health needs of the society is in effect what is meant by health manpower development.

Enlarging these objectives, under WHO guidance, we have seen most health educators emphasizing a shift of action from simply health care providers concerned with health problems to those imbued with enthusiasm for the emerging concepts of primary health care encouraging individuals increasingly to become aware that they are not simply passive receivers of a service where it exists, but that in fact wherever they may be, and whoever they are, man or woman, they are capable of being actively involved in matters regarding their own health. In this self-help, self-health approach they become aware of the issues involved, of the resources available, and function within the social and political sanctions of their community.

It may reasonably be said that understanding has at long last arrived that for any system of care to have impact on the health situation of a community the people themselves need to realize the problems and to collaborate fully in finding a solution. This concept in education for health is one in which health care providers and people both teach and learn from each other, changing roles constantly, devoted to the philosophy of the people being actively involved in the planning and maintenance of their own health and able to act in partnership with institutional health care providers.

This thrust of the WHO has emphasized not only the basic purpose of education for health, i.e., provision of knowledge, but goes further in seeking political aid and backing for all health-related activities.

By this approach, WHO argues, health is no longer the prerogative of any single group, but by virtue of its biopsychosocial and intersectoral nature it is the concern of all who are involved in socioeconomic and human development.

Under this thrust, men and women have become aware of their rights and privileges as human beings. Health science and technology can make a real impact *only* if people themselves become full partners in health protection and promotion.

The testing of the truth of the positions outlined in this discussion and the implementation of various approaches to training programs and community-based education have been carried out now for a decade or more. While most results suggest that the direction is methodologically sound, it is not the consideration of this chapter to give an analytical review of operations research and the management strategies at the present evolutionary stage of the "Health for All" Program. The nature of many of these endeavors is exemplified in the concluding bibliography.

One final issue, however, *does* need stressing. The ultimate challenge of "Health for All," to individuals and communities all over the world, needs attention to the *process* as well as to the *content* of health. Having learned that they can be responsible for their own health by changed behavior, societies and communities must continue and enlarge programs so that in a sense there is no end.* The successful fulfillment of primary health care must include *continuing education,* so that people may constantly face change, upheavals, even emergencies in their environment. Planning and implementing action for change is as much growing to develop their utmost physical and mental potential as simply avoiding illness or coping with disease. Promoting and protecting the quality of life includes preparing future generations to build and maintain a more just, equitable, and sociable, conscious, humane world. In these efforts, *continuing education* is the "will for health" and the keystone to securing the reasonable expectations of the biopsychosocial imperative—the harmonious evolution between man's biological environment and his psychosocial well-being.

Addendum: A Critical Case of Education for Health—The Multisectoral Fight against AIDS

The human immunodeficiency virus, HIV, the cause of AIDS, has become a major contemporary and social problem, the magnitude of which grows daily. Two keynote addresses given by Dr Hiroshi Nakajima, Director-General of the World Health Organization, lay emphasis

*WHO has published a manual that will help community health workers provide appropriate health education that uses local resources, and involves local people. Technical descriptions are given on health education methods appropriate for use with individuals, groups, and whole communities, and detailed guidance is given on how to use these methods, and how to adopt them to suit local needs. This publication is entitled *Education for Health: A Manual on Health Education in Primary Health Care,* Geneva, WHO, 1988. Such resources as *Games and Toys in the Teaching of Science and Technology,* Division of Science Technical and Environmental Education, UNESCO (Paris), 1988 are similarly of immense value in development, particularly in children and the early development of the young.

upon this disease complex and stress the critical need for complete and successful education for health.

In October 1988, speaking in State Department, Washington, D.C., Dr Nakajima said:

> The conquest of AIDS and HIV confronts your companies with fundamental biological problems that have never previously been successfully addressed. Too much speculative optimism was voiced before the difficulties were fully appreciated. It is to your immense credit that clinical studies involving more than forty different antiviral or immunomodulating drugs are already underway in this country alone.[1]
>
> The following month, at Acapulco, Mexico, Dr Nakajima observed: But another, slower revolution—more in the nature of an evolution—is taking place. I refer to the growing recognition of the part every individual can play in safeguarding his or her own well-being. The frightening spectre of AIDS, which casts a grim shadow on all too many lives today, may have brought one small benefit to mankind if it has made everybody sharply aware of the responsibility we have for our own and our family's health. . . .
>
> There must be very few literate people on earth today who have not received a warning about AIDS and how to prevent its spread. Since we have as yet neither vaccine, treatment, nor cure, our only real weapon against this lethal disease is health education. And WHO is in the forefront of the health education campaign, just as it is involved in coordinating the unprecedented efforts of biomedical scientists around the world to find answers to the virus.[2]

These statements by the Director-General put the problem of AIDS in perspective. Education for Health must be the first recourse to halt the disease. Upon this base the global strategy for the prevention and control of AIDS—developed by the WHO Global Program on AIDS (GPA)—has received the support of every nation in the world. It has been endorsed in resolutions adopted unanimously by the World Health Assembly (WHA 40.26); by the Economic and Social Council of the United Nations (E/1987/75); and by the United Nations General Assembly (42/8).[3]

Without Education for Health, every other component on AIDS programming—promoting, coordinating, maintaining prevention; research; technical and financial support; and national/international prevention and control programs can barely hope to succeed.

References

1. Nakajima H: Address to Fourteenth IFPMA Assembly, Washington, D.C., 5 October 1988, Department of State.
2. Nakajima H: Address at Symposium on *Primary Health Care: The Case of Mexico*, Acapulco, 12 November 1988. (WHO—The First 40 Years).

3. Global Programme on AIDS. *Management Structure and Advisory Bodies.* World Health Organization Document WHO/GPA/DIR/88.7.
4. SARAC Report. World Health Organization, Geneva, 1979.

Selected Bibliography

Abbatt FR, Mejia A: *Continuing the Education of Health Workers.* WHO, Geneva, 1988.

Bankowski Z, Fulop T: Health manpower out of balance—conflicts and prospects. *CIOMS,* 1987.

Bengtsson Bo (ed): *Rural Development Research—The Role of Power Relations.* SARAC Report, R4, 1979.

Bryant JH: *Medical Education and the Contemporary World.* US/Dept of Health, Education, and Welfare publication No./NIH/77-1232, 1976.

Cordes SM: Biopsychosocial imperatives from the rural perspective, in Day SB (ed): Biopsychosocial imperatives of health care. *Soc Sci Med* 1985; 21:12:1373–1379.

Cordes SM: Rural Health Care Delivery: *A Compilation of Recent and Ongoing Research.* AE and RS No 163, Department of Agricultural Economics and Rural Sociology, Pennsylvania State University, 1983.

Day SB: *Communication of Scientific Information.* Basel, S. Karger, 1975.

Day SB: *Health Communications.* New York, International Foundation, 1979.

Day SB: *Biopsychosocial Health.* New York, International Foundation, 1980.

Day SB: The Faculty of Medicine and Health Sciences, Province of Asir, Kingdom of Saudi Arabia. *The First Two Years.* Consultation and Planning Group, Vol I, Fac. Rep. 8/1.6.81.

Day SB: Clinical biopsychosocial practice and primary health care in eastern Nigeria. Soc Sci Med 1985; 21:12:1383–1389.

Engel GL: The clinical application of the biopsychosocial model. *Am J Psychiat* 1980, 137.

Flahault D, Roemer MI: *Leadership for Primary Health Care.* WHO. Public Health Papers, No 82, 1986.

Fulop T, Roemer MI: *International Development of Health Manpower Policy.* Geneva, WHO, 1982.

Fulop T: Health personnel for "Health for All"—Progress or stagnation. WHO *Chron* 40(5):194–199, 1986.

Greep JM, Schmidt HG: The network of community oriented, educational institutions for health. *World Health,* April 1984, 18–21.

Guilbert J-J: *Teacher Training Workshops in Education.* WHO/EDUC/85.185. Geneva, WHO, 1985.

Ikemi Y: The development of comprehensive medical care in Japan, in SB Day (ed): *Biopsychosocial Health.* New York, International Foundation, 1981, 75–81.

La-Anyane S: *Economics of Agricultural Development in Tropical Africa.* John Wiley, New York, 1985.

Lolas F: The emergence of the biopsychosocial approach. A model for third world health care systems. *Soc Sci Med* 1985; 21:12:1337.

Makany L: *Role of African Universities in the Promotion of Culture and Science as Basis for the Development of Africa.* Inauguration of the University of Botswana, 23 October 1982.

Nair CR (ed): *Agrohealth and Agromedicine—The Role for Integrated Aspects of Agrohealth towards the Mission of "Health for All" by the Year 2000.* WHO Collaborating Center, International Center for Health Sciences, Monograph. Nashville, 1987.

Network of Community Oriented Educational Institutions for Health Sciences. Publications office: University of Limburg, POB 616, Maastricht, Netherlands.

Nooman ZM, Refaat AH, Ezzat ES: *Experience in Community-Based Education at the Faculty of Medicine, Suez Canal University, Ismailia, Egypt.* Network Meeting, Geneva, 1987.

Neghme A: Essential teaching philosophy should be that of the biopsychosocial method. *Soc Sci Med* 1985, 21:12:1339.

Neghme A: *Education Medica En Crisis—Recados Para Los Universitarios.* Santiago De Chile, 1984.

Prywes M: Community Medicine—The "first-born" of a marriage between medical education and medical care. *Health Policy and Education* 1980, 1:291–300.

Rotem A, Barnoon S, Prywes M: Is integration of health services and manpower development possible? The Beer Sheba Case Study. *Health Policy* 1985; 5:223–239.

Sebai ZA: *The Health of the Family in Changing Arabia.* Tihama Publications (Jeddah), 1981.

Sebai ZA: Community health in Saudi Arabia. *Saudi Medical Journal,* 1982; 1.

Ransome-Kuti O: *Child Health Priorities in Nigeria.* Keynote address to the Annual Conference of the Paediatric Association of Nigeria, Calabar, 1983.

UNESCO: *Blueprint for the Future. UNESCO's Medium Term Plan 1984–1989.* UNESCO, 1984.

UNESCO: Document Series 29. *Games and Toys in the Teaching of Science and Technology.* Division of Science Technical and Environmental Education. UNESCO, Paris, 1988 (Technical Manual)

UNFSSTD: Report of the Second Beijing International Conference on Strategic Orientation of Science and Technology for National Development. UNFSSTD, New York, June 1986.

UNFSSTD: African Chairs of Technology Programme in Food Processing, Biotechnologies, and Nutrition and Health. Dakar, Senegal, March 1986.

World Health Organization: "Health for All" Series, I. Geneva, 1978.

World Health Assembly: Resolution WHA 30.43, 1977.

World Health Organization: *Primary Health Care.* Report of the International Conference on Primary Health Care, Alma-Ata, USSR, 6-12 September 1978. Geneva, 1978.

World Health Organization: "Health For All" Series, 3. WHO, Geneva, 1981.

World Health Organization: *Global Strategy for Health for All by the Year 2000.* Geneva, WHO, 1981.

World Health Organization: *Educational Handbook For Health Personnel.* Rev ed, J-J Guilbert. Geneva, WHO, 1981.

World Health Organization: *Guidelines for Training Community Health Workers in Nutrition.* Geneva, WHO, 1981.

World Health Organization: "Health For All" Series, No 8. *Seventh General Programme of Work Covering the Period 1984–1989.* Geneva, WHO, 1982.

World Health Organization: Seventh General Programme of Work Covering the period 1984-1989. *Programme 5, Health Manpower.* HMD/MTP/83.1. Geneva, WHO, 1983.

World Health Organization Technical Report Series, no 690. *New Approaches to Health Education in Primary Health Care.* WHO, Geneva, 1984.

World Health Organization: *Strengthening Ministries of Health for Primary Health Care.* WHO, Geneva, 1984.

World Health Organization: *The Role of Universities in the Strategies of Health for All.* WHO, Geneva, 1984.

World Health Organization Technical Report Series, No 746. *Community Based Education of Health Personnel.* WHO, Geneva, 1987.

World Health Organization: *Systems of Continuing Education—Priority to District Health Personnel.* 8338M/EPM/29 June 1988/Draft 3 (Unpublished). WHO, Geneva, 1988.

World Health Organization: *Education for Health—A Manual on Health Education in Primary Health Care.* WHO, Geneva, 1988. (Technical Manual).

Appendix

WHO International Health Regulations (1969)

Reprinted from *International Health Regulations (1969)*, Third Annotated Edition. Geneva, WHO, 1983.

PART I — DEFINITIONS

Article 1

For the purposes of these Regulations—

"*Aedes aegypti index*"[a] means the ratio, expressed as a percentage, between the number of houses in a limited well-defined area on the premises of which actual breeding-places of *Aedes aegypti* are found, and the total number of houses examined in that area;

"*aerosol dispenser*" means a dispenser holding a pressurized formulation which produces an insecticidal aerosol when the valve is opened;

"*aircraft*" means an aircraft making an international voyage;

"*airport*" means any airport designated by the Member State in whose territory it is situated as an airport of entry and departure for international air traffic, where the formalities incident to customs, immigration, public health,[b] animal and plant quarantine and similar procedures are carried out;

"*arrival*" of a ship, an aircraft, a train, or a road vehicle means—

(*a*) in the case of a seagoing vessel, arrival at a port;

(*b*) in the case of an aircraft, arrival at an airport;

(*c*) in the case of an inland navigation vessel, arrival either at a port or at a frontier post, as geographical conditions and treaties or arrangements among the States concerned, under Article 85 or under the laws and regulations in force in the territory of entry, may determine;

---

[a] If it is not practicable to examine all the houses in an area, examination should be made of a random sample of a size not less than that indicated in the table below:

CONFIDENCE INTERVAL FOR THE *AEDES AEGYPTI* INDEX OF ONE PER CENT. IN RELATION TO SIZE OF LOCALITY AND SAMPLE (95 PER CENT. PROBABILITY LEVEL)

Number of houses		Confidence interval
Locality	Sample	
700	500	0.7 to 1.7%
1000	700	0.7 to 1.5%
1500	1000	0.7 to 1.5%
2000	1000	0.7 to 1.6%
over 2000	1500	0.6 to 1.6%

A minimum of two inspections should be carried out; any additional inspection would increase the validity of the results. (WHO Official Records, No. 95, 1959, p. 474)

[b] The public health facilities would include those listed in Articles 14 and 18 of the International Health Regulations (1969). (WHO Official Records, No. 209, 1973, p. 74)

(*d*) in the case of a train or road vehicle, arrival at a frontier post;

"*baggage*" means the personal effects of a traveller or of a member of the crew;

"*container* (*freight container*)" [a] means an article of transport equipment—

(*a*) of a permanent character and accordingly strong enough to be suitable for repeated use;

(*b*) specially designed to facilitate the carriage of goods, by one or more modes of transport, without intermediate reloading;

(*c*) fitted with devices permitting its ready handling, particularly its transfer from one mode of transport to another;

(*d*) so designed as to be easy to fill and empty.

The term "*container* (*freight container*)" does not include vehicles or conventional packing;

"*crew*" means the personnel of a ship, an aircraft, a train, a road vehicle or other means of transport who are employed for duties on board;

"*day*" means an interval of twenty-four hours;

"*direct transit area*" [b] means a special area established in connexion with an airport, approved by the health authority concerned and under its direct supervision, for accommodating direct transit traffic and, in particular, for accommodating, in segregation, passengers and crews breaking their air voyage without leaving the airport;

"*Director-General*" means the Director-General of the Organization;

"*diseases subject to the Regulations*" (quarantinable diseases) means cholera, including cholera due to the *eltor* vibrio, plague, and yellow fever;

"*disinsecting*" means the operation in which measures are taken to kill the insect vectors of human disease present in ships, aircraft, trains, road vehicles, other means of transport, and containers;

"*epidemic*" means an extension of a disease subject to the Regulations by a multiplication of cases in an area;

"*free pratique*" means permission for a ship to enter a port, disembark and commence operation, or for an aircraft, after landing, to disembark and commence operation;

"*health administration*" means the governmental authority responsible over the whole of a territory to which these Regulations apply for the implementation of the health measures provided herein;

---

[a] Small parcels and boxes shall not be considered as containers. (WHO Official Records, No. 177, 1969, p. 554)

[b] (1) A direct transit area may be established in an airport which is not a sanitary airport. (WHO Official Records, No. 72, 1956, p. 36)

(2) Transfers of passengers between an airport and a direct transit area outside the precincts of the airport will be in conformity with the Regulations if they are made under the direct supervision and control of the health authority. (WHO Official Records, No. 56, 1954, p. 54)

"*health authority*" means the authority immediately responsible in its jurisdiction for the appropriate health measures permitted or prescribed by these Regulations;

"*imported case*" means an infected person arriving on an international voyage;

"*infected area*"[a] is defined on epidemiological principles by the health administration reporting the disease in its country and need not correspond to administrative boundaries. It is that part of its territory which, because of population characteristics, density and mobility and/or vector and animal reservoir potential, could support transmission of the reported disease;

"*infected person*" means a person who is suffering from a disease subject to the Regulations or who is subsequently shown to have been incubating such a disease;

"*in flight*" means the time elapsing between the closing of the doors of the aircraft before take-off and their opening on arrival;

"*in quarantine*" means that state or condition during which measures are applied by a health authority to a ship, an aircraft, a train, road vehicle, other means of transport or container, to prevent the spread of disease, reservoirs of disease or vectors of disease from the object of quarantine;

"*international voyage*" means—

(*a*) in the case of a ship or an aircraft, a voyage between ports or airports in the territories of more than one State, or a voyage between ports or airports in the territory or territories of the same State if the ship or aircraft has relations with the territory of any other State on its voyage but only as regards those relations;

(*b*) in the case of a person, a voyage involving entry into the territory of a State other than the territory of the State in which that person commences his voyage;

"*isolation*", when applied to a person or group of persons, means the separation of that person or group of persons from other persons, except the health staff on duty, in such a manner as to prevent the spread of infection;

"*medical examination*"[b] includes visit to and inspection of a ship, an aircraft, a train, road vehicle, other means of transport, and container, and the

---

[a] (1) Countries receiving travellers from infected areas should keep the measures applied to a necessary minimum. (WHO Official Records, No. 217, 1974, p. 55)

(2) A list of infected areas notified by health administrations is published in the Organization's *Weekly Epidemiological Record.*

(3) See notes to Article 3, pp. 10 and 11.

[b] "Preliminary examination" may include:

(1) the physical examination of any person, but the exercise of that right should depend on the circumstances of each individual case. (WHO Official Records, No. 56, 1954, p. 46)

(2) questioning travellers on their movements prior to disembarkation. (WHO Official Records, No. 87, 1958, p. 411)

(3) inspection of the passport, as being probably the best source of information when tracing the movements of a passenger during the course of a voyage which has involved changes in the mode of transportation. (WHO Official Records, No. 56, 1954, p. 57)

preliminary examination of persons, including scrutiny of vaccination certificates, but does not include the periodical inspection of a ship to ascertain the need for deratting;

"*Organization*" means the World Health Organization;

"*port*" means a seaport or an inland port;

"*ship*" means a seagoing or an inland navigation vessel making an international voyage;

"*suspect*" means a person who is considered by the health authority as having been exposed to infection by a disease subject to the Regulations and is considered capable of spreading that disease;

"*transferred case*" means an infected person whose infection originated in another area under the jurisdiction of the same health administration;

"*valid certificate*", when applied to vaccination, means a certificate conforming with the rules and the model laid down in Appendix 2.

PART II — NOTIFICATIONS AND EPIDEMIOLOGICAL INFORMATION

Article 2

For the application of these Regulations, each State recognizes the right of the Organization to communicate directly with the health administration of its territory or territories. Any notification or information sent by the Organization to the health administration shall be considered as having been sent to the State, and any notification or information sent by the health administration to the Organization shall be considered as having been sent by the State.

Article 3[a]

1. Each health administration shall notify the Organization by telegram or telex within twenty-four hours of its being informed that the first case of a disease subject to the Regulations, that is neither an imported case nor a

---

[a] (1) The notification of an infected area by a health administration must be limited to the territory of that health administration. The initial notification of the extent of the infected area may in certain cases be provisional in nature. When, on epidemiological investigation, redefinition of the infected area is indicated, the health administration should inform the Organization as soon as possible of any change in the initial notification. (WHO Official Records, No. 177, 1969, p. 554)

(2) In the absence of information on the origin of infection, as required under subparagraph 2 (*a*), a negative report is in conformity with the Regulations. It is then for the health administration to follow up the notification with such information as may later become available, as soon as possible. (WHO Official Records, No. 135, 1964, p. 32)

(3) In an effort to avoid delays, health administrations might consider having certain health authorities, e.g., those at towns and cities adjacent to a port or an airport, notify the Organization directly. (WHO Official Records, No. 135, 1964, p. 36, and No. 143, 1965, p. 45)

(4) See note to Article 1, definition of "infected area", p. 9.

transferred case, has occurred in its territory, and, within the subsequent twenty-four hours, notify the infected area.

2. In addition each health administration will notify the Organization by telegram or telex within twenty-four hours of its being informed:

(*a*) that one or more cases of a disease subject to the Regulations has been imported or transferred into a non-infected area—the notification to include all information available on the origin of infection;

(*b*) that a ship or aircraft has arrived with one or more cases of a disease subject to the Regulations on board—the notification to include the name of the ship or the flight number of the aircraft, its previous and subsequent ports of call, and the health measures, if any, taken with respect to the ship or aircraft.

3. The existence of the disease so notified on the establishment of a reasonably certain clinical diagnosis shall be confirmed as soon as possible by laboratory methods, as far as resources permit, and the result shall be sent immediately to the Organization by telegram or telex.

Reservations—Egypt, India, Pakistan
(for text, see Annex II, page 53).

Article 4[a]

1. Each health administration shall notify the Organization immediately of evidence of the presence of the virus of yellow fever, including the virus found in mosquitos or in vertebrates other than man, or the plague bacillus, in any part of its territory, and shall report the extent of the area involved.

2. Health administrations, when making a notification of rodent plague, shall distinguish wild rodent plague from domestic rodent plague and, in the case of the former, describe the epidemiological circumstances and the area involved.

Reservations—Egypt, India, Pakistan
(for text, see Annex II, page 53).

Article 5

Any notification required under paragraph 1 of Article 3 shall be promptly supplemented by information as to the source and type of the disease, the number of cases and deaths, the conditions affecting the spread of the disease, and the prophylactic measures taken.

---

[a] (1) See Article 1, definition of "infected area", p. 9.

(2) One of the following criteria should be used in determining activity of the virus in vertebrates other than man:

(i) the discovery of the specific lesions of yellow fever in the liver of vertebrates indigenous to the area or

(ii) the isolation of yellow fever virus from any indigenous vertebrates. (WHO Official Records, No. 64, 1955, p. 69)

(3) Measures need not normally be taken against an area which has been notified as infected with wild-rodent plague, unless there is evidence that the wild-rodent plague has infiltrated or is tending to infiltrate into the domestic rodent population, and thus threatens international traffic. (WHO Official Records, No. 56, 1954, p. 47, and No. 64, 1955, p. 38)

Article 6

1. During an epidemic the notifications and information required under Article 3 and Article 5 shall be followed by subsequent communications sent at regular intervals to the Organization.

2. These communications shall be as frequent and as detailed as possible. The number of cases and deaths shall be communicated at least once a week. The precautions taken to prevent the spread of the disease, in particular the measures which are being applied to prevent the spread of the disease to other territories by ships, aircraft, trains, road vehicles, other means of transport, and containers leaving the infected area, shall be stated. In the case of plague, the measures taken against rodents shall be specified. In the case of the diseases subject to the Regulations which are transmitted by insect vectors, the measures taken against such vectors shall also be specified.

Article 7[a]

1. The health administration for a territory in which an infected area has been defined and notified shall notify the Organization when that area is free from infection.

2. An infected area may be considered as free from infection when all measures of prophylaxis have been taken and maintained to prevent the recurrence of the disease or its spread to other areas, and when:

(*a*) in the case of plague or cholera, a period of time equal to at least twice the incubation period of the disease, as hereinafter provided, has elapsed since the last case identified has died, recovered or been isolated, and there is no epidemiological evidence of spread of that disease to any contiguous area;

(*b*) (i) in the case of yellow fever not transmitted by *Aedes aegypti*, three months have elapsed without evidence of activity of the yellow-fever virus;

(ii) in the case of yellow fever transmitted by *Aedes aegypti*, three months have elapsed since the occurrence of the last human case, or one month since that occurrence if the *Aedes aegypti* index has been continuously maintained below one per cent;

(*c*) (i) in the case of plague in domestic rodents, one month has elapsed since the last infected animal was found or trapped;

---

[a] (1) The period stipulated in paragraph 2 should begin when the last case is identified as a case, irrespective of the time at which the person may have been isolated. (WHO Official Records, No. 127, 1963, p. 33)

(2) The time-limits in paragraph 2 (*a*), equal to twice the incubation period of the disease, are minimum limits and health administrations may extend them before declaring an infected area in their territory free from infection and continue for a longer period their measures of prophylaxis to prevent the recurrence of the disease or its spread to other areas. (WHO Official Records, No. 72, 1956, p. 38, and No. 79, 1957, p. 499)

(ii) in the case of plague in wild rodents, three months have elapsed without evidence of the disease in sufficient proximity to ports and airports to be a threat to international traffic.

Reservations—India, Pakistan (for text, see Annex II, pages 53 and 54).

Article 8[a]

1. Each health administration shall notify the Organization of:

(*a*) the measures which it has decided to apply to arrivals from an infected area and the withdrawal of any such measures, indicating the date of application or withdrawal;

(*b*) any change in its requirements as to vaccination for any international voyage

2. Any such notification shall be sent by telegram or telex, and whenever possible in advance of any such change or of the application or withdrawal of any such measure.

3. Each health administration shall send to the Organization once a year, at a date to be fixed by the Organization, a recapitulation of its requirements as to vaccination for any international voyage.

4. Each health administration shall take steps to inform prospective travellers, through the co-operation of, as appropriate, travel agencies, shipping firms, aircraft operators or by other means, of its requirements and of any modifications thereto.

Article 9

In addition to the notifications and information required under Articles 3 to 8 inclusive, each health administration shall send to the Organization weekly:

(*a*) a report by telegram or telex of the number of cases of the diseases subject to the Regulations and deaths therefrom during the previous week in each of its towns and cities adjacent to a port or an airport, including any imported or transferred cases;

(*b*) a report by airmail of the absence of such cases during the periods referred to in subparagraphs (*a*), (*b*) and (*c*) of paragraph 2 of Article 7.

Article 10

Any notification and information required under Articles 3 to 9 inclusive shall also be sent by the health administration, on request, to any diplomatic mission or consulate established in the territory for which it is responsible.

---

[a] (1) The requirements of countries, as notified by health administrations, are published in *Vaccination Certificate Requirements for International Travel and Health Advice to Travellers*, a WHO publication. Amendments to this publication appear in the *Weekly Epidemiological Record.*

(2) Measures believed to be in excess of the Regulations shall be published by the Organization, accompanied by the phrase: "It appears that conformity of this measure with the Regulations may be open to question and the Organization is in communication with the health administration concerned." (WHO Official Records, No. 56, 1954, p. 55, and No. 79, 1957, p. 499)

Article 11[a]

1. The Organization shall send to all health administrations, as soon as possible and by the means appropriate to the circumstances, all epidemiological and other information which it has received under Articles 3 to 8 inclusive and paragraph (*a*) of Article 9 as well as information as to the absence of any returns required by Article 9. Communications of an urgent nature shall be sent by telegram, telex or telephone.

2. Any additional epidemiological data and other information available to the Organization through its surveillance programme shall be made available, when appropriate, to all health administrations.

3. The Organization may, with the consent of the government concerned, investigate an outbreak of a disease subject to the Regulations which constitutes a serious threat to neighbouring countries or to international health. Such investigation shall be directed to assist governments to organize appropriate control measures and may include on-the-spot studies by a team.

Article 12

Any telegram or telex sent, or telephone call made, for the purposes of Articles 3 to 8 inclusive and Article 11 shall be given the priority appropriate to the circumstances; in any case of exceptional urgency, where there is risk of the spread of a disease subject to the Regulations, the priority shall be the highest available under international telecommunication agreements.

Article 13[b]

1. Each State shall forward annually to the Organization, in accordance with Article 62 of the Constitution of the Organization, information concerning the occurrence of any case of a disease subject to the Regulations due to or carried by international traffic, as well as on the action taken under these Regulations or bearing upon their application.

2. The Organization shall, on the basis of the information required by paragraph 1 of this Article, of the notifications and reports required by these Regulations, and of any other official information, prepare an annual report on the functioning of these Regulations and on their effect on international traffic.

3. The Organization shall review the epidemiological trends of the diseases subject to the Regulations, and shall publish such data, not less than once a year, illustrated with maps showing infected and free areas of the world, and

---

[a] Notification to health administrations by means of the *Weekly Epidemiological Record* and the automatic telex reply service discharges the Organization's responsibilities for notification under Articles 11 (first sentence), 20, 21, 22, 69 and 85. (WHO Official Records, No. 56, 1954, pp. 55 and 66) (See also Annex IV)

[b] All health administrations should report, even negative information, on the occurrence of diseases subject to the Regulations and other matters relative to the functioning of the Regulations. (WHO Official Records, No. 217, 1974, p. 58, and No. 240, 1977, p. 45)

any other relevant information obtained from the surveillance programme of the Organization.

PART III — HEALTH ORGANIZATION

Article 14[a]

1. Each health administration shall ensure that ports and airports in its territory shall have at their disposal an organization and equipment adequate for the application of the measures provided for in these Regulations.

2. Every port and airport shall be provided with pure drinking-water and wholesome food supplied from sources approved by the health administration for public use and consumption on the premises or on board ships or aircraft. The drinking-water and food shall be stored and handled in such a manner as to ensure their protection against contamination. The health authority shall conduct periodic inspections of equipment, installations and premises, and shall collect samples of water and food for laboratory examinations to verify the observance of this Article. For this purpose and for other sanitary measures, the principles and recommendations set forth in the guides on these subjects published by the Organization shall be applied as far as practicable in fulfilling the requirements of these Regulations.

3. Every port and airport shall also be provided with an effective system for the removal and safe disposal of excrement, refuse, waste water, condemned food, and other matter dangerous to health.

Article 15

There shall be available to as many of the ports and airports in a territory as practicable an organized medical and health service with adequate staff, equipment and premises, and in particular facilities for the prompt isolation and care of infected persons, for disinfection, disinsecting and deratting, for bacteriological investigation, for the collection and examination of rodents for plague infection, for collection of water and food samples and their dispatch to a laboratory for examination, and for other appropriate measures provided for by these Regulations.

---

[a] (1) Microbiological sampling of drinking-water and food should be part of an overall sanitation programme. (WHO Official Records, No. 217, 1974, p. 58)

(2) All national health administrations should ensure the quality of food and water provided in airports and aircraft. (WHO Official Records, No. 240, 1977, p. 45)

(3) See the following WHO publications: *Guide to Ship Sanitation* (1967); *Vector Control in International Health* (1972); *Guide to Hygiene and Sanitation in Aviation*, 2nd ed., (1977); *Guidelines for Drinking-water Quality* are in preparation.

Article 16

The health authority for each port and airport shall:

(*a*) take all practicable measures to keep port and airport installations free of rodents;

(*b*) make every effort to extend rat-proofing to the port and airport installations.

Article 17

1. Each health administration shall ensure that a sufficient number of ports in its territory shall have at their disposal adequate personnel competent to inspect ships for the issue of the Deratting Exemption Certificates referred to in Article 53, and the health administration shall approve such ports for that purpose.

2. The health administration shall designate a number of these approved ports, depending upon the volume and incidence of its international traffic, as having at their disposal the equipment and personnel necessary to derat ships for the issue of the Deratting Certificates referred to in Article 53.

3. Each health administration which so designates ports shall ensure that Deratting Certificates and Deratting Exemption Certificates are issued in accordance with the requirements of the Regulations.

Article 18

1. Depending upon the volume of its international traffic, each health administration shall designate as sanitary airports a number of the airports in its territory, provided they meet the conditions laid down in paragraph 2 of this Article, and the provisions of Article 14.

2. Every sanitary airport shall have at its disposal:

(*a*) an organized medical service and adequate staff, equipment and premises;

(*b*) facilities for the transport, isolation, and care of infected persons or suspects;

(*c*) facilities for efficient disinfection and disinsecting, for the control of vectors and rodents, and for any other appropriate measure provided for by these Regulations;

(*d*) a bacteriological laboratory, or facilities for dispatching suspected material to such a laboratory;

(*e*) facilities within the airport or available to it for vaccination against yellow fever.

Article 19

1. Every port and the area within the perimeter of every airport shall be kept free from *Aedes aegypti* in its immature and adult stages and the mosquito vectors of malaria and other diseases of epidemiological significance in

international traffic. For this purpose active anti-mosquito measures shall be maintained within a protective area extending for a distance of at least 400 metres around the perimeter.

2. Within a direct transit area provided at any airport situated in or adjacent to an area where the vectors referred to in paragraph 1 of this Article exist, any building used as accommodation for persons or animals shall be kept mosquito-proof.

3. For the purposes of this Article, the perimeter of an airport means a line enclosing the area containing the airport buildings and any land or water used or intended to be used for the parking of aircraft.

4. Each health administration shall furnish data to the Organization once a year on the extent to which its ports and airports are kept free from vectors of epidemiological significance in international traffic.

Article 20[a]

1. Each health administration shall send to the Organization a list of the ports in its territory approved under Article 17 for the issue of:

(i) Deratting Exemption Certificates only and

(ii) Deratting Certificates and Deratting Exemption Certificates.

2. The health administration shall notify the Organization of any change which may occur from time to time in the list required by paragraph 1 of this Article.

3. The Organization shall send promptly to all health administrations the information received in accordance with this Article.

Article 21

1. The Organization shall, at the request of the health administration concerned, arrange to certify, after any appropriate investigation, that a sanitary airport in its territory fulfils the conditions required by the Regulations.

2. The Organization shall, at the request of the health administration concerned, and after appropriate investigation, certify that a direct transit area at an airport in a yellow-fever infected area in its territory fulfils the conditions required by the Regulations.

3. These certifications shall be subject to periodic review by the Organization, in co-operation with the health administration concerned, to ensure that the required conditions are fulfilled.

---

[a] Health administrations are urged to make from time to time a review of the ports designated under the Regulations in order to determine whether such designations meet the conditions of traffic. (WHO Official Records, No. 127, 1963, p. 35)

Article 22

1. Wherever the volume of international traffic is sufficiently important and whenever epidemiological conditions so require, facilities for the application of the measures provided for in these Regulations shall be made available at frontier posts on railway lines, on roads and, where sanitary control over inland navigation is carried out at the frontier, on inland waterways.

2. Each health administration shall notify the Organization when and where such facilities are provided.

3. The Organization shall send promptly to all health administrations the information received in accordance with this Article.

PART IV — HEALTH MEASURES AND PROCEDURE

Chapter I — General Provisions

Article 23

The health measures permitted by these Regulations are the maximum measures applicable to international traffic, which a State may require for the protection of its territory against the diseases subject to the Regulations.

Article 24[a]

Health measures shall be initiated forthwith, completed without delay, and applied without discrimination.

Article 25

1. Disinfection, disinsecting, deratting, and other sanitary operations shall be carried out so as:

(*a*) not to cause undue discomfort to any person, or injury to his health;

(*b*) not to produce any deleterious effect on the structure of a ship, an aircraft, or a vehicle, or on its operating equipment;

(*c*) to avoid all risk of fire.

2. In carrying out such operations on cargo, goods, baggage, containers and other articles, every precaution shall be taken to avoid any damage.

3. Where there are procedures or methods recommended by the Organization they should be employed.

---

[a] There are no provisions of the Regulations which exempt travellers with diplomatic status from the application of the Regulations. Health measures—e.g., examination of vaccination certificates—carried out in accordance with the Regulations have as their object the protection of health and are to be dissociated from other measures of an administrative or police nature regulating entry into and sojourn in a country and from which persons with diplomatic status may be exempt. As a consequence, the Regulations are applicable to travellers with diplomatic status and, depending on the circumstances, such travellers may be placed under medical surveillance or isolation if, for example, they do not possess the necessary certificates of vaccination. (WHO Official Records, No. 143, 1965, p. 49)

Article 26[a]

1. A health authority shall, when so requested, issue free of charge to the carrier a certificate specifying the measures applied to a ship, aircraft, train, road vehicle, other means of transport, or container, the parts thereof treated, the methods employed, and the reasons why the measures have been applied. In the case of an aircraft this information shall, on request, be entered instead in the Health Part of the Aircraft General Declaration.

2. Similarly, a health authority shall, when so requested, issue free of charge:

(*a*) to any traveller a certificate specifying the date of his arrival or departure and the measures applied to him and his baggage;

(*b*) to the consignor, the consignee, and the carrier, or their respective agents, a certificate specifying the measures applied to any goods.

Article 27[b]

1. A person under surveillance shall not be isolated and shall be permitted to move about freely. The health authority may require him to report to it, if necessary, at specified intervals during the period of surveillance. Except as limited by the provisions of Article 64, the health authority may also subject such a person to medical investigation and make any inquiries which are necessary for ascertaining his state of health.

2. When a person under surveillance departs for another place, within or without the same territory, he shall inform the health authority, which shall immediately notify the health authority for the place to which the person is proceeding. On arrival the person shall report to that health authority which may apply the measure provided for in paragraph 1 of this Article.

Article 28

Except in case of an emergency constituting a grave danger to public health, a ship or an aircraft, which is not infected or suspected of being infected with a disease subject to the Regulations, shall not on account of any other epidemic disease be refused free pratique by the health authority for a port or an airport; in particular it shall not be prevented from discharging or loading cargo or stores, or taking on fuel or water.

Article 29

A health authority may take all practicable measures to control the discharge from any ship of sewage and refuse which might contaminate the waters of a port, river or canal.

---

[a] See note to Article 46, p. 25.

[b] Enforcement of surveillance must rely on national legislation. (WHO Official Records, No. 56, 1954, p. 56, and No. 143, 1965, p. 49)

Chapter II — Health Measures on Departure

Article 30[a]

1. The health authority for a port or an airport or for the area in which a frontier post is situated shall take all practicable measures:

(*a*) to prevent the departure of any infected person or suspect;

(*b*) to prevent the introduction on board a ship, an aircraft, a train, a road vehicle, other means of transport, or container, of possible agents of infection or vectors of a disease subject to the Regulations.

2. The health authority in an infected area may require a valid vaccination certificate from departing travellers.

3. The health authority referred to in paragraph 1 of this Article may, when it considers it necessary, medically examine any person before his departure on an international voyage. The time and place of this examination shall be arranged to take into account any other formalities, so as to facilitate his departure and to avoid delay.

4. Notwithstanding the provisions of subparagraph (*a*) of paragraph 1 of this Article, a person on an international voyage who on arrival is placed under surveillance may be allowed to continue his voyage. The health authority shall, in accordance with Article 27, notify by the most expeditious means the health authority for the place to which he is proceeding.

Chapter III — Health Measures Applicable between Ports or Airports of Departure and Arrival

Article 31

No matter capable of causing any epidemic disease shall be thrown or allowed to fall from an aircraft when it is in flight.

---

[a] (1) Health administrations are urged to take all practical measures to inform the travelling public and travel agencies of the vaccination requirements of all countries to which a traveller is proceeding. They should advise travellers that these requirements are related not only to the health conditions prevailing in the country of departure but also to conditions in countries in which the traveller disembarks or transits during his journey, except in so far as he follows the provisions of Article 34. (WHO Official Records, No. 127, 1963, p. 45, and No. 143, 1965, p. 49)

(2) "Operators shall take precautions to the end that passengers hold any control documents required by Contracting States." (Standard 3.36, eighth edition of the ICAO Annex 9 to the Convention on International Civil Aviation; WHO Official Records, No. 143, 1965, p. 49)

(3) "Public authorities should invite shipowners to take all reasonable precautions to the end that passengers hold any control documents required by Contracting Governments." (Recommended Practice 3.15.1, Convention on Facilitation of International Maritime Traffic, Inter-Governmental Maritime Consultative Organization, 1965)

(4) Health administrations should take the steps necessary for embassies abroad to be informed of their country's health requirements, so that potential travellers could obtain up-to-date information. Airlines and travel agents should continue to improve their efforts to inform their customers of the health requirements of countries to be visited. (WHO Official Records, No. 217, 1974, pp. 55 and 63, and No. 240, 1977, p. 60)

(5) See Article 83, p. 36

Article 32

1. No health measure shall be applied by a State to any ship which passes through waters within its jurisdiction without calling at a port or on the coast.

2. If for any reason such a call is made, the laws and regulations in force in the territory may be applied without exceeding, however, the provisions of these Regulations.

Article 33

1. No health measure, other than medical examination, shall be applied to a healthy ship, as specified in Part V, which passes through a maritime canal or waterway in the territory of a State on its way to a port in the territory of another State, unless such ship comes from an infected area or has on board any person coming from an infected area, within the incubation period of the disease with which the area is infected.

2. The only measure which may be applied to such a ship coming from such an area or having such a person on board is the stationing on board, if necessary, of a sanitary guard to prevent all unauthorized contact between the ship and the shore, and to supervise the application of Article 29.

3. A health authority shall permit any such ship to take on, under its control, fuel, water and stores.

4. An infected or suspected ship which passes through a maritime canal or waterway may be treated as if it were calling at a port in the same territory.

Article 34[a]

Notwithstanding any provision to the contrary in these Regulations except Article 69, no health measure, other than medical examination, shall be applied to:

(*a*) passengers and crew on board a healthy ship from which they do not disembark;

(*b*) passengers and crew from a healthy aircraft who are in transit through a territory and who remain in a direct transit area of an airport of that territory, or, if the airport is not yet provided with such an area, who submit to the measures for segregation prescribed by the health authority in order to prevent the spread of disease; if such persons are obliged to leave the airport at which they disembark solely in order to continue their voyage from another airport in the vicinity of the first airport, no such measure shall be applied to them if the transfer is made under the control of the health authority or authorities.

---

[a] See notes to Article 1, definition of "medical examination", p. 9.

Chapter IV — Health Measures on Arrival

Article 35[a]

Whenever practicable States shall authorize granting of free pratique by radio to a ship or an aircraft when on the basis of information received from it prior to its arrival, the health authority for the intended port or airport of arrival is of the opinion that its arrival will not result in the introduction or spread of a disease subject to the Regulations.

Article 36[b]

1. The health authority for a port, an airport, or a frontier station may subject to medical examination on arrival any ship, aircraft, train, road vehicle, other means of transport, or container, as well as any person arriving on an international voyage.

2. The further health measures which may be applied to the ship, aircraft, train, road vehicle, other means of transport, and container shall be determined by the conditions which existed on board during the voyage or which exist at the time of the medical examination, without prejudice, however, to the measures which are permitted by these Regulations to be applied to the ship, aircraft, train, road vehicle, other means of transport, and container if it arrives from an infected area.

3. Where a health administration has special problems which could constitute a grave danger to public health, it may require a person on an international voyage to give on arrival a destination address in writing.

Article 37

The application of the measures provided for in Part V which depend on arrival from an infected area as notified by the health administration concerned shall be limited to the ship, aircraft, train, road vehicle, or other means of transport, person, container or article as the case may be, arriving from such an area, provided that the health authority for the infected area is taking all measures necessary for checking the spread of the disease and is applying the measures provided for in paragraph 1 of Article 30.

---

[a] (1) Officers in command of aircraft and ships should make known as long as possible before arrival to airport and port authorities any case of illness on board, in the interests of the patient and the health authority and to facilitate the clearance of the aircraft or ship. (WHO Official Records, No. 209, 1973, p. 78)

(2) As radio pratique has been extensively used without endangering public health, serious consideration should be given to expanding that practice. (WHO Official Records, No. 217, 1974, p. 64)

[b] See notes to Article 1, definition of "medical examination", p. 9.

Article 38[a]

On arrival of a ship, an aircraft, a train, a road vehicle, or other means of transport, an infected person on board may be removed and isolated by the health authority. Such removal by the health authority shall be compulsory if it is required by the person in charge of the means of transport.

Article 39

1. Apart from the provisions of Part V, a health authority may place under surveillance any suspect on an international voyage arriving by whatever means from an infected area. Such surveillance may be continued until the end of the appropriate period of incubation specified in Part V.

2. Except where specifically provided for in these Regulations, isolation shall not be substituted for surveillance unless the health authority considers the risk of transmission of the infection by the suspect to be exceptionally serious.

Article 40

Any health measure, other than medical examination, which has been applied at a previous port or airport shall not be repeated at a subsequent port or airport, unless:

(*a*) after the departure of a ship or an aircraft from the port or airport where the measures were applied, an incident of epidemiological significance calling for a further application of any such measure has occurred either in that port or airport or on board the ship or aircraft;

(*b*) the health authority for the subsequent port or airport has ascertained on the basis of definite evidence that the individual measure so applied was not substantially effective.

Article 41

Subject to Article 73, a ship or an aircraft shall not be prevented for health reasons from calling at any port or airport. If the port or airport is not equipped for applying the health measures which are permitted by these Regulations and which in the opinion of the health authority for the port or airport are required, such ship or aircraft may be ordered to proceed at its own risk to the nearest suitable port or airport convenient to the ship or aircraft.

Article 42

An aircraft shall not be considered as having come from an infected area if it has landed only in such an area at any sanitary airport which is not itself an infected area.

Reservations—India, Pakistan (for text, see Annex II, pages 53 and 54).

---

[a] Compulsory removal of infected persons should not be insisted upon in ports where adequate facilities for the reception of such persons cannot be expected to be available. (WHO Official Records, No. 64, 1955, p. 34)

Article 43

Any person on board a healthy aircraft which has landed in an infected area, and the passengers and crew of which have complied with the conditions laid down in Article 34, shall not be considered as having come from such an area.

Reservations—India, Pakistan (for text, see Annex II, pages 53 and 54).

Article 44

1. Except as provided in paragraph 2 of this Article, any ship or aircraft, which is unwilling to submit to the measures required by the health authority for the port or airport in accordance with these Regulations, shall be allowed to depart forthwith, but it shall not during its voyage call at any other port or airport in the same territory. Such a ship or an aircraft shall nevertheless be permitted, while in quarantine, to take on fuel, water and stores. If, on medical examination, such a ship is found to be healthy, it shall not lose the benefit of Article 33.

2. A ship or an aircraft arriving at a port or an airport situated in an area where the vector of yellow fever is present shall not, in the following circumstances, be allowed to depart and shall be subject to the measures required by the health authority in accordance with these Regulations:

(*a*) if the aircraft is infected with yellow fever;

(*b*) if the ship is infected with yellow fever, and *Aedes aegypti* have been found on board, and the medical examination shows that any infected person has not been isolated in good time.

Article 45

1. If, for reasons beyond the control of the pilot in command, an aircraft lands elsewhere than at an airport, or at an airport other than the airport at which the aircraft was due to land, the pilot in command or other person in charge shall make every effort to communicate without delay with the nearest health authority or any other public authority.

2. As soon as the health authority has been informed of the landing it may take such action as is appropriate, but in no case shall it exceed the measures permitted by these Regulations.

3. Subject to paragraph 5 of this Article, and except for the purpose of communicating with any such health or public authority or with the permission of any such authority, no person on board the aircraft shall leave its vicinity and no cargo shall be removed from that vicinity.

4. When any measure required by the health authority has been completed, the aircraft may, so far as health measures are concerned, proceed either to the airport at which it was due to land, or, if for technical reasons it cannot do so, to a conveniently situated airport.

5. The pilot in command or other person in charge may take such emergency measures as may be necessary for the health and safety of passengers and crew.

Chapter V—Measures concerning the International Transport of Cargo, Goods, Baggage, and Mail

Article 46[a]

1. Cargo and goods shall be submitted to the health measures provided for in these Regulations only when coming from infected areas and when the health authority has reason to believe that the cargo and goods may have become contaminated by the agent of a disease subject to the Regulations or may serve as a vehicle for the spread of any such disease.

2. Goods, other than live animals, in transit without transhipment shall not be subject to health measures or detained at any port, airport, or frontier.

3. The issue of a certificate of disinfection of merchandise which is the subject of trade between two countries may be governed by bilateral agreements between the exporting and the importing countries.

Article 47

Except in the case of an infected person or suspect, baggage may be disinfected or disinsected only in the case of a person carrying infectious material or insect vectors of a disease subject to the Regulations.

Article 48

1. Mail, newspapers, books, and other printed matter shall not be subject to any health measure.

2. Postal parcels may be subject to health measures only if they contain:

   (*a*) any of the foods referred to in Article 63 which the health authority has reason to believe comes from a cholera-infected area;

   (*b*) linen, wearing apparel, or bedding, which has been used or soiled and to which the provisions of Part V are applicable;

   (*c*) infectious material; or

   (*d*) living insects and other animals capable of being a vector of human disease if introduced or established.

---

[a] The duty of the health authority at the port of export is to take all practicable measures under the terms of paragraph 1 (*b*) of Article 30 to prevent the introduction on board a ship, an aircraft, a train, a road vehicle or other means of transport of possible agents of infection or vectors of a disease subject to the Regulations. Whenever disinfection has been carried out by the health authority, it is required to furnish a certificate to that effect, if requested to do so, in accordance with the terms of paragraph 2 (*b*) of Article 26. If no measures have been carried out, the implication is that the health authority did not consider them necessary, but it is not required under Article 26 to furnish a certificate to that effect. (WHO Official Records, No. 56, 1954, p. 47)

Article 49

A health administration shall ensure as far as practicable that containers used in international traffic by rail, road, sea or air shall, in packing, be kept free of infectious material, vectors or rodents.

PART V — SPECIAL PROVISIONS RELATING TO EACH OF THE DISEASES SUBJECT TO THE REGULATIONS

Chapter I — Plague

Article 50

For the purposes of these Regulations the incubation period of plague is six days.

Article 51

Vaccination against plague shall not be required as a condition of admission of any person to a territory.

Article 52

1. Each State shall employ all means in its power to diminish the danger from the spread of plague by rodents and their ectoparasites. Its health administration shall keep itself constantly informed by systematic collection and regular examination of rodents and their ectoparasites of the conditions in any area, especially any port or airport, infected or suspected of being infected by rodent plague.

2. During the stay of a ship or an aircraft in a port or an airport infected by plague, special care shall be taken to prevent the introduction of rodents on board.

Article 53[a]

1. Every ship shall be either:

(*a*) permanently kept in such a condition that it is free of rodents and the plague vector; or

(*b*) periodically deratted.

---

[a] (1) Deratting Certificates and Deratting Exemption Certificates are valid for a maximum of six months but, under certain conditions, the validity of such certificates may be extended only once by a period of one month. (WHO Official Records, No. 79, 1957, p. 502, No. 87, 1958, p. 404, and No. 95, 1959, p. 482)

(2) If inspection of a ship, carried out at the end of the period of validity of its Deratting Exemption Certificate, proves that the ship is still entitled to a Deratting Exemption Certificate, a new certificate should be issued. Periodic deratting of ships is not necessary if inspection proves that the ship is entitled to a Deratting Exemption Certificate. (WHO Official Records, No. 87, 1958, p. 405)

(3) There is no provision in the Regulations for endorsement by a port health authority of a valid Deratting Certificate or Deratting Exemption Certificate to the effect that inspection of the ship has confirmed the accuracy of the information given on the certificate. (WHO Official Records, No. 79, 1957, p. 502)

2. A Deratting Certificate or a Deratting Exemption Certificate shall be issued only by the health authority for a port approved for that purpose under Article 17. Every such certificate shall be valid for six months, but this period may be extended by one month for a ship proceeding to such a port if the deratting or inspection, as the case may be, would be facilitated by the operations due to take place there.

3. Deratting Certificates and Deratting Exemption Certificates shall conform with the model specified in Appendix 1.

4. If a valid certificate is not produced, the health authority for a port approved under Article 17, after inquiry and inspection, may proceed in the following manner:

(*a*) If the port has been designated under paragraph 2 of Article 17, the health authority may derat the ship or cause the deratting to be done under its direction and control. It shall decide in each case the technique which should be employed to secure the extermination of rodents on the ship. Deratting shall be carried out so as to avoid as far as possible damage to the ship and to any cargo and shall not take longer than is absolutely necessary. Wherever possible deratting shall be done when the holds are empty. In the case of a ship in ballast, it shall be done before loading. When deratting has been satisfactorily completed, the health authority shall issue a Deratting Certificate.

(*b*) At any port approved under Article 17, the health authority may issue a Deratting Exemption Certificate if it is satisfied that the ship is free of rodents. Such a certificate shall be issued only if the inspection of the ship has been carried out when the holds are empty or when they contain only ballast or other material, unattractive to rodents, of such a nature or so disposed as to make a thorough inspection of the holds possible. A Deratting Exemption Certificate may be issued for an oil tanker with full holds.

5. If the conditions under which a deratting is carried out are such that, in the opinion of the health authority for the port where the operation was performed, a satisfactory result cannot be obtained, the health authority shall make a note to that effect on the existing Deratting Certificate.

Article 54

In exceptional circumstances of an epidemiological nature, when the presence of rodents is suspected on board, an aircraft may be disinsected and deratted

Article 55

Before departure on an international voyage from an area where there is an epidemic of pulmonary plague, every suspect shall be placed in isolation by the health authority for a period of six days, reckoned from the date of the last exposure to infection.

Article 56

1. A ship or an aircraft on arrival shall be regarded as infected if:

(*a*) It has a case of human plague on board;

(*b*) a plague-infected rodent is found on board.

A ship shall also be regarded as infected if a case of human plague has occurred on board more than six days after embarkation.

2. A ship on arrival shall be regarded as suspected if:

(*a*) it has no case of human plague on board, but such a case has occurred on board within the first six days after embarkation;

(*b*) there is evidence of an abnormal mortality among rodents on board of which the cause is not yet known;

(*c*) it has a person on board who has been exposed to pulmonary plague and has not met the requirements of Article 55.

3. Even when coming from an infected area or having on board a person coming from an infected area, a ship or an aircraft on arrival shall be regarded as healthy if, on medical examination, the health authority is satisfied that the conditions specified in paragraphs 1 and 2 of this Article do not exist.

Article 57

1. On arrival of an infected or suspected ship or an infected aircraft, the following measures may be applied by the health authority:

(*a*) disinsecting of any suspect and surveillance for a period of not more than six days reckoned from the date of arrival;

(*b*) disinsecting and, if necessary, disinfection of:

(i) any baggage of any infected person or suspect; and

(ii) any other article such as used bedding or linen, and any part of the ship or aircraft, which is considered to be contaminated.

2. On arrival of a ship, an aircraft, a train, road vehicle or other means of transport having on board a person suffering from pulmonary plague, or if there has been a case of pulmonary plague on board a ship within the period of six days before its arrival, the health authority may, in addition to the measures required by paragraph 1 of this Article, place the passengers and crew of the ship, aircraft, train, road vehicle or other means of transport in isolation for a period of six days, reckoned from the date of the last exposure to infection.

3. If there is rodent plague on board a ship, or in its containers, it shall be disinsected and deratted, if necessary in quarantine, in the manner provided for in Article 53 subject to the following provisions:

(*a*) the deratting shall be carried out as soon as the holds have been emptied;

(*b*) one or more preliminary derattings of a ship with the cargo *in situ*, or during its unloading, may be carried out to prevent the escape of infected rodents;

(*c*) if the complete destruction of rodents cannot be secured because only part of the cargo is due to be unloaded, a ship shall not be prevented from unloading that part, but the health authority may apply any measures, including placing the ship in quarantine, which it considers necessary to prevent the escape of infected rodents.

4. If a rodent infected with plague is found on board an aircraft, the aircraft shall be disinsected and deratted, if necessary in quarantine.

Article 58

A ship shall cease to be regarded as infected or suspected, or an aircraft shall cease to be regarded as infected, when the measures required by the health authority in accordance with Articles 38 and 57 have been effectively carried out, or when the health authority is satisfied that the abnormal mortality among rodents is not due to plague. The ship or aircraft shall thereupon be given free pratique.

Article 59

On arrival, a healthy ship or aircraft shall be given free pratique, but, if it has come from an infected area, the health authority may:

(*a*) place under surveillance any suspect who disembarks, for a period of not more than six days, reckoned from the date on which the ship or aircraft left the infected area;

(*b*) require the destruction of rodents on board a ship and disinsecting in exceptional cases and for well-founded reasons which shall be communicated in writing to the master.

Article 60

If, on arrival of a train or a road vehicle, a case of human plague is discovered, the measures provided for in Article 38 and in paragraphs 1 and 2 of Article 57 may be applied by the health authority, disinsecting and, if necessary, disinfection being applied to any part of the train or road vehicle which is considered to be contaminated.

Chapter II — Cholera[a]

Article 61

For the purposes of these Regulations the incubation period of cholera is five days.

---

[a] (1) Vaccination, while it provides limited individual protection to the traveller, is irrelevant to the problem of protecting a community from importation of the vibrio. (WHO Official Records, No. 209, 1973, p. 91, and No. 240, 1977, p. 53)

(2) Restrictive measures would not prevent the international spread of the disease. (WHO Official Records, No. 217, 1974, p. 60)

Article 62

1. If on arrival of a ship, aircraft, train, road vehicle or other means of transport a case of cholera is discovered, or a case has occurred on board, the health authority (*a*) may apply surveillance or isolation of suspects among passengers or crew for a period not to exceed five days reckoned from the date of disembarkation; (*b*) shall be responsible for the supervision of the removal and safe disposal of any water, food (excluding cargo), human dejecta, waste water including bilge water, waste matter, and any other matter which is considered to be contaminated, and shall be responsible for the disinfection of water tanks and food handling equipment.

2. Upon accomplishment of (*b*) the ship, aircraft, train, road vehicle or other means of transport shall be given free pratique.

Article 63[a]

Foodstuffs carried as cargo on board ships, aircraft, trains, road vehicles or other means of transport in which a case of cholera has occurred during the journey, may not be subjected to bacteriological examination except by the health authorities of the country of final destination.

Article 64

1. No person shall be required to submit to rectal swabbing.

2. A person on an international voyage, who has come from an infected area within the incubation period of cholera and who has symptoms indicative of cholera, may be required to submit to stool examination.

Chapter III — Yellow Fever

Article 65

For the purposes of these Regulations the incubation period of yellow fever is six days.

Article 66

1. Vaccination against yellow fever may be required of any person leaving an infected area on an international voyage.

2. If such a person is in possession of a certificate of vaccination against yellow fever which is not yet valid, he may nevertheless be permitted to depart, but the provisions of Article 68 may be applied to him on arrival.

3. A person in possession of a valid certificate of vaccination against yellow fever shall not be treated as a suspect, even if he has come from an infected area.

---

[a] The previous text of this article referred expressly to the following foodstuffs: fish, shellfish, fruit vegetables or beverages.

4. The yellow-fever vaccine used must be approved by the Organization, and the vaccinating centre must have been designated by the health administration for the territory in which it is situated. The Organization shall be assured that the vaccines used for this purpose continue to be of suitable quality.

Article 67[a]

1. Every person employed at a port or an airport situated in an infected area, and every member of the crew of a ship or an aircraft using any such port or airport, shall be in possession of a valid certificate of vaccination against yellow fever.

2. Every aircraft leaving an airport situated in an infected area shall be disinsected in accordance with Article 25, using methods recommended by the Organization, and details of the disinsecting shall be included in the Health Part of the Aircraft General Declaration, unless this part of the Aircraft General Declaration is waived by the health authority of the airport of arrival. States concerned shall accept disinsecting of aircraft by the approved vapour disinsecting system carried out in flight.

3. Every ship leaving a port in an area where *Aedes aegypti* still exists and bound for an area where *Aedes aegypti* has been eradicated shall be kept free of *Aedes aegypti* in its immature and adult stages.

4. An aircraft leaving an airport where *Aedes aegypti* exists and bound for an area where *Aedes aegypti* has been eradicated shall be disinsected in accordance with Article 25, using methods recommended by the Organization.

Article 68

A health authority in an area where the vector of yellow fever is present may require a person on an international voyage, who has come from an infected area and is unable to produce a valid certificate of vaccination against yellow fever, to be isolated until his certificate becomes valid, or until a period of not more than six days reckoned from the date of last possible exposure to infection has elapsed, whichever occurs first.

Article 69

1. A person coming from an infected area who is unable to produce a valid certificate of vaccination against yellow fever and who is due to proceed on an international voyage to an airport in an area where the vector of yellow fever is present and at which the means for securing segregation provided for in Article 34 do not yet exist, may, by arrangement between the health administrations for the territories in which the airports concerned are situated, be prevented

---

[a] The recommendations concerning the disinsecting of aircraft contained in Annex VI to the Second Annotated Edition of the Regulations are under review in the light of technical developments. Current information may be obtained from the Division of Vector Biology and Control, World Health Organization.

from proceeding from an airport at which such means are available, during the period provided for in Article 68.

2. The health administrations concerned shall inform the Organization of any such arrangement, and of its termination. The Organization shall immediately send this information to all health administrations.

Article 70[a]

1. On arrival, a ship shall be regarded as infected if it has a case of yellow fever on board, or if a case has occurred on board during the voyage. It shall be regarded as suspected if it has left an infected area less than six days before arrival, or, if arriving within thirty days of leaving such an area, the health authority finds *Aedes aegypti* or other vectors of yellow fever on board. Any other ship shall be regarded as healthy.

2. On arrival, an aircraft shall be regarded as infected if it has a case of yellow fever on board. It shall be regarded as suspected if the health authority is not satisfied with a disinsecting carried out in accordance with paragraph 2 of Article 67 and it finds live mosquitos on board the aircraft. Any other aircraft shall be regarded as healthy.

Article 71

1. On arrival of an infected or suspected ship or aircraft, the following measures may be applied by the health authority:

(*a*) in an area where the vector of yellow fever is present, the measures provided for in Article 68 to any passenger or member of the crew who disembarks and is not in possession of a valid certificate of vaccination against yellow fever;

(*b*) inspection of the ship or aircraft and destruction of any *Aedes aegypti* or other vectors of yellow fever on board; in an area where the vector of yellow fever is present, the ship may, until such measures have been carried out, be required to keep at least 400 metres from land.

2. The ship or aircraft shall cease to be regarded as infected or suspected when the measures required by the health authority in accordance with Article 38 and with paragraph 1 of this Article have been effectively carried out, and it shall thereupon be given free pratique.

Article 72

On arrival of a healthy ship or aircraft coming from an infected area, the measures provided for in subparagraph (*b*) of paragraph 1 of Article 71 may be applied. The ship or aircraft shall thereupon be given free pratique.

---

[a] The two conditions indicated in paragraph 2 must be fulfilled before a health authority may consider an aircraft as suspected. (WHO Official Records, No. 118, 1962, p. 49)

Article 73

A State shall not prohibit the landing of an aircraft at any sanitary airport in its territory if the measures provided for in paragraph 2 of Article 67 are applied, but, in an area where the vector of yellow fever is present, aircraft coming from an infected area may land only at airports specified by the State for that purpose.

Article 74

On arrival of a train, a road vehicle, or other means of transport in an area where the vector of yellow fever is present, the following measures may be applied by the health authority:

(*a*) isolation, as provided for in Article 68, of any person coming from an infected area, who is unable to produce a valid certificate of vaccination against yellow fever;

(*b*) disinsecting of the train, road vehicle or other means of transport if it has come from an infected area.

Article 75

In an area where the vector of yellow fever is present the isolation provided for in Article 38 and in this Chapter shall be in mosquito-proof accommodation.

PART VI — HEALTH DOCUMENTS

Article 76

Bills of health, with or without consular visa, or any certificate, however designated, concerning health conditions of a port or an airport, shall not be required from any ship or aircraft.

Article 77

1. The master of a seagoing vessel making an international voyage, before arrival at its first port of call in a territory, shall ascertain the state of health on board, and, except when a health administration does not require it, he shall, on arrival, complete and deliver to the health authority for that port a Maritime Declaration of Health which shall be countersigned by the ship's surgeon if one is carried.

2. The master, and the ship's surgeon if one is carried, shall supply any information required by the health authority as to health conditions on board during the voyage.

3. A Maritime Declaration of Health shall conform with the model specified in Appendix 3.

4. A health administration may decide:

(*a*) either to dispense with the submission of the Maritime Declaration of Health by all arriving ships; or

(*b*) to require it only if the ship arrives from certain stated areas, or if there is positive information to report.

In either case, the health administration shall inform shipping operators.

Article 78

1. The pilot in command of an aircraft, on landing at the first airport in a territory, or his authorized agent, shall complete and deliver to the health authority for that airport the Health Part of the Aircraft General Declaration which shall conform with the model specified in Appendix 4, except when a health administration does not require it.

2. The pilot in command of an aircraft, or his authorized agent, shall supply any information required by the health authority as to health conditions on board during the voyage.

3. A health administration may decide:

(*a*) either to dispense with the submission of the Health Part of the Aircraft General Declaration by all arriving aircraft; or

(*b*) to require it only if the aircraft arrives from certain stated areas, or if there is positive information to report.

In either case, the health administration shall inform aircraft operators.

Article 79[a]

1. The certificates specified in Appendices 1 and 2 shall be printed in English and in French. An official language of the territory of issue may be added.

2. The certificates referred to in paragraph 1 of this Article shall be completed in English or in French. Completion in another language in addition is not excluded.

3. International certificates of vaccination must be signed in his own hand by a medical practitioner or other person authorized by the national health administration; his offical stamp is not an accepted substitute for his signature.

---

[a] (1) A certificate not printed in the proper form or not completed in the English or French language is not a valid certificate under the Regulations. (WHO Official Records, No. 102, 1960, p. 48, and No. 118, 1962, p. 54)

(2) The date on certificates of vaccination should be recorded in the following sequence: day, month, year—the month to be written in letters and not in figures (example: 5 January 1982). (WHO Official Records, No. 56, 1954, p. 54, and No. 118, 1962, p. 54)

(3) Health administrations should take all reasonable steps to ensure that the certificates issued in their territories are in conformity with the Regulations and the interpretations thereon of the Health Assembly, and particularly that certificates are fully completed and all entries on them are legible. (WHO Official Records, No. 102, 1960, p. 50, and No. !18, 1962, p. 54)

See also the notes to Appendix 2 (p. 45).

For model of a correctly completed certificate, see Annex VI, pp. 64-65.

4. International certificates of vaccination are individual certificates and shall in no circumstances be used collectively. Separate certificates shall be issued for children.

5. No departure shall be made from the model of the certificate specified in Appendix 2, and no photograph shall be included.

6. A parent or guardian shall sign the international certificate of vaccination when the child is unable to write. The signature of an illiterate shall be indicated in the usual manner by his mark and the indication by another that this is the mark of the person concerned.

7. If a vaccinator is of the opinion that vaccination is contraindicated on medical grounds he shall provide the person with reasons, written in English or French, underlying that opinion, which health authorities should take into account.

Article 80

A vaccination document issued by the Armed Forces to an active member of those Forces shall be accepted in lieu of an international certificate in the form shown in Appendix 2 if:

(*a*) it embodies medical information substantially the same as that required by such form; and

(*b*) it contains a statement in English or in French recording the nature and date of the vaccination and to the effect that it is issued in accordance with this Article.

Article 81[a]

No health document, other than those provided for in these Regulations, shall be required in international traffic.

Reservations—India, Pakistan (for text, see Annex II, pages 53 and 54).

PART VII — CHARGES

Article 82[b]

1. No charge shall be made by a health authority for:

(*a*) any medical examination provided for in these Regulations, or any supplementary examination, bacteriological or otherwise, which may be required to ascertain the state of health of the person examined;

(*b*) any vaccination of a person on arrival and any certificate thereof.

[a] No health certificate may be required from persons on an international voyage. In the case of travellers who, though not immigrants, are nevertheless intending to reside in a country for a protracted period (such as students), the provision of a health certificate should preferably be a condition of the granting of the visa rather than be required as a travel document on arrival. (WHO Official Records, No. 72, 1956, p. 37)

[b] (1) It is not permissible to exact or receive payment for medical examination carried out at any time of the day or night. The terms of Article 24 require that health measures shall be initiated forthwith and

(*continued on next page*)

2. Where charges are made for applying the measures provided for in these Regulations, other than the measures referred to in paragraph 1 of this Article, there shall be in each territory only one tariff for such charges and every charge shall:

(*a*) conform with this tariff;

(*b*) be moderate and not exceed the actual cost of the service rendered;

(*c*) be levied without distinction as to the nationality, domicile, or residence of the person concerned, or as to the nationality, flag, registry or ownership of the ship, aircraft, train, road vehicle, other means of transport, and containers. In particular, there shall be no distinction made between national and foreign persons, ships, aircraft, trains, road vehicles, other means of transport, and containers.

3. The levying of a charge for the transmission of a message relating to provisions of these Regulations by radio may not exceed the normal charge for radio messages.

4. The tariff, and any amendment thereto, shall be published at least ten days in advance of any levy thereunder and notified immediately to the Organization.

PART VIII — VARIOUS PROVISIONS

Article 83[a]

1. Every aircraft leaving an airport situated in an area where transmission of malaria or other mosquito-borne disease is occurring, or where insecticide-resistant mosquito vectors of disease are present, or where a vector species is

---

(*continued from previous page*)

completed without delay. Arrangements should be made to enable quarantine services to do this at all times, particularly in airports and the larger ports. (WHO Official Records, No. 56, 1954, p. 56, and No. 72, 1956, p. 37)

(2) An aircraft operator, as the employer of the disembarking crew, might be held responsible for isolation expenses of its own employees (crew). However, isolation expenses for other international travellers cannot be the subject of a charge against the carrier; these expenses are for the traveller himself or for the country of disembarkation to pay. (WHO Official Records, No. 135, 1964, p. 39, and No. 143, 1965, p. 57)

(3) Fines such as those imposed on a ship for not hoisting on arrival a flag requesting free pratique, and any other charges not covered by the Regulations, such as port dues, are matters of maritime practice and the Regulations are not applicable. (WHO Official Records, No. 72, 1956, p. 37)

[a] (1) Health administrations of countries which are approaching or have already reached the phases of consolidation or maintenance of a malaria eradication programme may need to take measures to prevent the importation of malaria. (WHO Official Records, No. 87, 1958, p. 413)

(2) (i) Persons originating in malarious areas and proceeding to areas from which malaria has been eradicated and where conditions for transmission persist (recipient areas) who would probably live in towns and therefore present little danger for transmission, should be advised to take sporontocidal treatment if they plan to spend nights in the countryside. A suitable information or warning card should be given to these individuals on entry.

(ii) The medical officers responsible for crews of ships and aircraft should be adequately trained in the diagnosis and treatment of malaria and in measures of personal prophylaxis. Operators and shipowners should ensure that all members of crews of ships and aircraft touching ports and airports in malarious areas are subjected to supervised suppressant treatment during a suitable period of time. (WHO Official Records, No. 135, 1964, p. 34) present that has been eradicated in the area where the airport of destination of the aircraft is situated, shall be disinsected in accordance with Article 25 using the methods recommended by the Organization. States concerned shall accept disinsecting of aircraft by the approved vapour disinsecting system carried out in flight. Every ship leaving a port in the situation referred to above shall be kept free from the immature and adult stages of the mosquito concerned.

2. On arrival at an airport in an area where malaria or other mosquito-borne disease could develop from imported vectors, or where a vector species has been eradicated that is present in the area in which the airport of origin is located, the aircraft mentioned in paragraph 1 of this Article may be disinsected in accordance with Article 25 if the health authority is not provided with satisfactory evidence that disinsecting has been carried out in accordance with paragraph 1 of this Article. Every ship arriving in a port in the situation referred to above should be treated and freed, under the control of the health authority, from the immature and adult stages of the mosquito concerned.

3. As far as practicable, and where appropriate, a train, road vehicle, other means of transport, container, or boat used for international coastal traffic or for international traffic on inland waterways, shall be kept free of insect vectors of human disease.

Article 84[b]

1. Migrants, nomads, seasonal workers or persons taking part in periodic mass congregations, and any ship, in particular small boats for international coastal traffic, aircraft, train, road vehicle or other means of transport carrying

---

(3) Persons on an international voyage (other than those mentioned in Article 84) should not be subjected to any special measures in respect of malaria. Special attention should be given to individuals or groups of travellers specified under Article 84. (WHO Official Records, No. 87, 1958, p. 413, and No. 135, 1964, p. 34)

(4) Efforts to disseminate information on malaria risk to travellers, through physicians, travel agents, airlines, shipping companies and other appropriate means, should be intensified. (WHO Official Records, No. 217, 1974, p. 63)

(5) The *Weekly Epidemiological Record* publishes every year information on the malaria situation in the world, particularly referring to malaria-free countries/areas, incidence of the disease in malarious countries/areas, malaria imported into malaria-free countries/areas, occurrence of drug resistant malaria, and including a map showing the malaria distribution in the world.

(6) The recommendations concerning the disinsecting of aircraft, contained in Annex VI to the Second Annotated Edition of the Regulations, are under review in the light of technical developments. Current information may be obtained from the Division of Vector Biology and Control, World Health Organization. For special measures applicable to certain categories of travellers, see Article 84.

[b] (1) (i) To prevent the introduction of malaria into recipient areas, special measures should be applied to individuals or groups of persons specified under Article 84 arriving from areas where malaria transmission occurs.

(ii) Appropriate steps should be taken against mosquitos in frontier zones in the centres where the above-mentioned groups assemble.

(iii) In international frontier zones, common control measures should be adopted by the countries concerned to avoid the carrying of malaria from one country to another.

(iv) Full exchange of information on the movement of population groups and on the susceptibility and resistance of anopheline vectors to insecticides should be instituted. (WHO Official Records, No. 135, 1964, p. 33)

(2) For WHO recommended standards of hygiene on ships and aircraft carrying persons taking part in periodic mass congregations, see Annex V, page 61.

them, may be subjected to additional health measures conforming with the laws and regulations of each State concerned, and with any agreement concluded between any such States.

2. Each State shall notify the Organization of the provisions of any such laws and regulations or agreement.

3. The standards of hygiene on ships and aircraft carrying persons taking part in periodic mass congregations shall not be inferior to those recommended by the Organization.

Article 85

1. Special treaties or arrangements may be concluded between two or more States having certain interests in common owing to their health, geographical, social or economic conditions, in order to facilitate the application of these Regulations, and in particular with regard to:

(*a*) the direct and rapid exchange of epidemiological information between neighbouring territories;

(*b*) the health measures to be applied to international coastal traffic and to international traffic on inland waterways, including lakes;

(*c*) the health measures to be applied in contiguous territories at their common frontier;

(*d*) the combination of two or more territories into one territory for the purposes of any of the health measures to be applied in accordance with these Regulations;

(*e*) arrangements for carrying infected persons by means of transport specially adapted for the purpose.

2. The treaties or arrangements referred to in paragraph 1 of this Article shall not be in conflict with the provisions of these Regulations.

3. States shall inform the Organization of any such treaty or arrangement which they may conclude. The Organization shall send immediately to all health administrations information concerning any such treaty or arrangement.

PART IX — FINAL PROVISIONS

Article 86

1. These Regulations, subject to the provisions of Article 88 and the exceptions hereinafter provided, replace, as between the States bound by these Regulations and as between these States and the Organization, the provisions of the following existing International Sanitary Conventions, Regulations and similar agreements:

(*a*) International Sanitary Convention, signed in Paris, 3 December 1903;

(*b*) Pan American Sanitary Convention, signed in Washington, 14 October 1905;

(*c*) International Sanitary Convention, signed in Paris, 17 January 1912;

(*d*) International Sanitary Convention, signed in Paris, 21 June 1926;

(*e*) International Sanitary Convention for Aerial Navigation, signed at The Hague, 12 April 1933;

(*f*) International Agreement for dispensing with Bills of Health, signed in Paris, 22 December 1934;

(*g*) International Agreement for dispensing with Consular Visas on Bills of Health, signed in Paris, 22 December 1934;

(*h*) Convention modifying the International Sanitary Convention of 21 June 1926, signed in Paris, 31 October 1938;

(*i*) International Sanitary Convention, 1944, modifying the International Sanitary Convention of 21 June 1926, opened for signature in Washington, 15 December 1944;

(*j*) International Sanitary Convention for Aerial Navigation, 1944, modifying the International Sanitary Convention of 12 April 1933, opened for signature in Washington, 15 December 1944;

(*k*) Protocol of 23 April 1946 to prolong the International Sanitary Convention, 1944, signed in Washington;

(*l*) Protocol of 23 April 1946 to prolong the International Sanitary Convention for Aerial Navigation, 1944, signed in Washington;

(*m*) International Sanitary Regulations, 1951, and the Additional Regulations of 1955, 1956, 1960, 1963 and 1965.

2. The Pan American Sanitary Code, signed at Habana, 14 November 1924, remains in force with the exception of Articles 2, 9, 10, 11, 16 to 53 inclusive, 61, and 62, to which the relevant part of paragraph 1 of this Article shall apply.

Article 87

1. The period provided in execution of Article 22 of the Constitution of the Organization for rejection or reservation shall be nine months from the date of the notification by the Director-General of the adoption of these Regulations by the World Health Assembly.

2. Such period may, by notification to the Director-General, be extended to eighteen months with respect to overseas or other outlying territories for whose international relations the State may be responsible.

3. Any rejection or reservation received by the Director-General after the expiry of the periods referred to in paragraph 1 or 2 of this Article shall have no effect.

Article 88

1. If any State makes a reservation to these Regulations, such reservation shall not be valid unless it is accepted by the World Health Assembly, and these Regulations shall not enter into force with respect to that State until such reservation has been accepted by the Assembly or, if the Assembly objects to it

on the ground that it substantially detracts from the character and purpose of these Regulations, until it has been withdrawn.

2. A rejection in part of the Regulations shall be considered as a reservation.

3. The World Health Assembly may, as a condition of its acceptance of a reservation, request the State making such reservation to undertake that it will continue to fulfil any obligation or obligations corresponding to the subject-matter of such reservation, which such State has previously accepted under the existing conventions, regulations and similar agreements listed in Article 86.

4. If a State makes a reservation which in the opinion of the World Health Assembly detracts to an insubstantial extent from an obligation or obligations previously accepted by that State under the existing conventions, regulations and similar agreements listed in Article 86, the Assembly may accept such reservation without requiring as a condition of its acceptance an undertaking of the kind referred to in paragraph 3 of this Article.

5. If the World Health Assembly objects to a reservation, and that reservation is not then withdrawn, these Regulations shall not enter into force with respect to the State which has made such a reservation. Any existing conventions, regulations and similar agreements listed in Article 86 to which such State is already a party consequently remain in force as far as such State is concerned.

Article 89

A rejection, or the whole or part of any reservation, may at any time be withdrawn by notifying the Director-General.

Article 90

1. These Regulations shall come into force on the first day of January 1971.

2. Any State which becomes a Member of the Organization after that date and which is not already a party hereto may notify its rejection of, or any reservation to, these Regulations within a period of three months from the date on which that State becomes a Member of the Organization. Unless rejected, these Regulations shall come into force with respect to that State, subject to the provisions of Article 88 upon expiry of that period.

Article 91

1. Any State not a Member of the Organization, which is a party to any conventions, regulations and similar agreements listed in Article 86 or to which the Director-General has notified the adoption of these Regulations by the World Health Assembly, may become a party hereto by notifying its acceptance to the Director-General and, subject to the provisions of Article 88, such acceptance shall become effective upon the date of coming-into-force of these Regulations, or, if such acceptance is notified after that date, three months after the date of receipt by the Director-General of the notification of acceptance.

2. For the purpose of the application of these Regulations Articles 23, 33, 62, 63 and 64 of the Constitution of the Organization shall apply to any non-Member State which becomes a party to these Regulations.

3. Any non-Member State which has become a party to these Regulations may at any time withdraw from participation in these Regulations, by means of a notification addressed to the Director-General which shall take effect six months after he has received it. The State which has withdrawn shall, as from that date, resume application of the provisions of any conventions, regulations and similar agreements listed in Article 86 to which it was previously a party.

Article 92

The Director-General shall notify all Members and Associate Members, and also other parties to any conventions, regulations and similar agreements listed in Article 86 of the adoption by the World Health Assembly of these Regulations. The Director-General shall also notify these States as well as any other State, which has become a party to these Regulations, of any additional Regulations amending or supplementing these Regulations, of any notification received by him under Articles 87, 89, 90 and 91 respectively, as well as of any decision taken by the World Health Assembly under Article 88.

Article 93

1. Any question or dispute concerning the interpretation or application of these Regulations or of any Regulations supplementary to these Regulations may be referred by any State concerned to the Director-General who shall attempt to settle the question or dispute. If such question or dispute is not thus settled, the Director-General on his own initiative, or at the request of any State concerned, shall refer the question or dispute to the appropriate committee or other organ of the Organization for consideration.

2. Any State concerned shall be entitled to be represented before such committee or other organ.

3. Any such dispute which has not been thus settled may, by written application, be referred by any State concerned to the International Court of Justice for decision.

Article 94

1. The English and French texts of these Regulations shall be equally authentic.

2. The original texts of these Regulations shall be deposited in the archives of the Organization. Certified true copies shall be sent by the Director-General to all Members and Associate Members, and also to other parties to one of the conventions, regulations and similar agreements listed in Article 86. Upon the entry-into-force of these Regulations, certified true copies shall be delivered by the Director-General to the Secretary-General of the United Nations for registration in accordance with Article 102 of the Charter of the United Nations.

Index

Prepared by Ctibor Votrubec, Associate Professor of Medical Geography, Institute of Tropical Health, Postgraduate Medical School, Prague, Czechoslovakia.

MIX
Papier aus verantwortungsvollen Quellen
Paper from responsible sources
FSC® C105338
FSC
www.fsc.org

If you have any concerns about our products,
you can contact us on
ProductSafety@springernature.com

In case Publisher is established outside the EU,
the EU authorized representative is:
Springer Nature Customer Service Center GmbH
Europaplatz 3, 69115 Heidelberg, Germany

Printed by Libri Plureos GmbH
in Hamburg, Germany